T0302151

Psychiatric and Behavioral Disorders in Intellectual and Developmental Disabilities

Third Edition

Psychiatric and Behavioral Disorders in Intellectual and Developmental Disabilities

Third Edition

Edited by

Colin Hemmings, BSc, MBBS, MSc, MA, MD(Res), MRCPsych
Maudsley Hospital, London, UK

Nick Bouras, MD, PhD, FRCPsych
Institute of Psychiatry, Psychology and Neuroscience, King's College London, and Maudsley International, London, UK

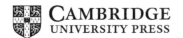

CAMBRIDGE
UNIVERSITY PRESS

University Printing House, Cambridge CB2 8BS, United Kingdom

One Liberty Plaza, 20th Floor, New York, NY 10006, USA

477 Williamstown Road, Port Melbourne, VIC 3207, Australia

314-321, 3rd Floor, Plot 3, Splendor Forum, Jasola District Centre, New Delhi - 110025, India

79 Anson Road, #06-04/06, Singapore 079906

Cambridge University Press is part of the University of Cambridge.

It furthers the University's mission by disseminating knowledge in the pursuit of
education, learning and research at the highest international levels of excellence.

www.cambridge.org
Information on this title: www.cambridge.org/9781107645943

© Cambridge University Press 2016

First published 2016
First edition 1999
Second edition 2007

A catalogue record for this publication is available from the British Library

Library of Congress Cataloging in Publication data
Psychiatric and behavioural disorders in developmental disabilities and mental retardation
Psychiatric and behavioral disordes in intellectual an developmental disabilities / edited by
Colin Hemmings, Maudsley Hospital, London, UK, Nick Bouras, Institute of Psychiatry, Psychology,
Neuroscience, King's College London and Maudsley International, London, UK.–Third edition.
    pages cm
Revision of: Psychiatric and behavioural disorders in developmental disabilities and mental
retardation. 1999.
ISBN 978-1-107-64594-3 (Paperback)
1. People with mental disabilities–Mentalhealth.
2. People with mental disabilities–Mental health services. I. Hemmings,Colin. II. Bouras,
Nick. III. Title.
RC451.4.M47P77 2015
362.4–dc23   2015013887

ISBN 978-1-107-64594-3 Paperback

....

Contents

List of contributors vii
Preface xi

Section 1: Foundations

1 **Historical and international perspectives of services** 1
Nick Bouras

2 **Classification and diagnosis** 15
Marco O. Bertelli, Luis Salvador-Carulla, and James Harris

3 **The epidemiology of psychiatric disorders in adults with intellectual disabilities** 34
Jason Buckles

4 **Assessment instruments and rating scales** 45
Heidi Hermans

Section 2: Mental disorders

5 **Dementias** 55
Jennifer Torr

6 **Schizophrenia spectrum disorders** 65
Rory Sheehan, Lucy Fodor-Wynne, and Angela Hassiotis

7 **Mood disorders** 78
Anna M. Palucka, Pushpal Desarkar, and Yona Lunsky

8 **Anxiety disorders** 89
Jane McCarthy and Eddie Chaplin

9 **Stress, traumatic, and bereavement reactions** 99
Philip Dodd and Fionnuala Kelly

10 **Personality disorders** 109
William R. Lindsay and Regi Alexander

11 **Mental illness with intellectual disabilities and autism spectrum disorders** 119
Trine L. Bakken, Sissel B. Helvershou, Siv Helene Høidal, and Harald Martinsen

12 **Attention-deficit/hyperactivity disorder (ADHD)** 129
Elizabeth Evans and Julian Trollor

Section 3: Interventions

13 **Psychopharmacology** 139
Stephen Ruedrich

14 **Psychodynamic psychotherapy** 151
Nigel Beail

15 **Cognitive-behavioral therapy** 161
Dave Dagnan

16 **Behavioral approaches** 171
Betsey A. Benson

Section 4: Special topics

17 **Psychopathology of children with intellectual disabilities** 181
Bruce Tonge

18 **Behavioral phenotypes/genetic syndromes** 196
Robert M. Hodapp, Nathan A. Dankner, and Elisabeth M. Dykens

19 **Offending behavior** 207
John L. Taylor and William R. Lindsay

20 **Problem behaviors and the interface with psychiatric disorders** 224
Sally-Ann Cooper

21 **The interface between medical and psychiatric disorders** 231
Jessica A. Hellings and Seema Jain

22 **Epilepsy** 242
Frank M. C. Besag

Section 5: Services

23 **Specialized and mainstream mental health services** 252
Johanna Lake, Carly McMorris, and Yona Lunsky

24 **Service users' and carers' experiences of mental health services** 262
Katrina Scior

25 **Carer and family perspectives** 269
Gemma L. Unwin, Shoumitro Deb, and John Rose

Section 6: Reflections

26 **Reflections** 279
Colin Hemmings

Index 289

Contributors

Regi Alexander, MBBS, DPM, FRCPsych
Honorary Senior Lecturer, Norwich
Medical School, University of East Anglia
and Consultant Psychiatrist, St. John's
House, Partnerships in Care LD Services,
Diss, Norfolk, UK

Trine L. Bakken, PhD, MHSc, RN
Head of Regional Competence Unit for
Mental Health and Intellectual Disabilities/
Autism, Oslo University Hospital, Oslo,
Norway

Nigel Beail, MSc, PhD, FBPsS, CPsychol, FIPD
HCPC Registered Clinical Psychologist;
Consultant and Head of Psychological
Services, Adult Learning Disabilities
Specialist Health Services; Professional
Head of Psychological Services at the
Barnsley Business Delivery Unit, South
West Yorkshire Partnership NHS
Foundation Trust; and Professor of
Psychology at the Clinical Psychology Unit,
Department of Psychology, University of
Sheffield, Sheffield, UK

Betsey A. Benson, PhD
Associate Professor of Clinical Psychiatry
and Psychology, Ohio State University
Nisonger Center, Columbus, OH, USA

Marco O. Bertelli, MD
Scientific Director, CREA (Research and
Clinical Center), Fondazione San
Sebastiano, Florence, Italy

Frank M. C. Besag, FRCP, FRCPsych, FRCPCH
Professor and Consultant
Neuropsychiatrist, Child and Adolescent
Mental Health Service, Learning Disability
Team (CAMHS LD), East London NHS
Foundation Trust, Bedford, UK

Nick Bouras, MD, PhD, FRCPsych
Emeritus Professor of Psychiatry at the
Institute of Psychiatry, Psychology,
Neuroscience, David Goldberg Centre,
King's College London, and Programme
Director of Maudsley International,
London, UK

Jason Buckles, MA, LPCC
Doctoral Candidate at the University of
New Mexico, Department of Educational
Specialties, Albuquerque, NM, and
Statewide Clinical Director at the New
Mexico Department of Health,
Developmental Disabilities Supports
Division, Bureau of Behavioral Support,
Albuquerque, NM, USA

Eddie Chaplin, PhD, MSc, RMN
Research Lead at South London and
Maudsley NHS Trust and Institute of
Psychiatry, Psychology, and Neuroscience,
London, UK

Sally-Ann Cooper, MBBS, MD, FRCPsych
Professor of Learning Disabilities and
Deputy Director at the Institute of Health
and Wellbeing, Gartnavel Royal Hospital,
Glasgow, UK

Dave Dagnan, PhD
Consultant Clinical Psychologist/Clinical
Director, Cumbria Partnership NHS
Foundation Trust, Community Learning
Disability Services, Workington, UK

Nathan A. Dankner, MS
Graduate Student, Vanderbilt University,
Nashville, TN, USA

Shoumitro Deb, MBBS, FRCPsych, MD
Clinical Professor of Neuropsychiatry,
Imperial College London, Division of

Brain Sciences, Department of Medicine, London, UK

Pushpal Desarkar, MD, DPM
Staff Psychiatrist and Assistant Professor of Psychiatry, Centre for Addiction and Mental Health, University of Toronto, Toronto, ON, Canada

Philip Dodd, MB, MSc, MRCPsych, MA, MD
Director of Psychiatry/Clinical Senior Lecturer, St. Michael's House, Intellectual Disability Service, Dublin/University of Dublin, Trinity College, Dublin, Ireland

Elisabeth M. Dykens, PhD
Professor of Psychology and Human Development, Professor of Psychiatry, Professor of Pediatrics, Director and Annette Schaffer Eskind Professor, Vanderbilt Kennedy Center, Nashville, TN, USA

Elizabeth Evans, PhD
Lecturer at the Department of Developmental Disability Neuropsychiatry, School of Psychiatry, University of New South Wales, NSW, Australia

Lucy Fodor-Wynne
Honorary Research Assistant, University College London, and Research Assistant, Hertfordshire Partnership University NHS Foundation Trust, Hatfield, UK

James Harris, MD
Director, Developmental Neuropsychiatry, Professor of Psychiatry and Behavioral Sciences, Mental Health, and Pediatrics, The Johns Hopkins University School of Medicine and Bloomberg School of Public Health, Baltimore, MD, USA

Angela Hassiotis, MA, PhD
Professor of Psychiatry of Intellectual Disability in the Division of Psychiatry, Faculty of Brain Sciences at UCL, and Honorary Consultant Psychiatrist at the Camden Learning Disability Service, London, UK

Jessica A. Hellings, MB, BCh, MMedPsych(SA)
Program Director at The Ohio State University Nisonger Center, Columbus, OH, USA

Sissel B. Helvershou, PhD and Licensed Specialist in Clinical Psychology
Researcher at NevSom – Norwegian Center of Expertise for Neurodevelopmental Disorders and Hypersomnias, Oslo University Hospital, Oslo, Norway

Colin Hemmings, BSc, MBBS, MSc, MA, MD(Res), MRCPsych
Consultant Psychiatrist in Intellectual Disabilities at the Maudsley Hospital, London, UK

Heidi Hermans, PhD
Psychologist/Researcher, Erasmus MC, University Medical Center Rotterdam, Rotterdam, the Netherlands

Robert M. Hodapp, PhD
Professor, Department of Special Education, Vanderbilt University, Nashville, TN, USA

Siv Helene Høidal, MD
Head Psychiatrist, Regional Department for Adults with Intellectual Disabilities/ Autism, Oslo University Hospital, Oslo, Norway

Seema Jain
MD Candidate at The Ohio State University College of Medicine, Columbus, OH, USA

Fionnuala Kelly, MB, MRCPsych
Consultant Psychiatrist/Clinical Senior Lecturer, Daughters of Charity Intellectual Disability Service, Dublin/ University of Dublin, Trinity College, Dublin, Ireland

Johanna Lake, MSc, PhD
Postdoctoral Fellow, Centre for Addiction and Mental Health, Toronto, ON, Canada

William R. Lindsay, PhD, FBPS, FIASSID, FAcSS
Consultant Forensic Clinical Psychologist
and Head of Research for Danshell, The
Danshell Group and the University of
Abertay, Dundee, UK

Yona Lunsky, PhD, CPsych
Clinician Scientist and Associate Professor
of Psychiatry, Centre for Addiction and
Mental Health, University of Toronto,
Toronto, ON, Canada

Harald Martinsen, Licensed Psychologist
Professor Emeritus, University of Oslo,
Oslo, Norway

Jane McCarthy MD, MRCGP, FRCPsych
Consultant Psychiatrist, East London NHS
Foundation Trust and King's College
London, London, UK

Carly McMorris, MA
PhD Candidate, York University, Toronto,
ON, Canada

Anna M. Palucka, PhD, CPsych
Psychologist and Assistant Professor of
Psychiatry, Centre for Addiction and
Mental Health, University of Toronto,
Toronto, ON, Canada

John Rose, PhD, MClinPsy
Professor, School of Psychology, University
of Birmingham, and Academic
Department, St. Andrews, Cliftonville,
Northampton, UK

Stephen Ruedrich, MD
L. Douglas Lenkoski Professor and Vice
Chair of Psychiatry, Case Western Reserve
University School of Medicine, University
Hospitals of Cleveland, Cleveland, OH, USA

Luis Salvador-Carulla, MD, PhD
Professor of Disability and Mental Health
and Head, Mental Health Policy Unit,
Brain and Mind Research Institute,
University of Sydney, Australia

Katrina Scior, DClinPsy, PhD
Senior Lecturer in Clinical
Psychology, University College
London, London, UK

Rory Sheehan, MBChB, MRCPsych
Specialist Registrar and Academic Clinical
Fellow in Psychiatry of Intellectual
Disabilities, Mental Health Sciences
Unit, University College London, and
Camden Learning Disabilities Service,
London, UK

John L. Taylor, BSc, MPhil, DPsychol, CPsychol, CSi, AFBPsS
Professor of Clinical Psychology at
Northumbria University, Newcastle-
upon-Tyne, and Consultant Clinical
Psychologist, Northumberland
Tyne & Wear NHS Foundation
Trust, UK

Bruce Tonge, MBBS, FRANZCP, DPM, MRCPsych
Emeritus Professor at the Department
of Psychiatry, Monash University,
Monash Medical Centre, Clayton, VIC,
Australia

Jennifer Torr, MBBS, MMed(Psych), FRANZCP
Adjunct Senior Lecturer at the Centre
for Developmental Health Victoria,
Monash University, Notting Hill, VIC,
Australia

Julian Trollor, MBBS, FRANZCP, MD
Chair of Intellectual Disability Mental
Health and Professor, School of Psychiatry
at UNSW Australia, Sydney, NSW,
Australia

Gemma L. Unwin, PhD, BSc
Research Fellow, School of Psychology,
University of Birmingham,
Birmingham, UK

Preface

This is the third edition of *Psychiatric and Behavioral Disorders in Intellectual and Developmental Disabilities.* It is the update of a book that was first published in 1999 (Bouras, 1999), with the second edition published in 2007 (Bouras and Holt, 2007), and it has become widely known and highly regarded in this field. Like the earlier editions, this new edition is primarily focused on intellectual disabilities (ID), as defined by the standard classification systems, but also includes content on other developmental disabilities. It focuses clearly on mental health aspects of ID rather than on broader health issues, but the focus is on mental ill-health in its widest sense to include significant behavioral problems. It provides the essential concepts and facts for all those involved in the mental health care of people with ID. It brings together the research findings and includes concise chapters on all of the key topics by a multiprofessional team of contributors. The international authors provide arguably the most worldwide perspective of the research in the mental health of ID field. In reviewing each area, the authors have included advances since the last edition and many have offered pointers to further progress. In addition, this book also provides useful principles for clinical practice including those underpinning assessment, management, and service delivery and is a comprehensive resource on which these can be based.

The book is divided into sections including *foundations, mental disorders, interventions, special topics,* and *services.* The *foundations* section is essential reading for the basic concepts of this field. Firstly, the context is always needed to make best sense of the current situation and evidence. Nick Bouras has been one of the leading influences in the study and practice of the mental health aspects of ID. He contributes the chapter on *historical and international perspectives*, which sets out the context of where the field is now, well into the 21st century. Understanding the key concepts that underpin clinical practice is vital for clinicians and researchers, and managers of services for people with ID, in order to maintain the clear focus of what is needed amidst all the competing demands and agendas. Of key importance is the current position of deinstutionalization in most high-income countries, driven at least in part by the normalization philosophy. It is by now well known that for a large period of history mental health problems were not considered in people with ID. It is also well known now that, converse to many expectations, the prevalence of mental health and behavioral problems was not decreased by deinstitutionalization in the latter part of the 20th century. Lessons can, thus, be drawn from history for those countries still yet to undergo the deinstitutionalization process. For example, this chapter highlights how in the UK, the development of the "community learning disabilities teams" were not as radical as they perhaps may have seemed to be. These new teams, in many ways, recreated the workings of the mental asylums by being set up as a "one-stop shop." Although seemingly comprehensive on one hand, on the other they led to some blurring of focus in an attempt to meet all the various needs of people with ID. In particular this contributed towards a disconnection with generic mental health services, meaning that people with mental health problems often fall in the gaps between services. The chapter helps to show the inevitably temporal nature of service design and the trends in this field, for example, the relatively recent increased recognition and emphasis on autism spectrum disorders.

The extended chapter in two parts by Marco O. Bertelli, Luis Salvador-Carulla, and James Harris on (i) *classification* and (ii) *diagnosis* of ID provides the core to which all the other chapters are related. They describe the process of moving from ICD-10 and DSM-IV conceptualizations to ICD-11 (unpublished at the time this book goes to print) and DSM-5. The place of ID in standard classification systems is crucial, not least to determine the relationship and connectedness of this specialist field with "mainstream" mental health. Although modified classification systems have been and are useful for advancing understanding of the atypical presentations seen in people with less than typical IQ, it is notable that they have not been adopted uniformly. The authors describe how the terminology between Intellectual Developmental Disorder (IDD) and ID in DSM-5 was developed and describe how the previously labeled *mental retardation* was simultaneously conceptualized as both a disability and a health (mental) disorder. Of note too is the relative shift in emphasis in the new DSM-5 from impairments in intellectual functioning to those in social functioning for the diagnosis of ID/IDD. Also highlighted is the recognition that the emphasis on the global IQ score is misleading owing to the large variations in specific functioning between people often found at a particular overall IQ score.

In his chapter on *epidemiology*, Jason Buckles writes a comprehensive review of the epidemiological evidence in recent years. The longstanding problems in agreeing criteria for definition and classification have been well documented. Even what should and what should not be included as a psychiatric disorder is not yet consistently agreed upon. The problems of both underdiagnosing and overdiagnosing in people with ID is highlighted, including the non-clinical influences on the diagnostic process. However, despite this, we are now further forward, allowing comparisons to be made between studies with more credibility. The author systematically examines each point in the process of epidemiological research and describes ways to progress still further despite all the difficulties. Also intimately related to these preceding chapters is the *assessment instruments and rating scales* chapter by Heidi Hermans. This includes guidance on selecting the most suitable rating instrument and includes some recent developments focusing on empowerment and digitalization.

The next section of the book contains chapters on the major types of *mental disorders*. First, Jennifer Torr reviews the *dementias* in people with ID. This topic is of continually growing importance as more and people with ID live longer lives owing to improved treatments and living standards. Rory Sheehan, Lucy Fodor-Wynne, and Angela Hassiotis contribute the chapter on the *schizophrenia spectrum disorders*. The authors have included a review of more recent findings, helping to understand better the nature of the link between ID and the schizophrenias. The chapter on *mood disorders* by Anna M. Palucka, Pushpal Desarkar, and Yona Lunsky describes how in more recent years more is known about the links between the affective disorders and suicide and traumatic events. Jane McCarthy and Eddie Chaplin in their chapter describe the *anxiety disorders* and highlight some of the recent evidence exploring the risk factors for these, including autism, physical health problems, social exclusion, and negative life events. Again, more evidence has been forthcoming in recent years of the many genetic links with anxiety disorders.

In a very welcome new addition for this edition, Philip Dodd and Fionnuala Kelly have written a chapter on *stress, traumatic, and bereavement reactions*, which are well recognized to be of major clinical importance by all working with people with ID, and yet not always or easily captured in standard classification systems. This chapter links the developments in stress and trauma in people with ID, including post-traumatic stress disorder and bereavement reactions. It clarifies recent terminologies used with research in the ID and the non-ID populations. William R. Lindsay and Regi Alexander next review *personality disorders* in ID. More recent evidence has looked at the prevalence of personality disorder and associated risks in forensic populations and also investigated the use of dialectical behavior therapy for people with ID.

In another important new chapter addition for this new edition of the book, Trine L. Bakken, Sissel B. Helvershou, Siv Helene Høidal, and Harald Martinsen consider the complex topic of *mental illness in people with ID and autism spectrum disorders*. Much of the recent research on the confounding between autism and mental illness that can occur and the identification of psychopathology in autism has been done by the authors themselves. The chapter by Elizabeth Evans and Julian Trollor on *ADHD in people with ID* includes a review of evidence regarding the family and educational interventions that are crucial in the management of ADHD in ID. The authors also include various guidelines that have been published by leading authorities since the last edition of this book.

The section on *interventions* contains four chapters. The chapter by Stephen Ruedrich on *psychopharmacology* includes a review of research into medication use for behavioral problems, in genetic syndromes, and for autism spectrum disorders. It will be directly useful for clinical practice, drawing on recent medication guidelines. The following chapters then include reviews of the modifications and use to date of *psychodynamic psychotherapy* (Nigel Beail) and *cognitive-behavioral therapy* (Dave Dagnan). This clinical use of the psychotherapies, and the tentatively positive research findings so far, continue to slowly confound some previously pessimistic views that these psychotherapies could not be modified to be made applicable for people with ID. These chapters show that a key to progress is publication of evidence, to include case studies where larger-scale studies are not yet possible or feasible, and also to publish reflections on clinical practice. Betsey A. Benson then contributes the chapter on *behavioral approaches*. Evidence has grown of effective behavioral treatments for people with ID, with multiple new studies since the last edition. However, there remain many stumbling blocks between the research findings and the translation of them into practice, and one of the most important of these seems to be in staff training.

The *special topics* section chapter on the *psychopathology of children with ID* by Bruce Tonge will be of particular interest to clinicians in child and adolescent services, as it includes several case studies and evidence-based guidance on clinical assessment. The chapter on *behavioral phenotypes/genetic syndromes* by Robert M. Hodapp, Nathan A. Dankner, and Elisabeth M. Dykens is of great interest because there has been so much recent advancement in the field of genetics. The authors highlight that findings are becoming more nuanced, for example regarding subsets of people with specific conditions or to phenotypic variants caused by quite closely related genetic changes.

In the next chapter John Taylor and William R. Lindsay review *offending behavior* in people with ID. In this chapter they include recent evidence showing that risk assessment instruments used and evaluated in the non-ID population can also be used with similar accuracy with offenders with ID. They also include recent research on psychological interventions, both individual and group-based, for the reduction of anger and aggression in offenders with ID. Sally-Ann Cooper writes the chapter on *problem behaviors and the interface with psychiatric disorders.* The author reviews some of the statistical analyses, including factor analyses, which have been employed to look at the relationships between mental health problems and problem behaviors. The chapter on *the interface between medical and psychiatric disorders* is authored by Jessica A. Hellings and Seema Jain. The comorbidity, service need, and assessment problems from this interface described by the authors are of crucial importance for assessment and treatment of psychiatric and behavioral disorders in people with ID. In the chapter on *epilepsy*, Frank M.C. Besag reviews the relationship between epilepsy and ID, and then the complicated triad between epilepsy, ID, and mental health problems. Recent evidence on the associations with specific chromosomal abnormalities and epilepsy and ID are included.

In the section on *services*, Johanna Lake, Carly McMorris, and Yona Lunsky have written the chapter on *specialist and mainstream mental health services* for people with ID. They summarize what has been learnt about the outcomes of people using these services and consider the main models of service delivery. They highlight the emerging literature recently regarding hybrid service configurations. The following two new addition chapters highlight the importance of clinicians remembering who the services are really for. People with ID and their carers and families are increasingly acknowledged to have the right to a major say in the services they receive. Many of the research studies reported in these next two chapters have, thus, been completed since the last edition of this book. Katrina Scior has written a new addition chapter on *service users' and carers' experiences of mental health services,* which includes evidence that has emerged regarding the importance of staff attitudes for the experiences of people with ID receiving mental health services. Gemma L. Unwin, Shoumitro Deb, and John Rose contribute with another new addition chapter on *carer and family perspectives.* Research findings on positive aspects of caring are included as well as the evidence on the risk of carer stress and burnout.

Finally, there is a *reflections* chapter by Colin Hemmings, which considers all of the preceding chapters in this book as a whole and reflects on some of the ongoing debates and trends in this field. It outlines some of the ways the field could develop, including in services and research, towards the time when a further edition of this book will be necessary.

References

Bouras, N. (ed.) (1999). *Psychiatric and Behavioural Disorders in Developmental Disabilities and Mental Retardation.* Cambridge: Cambridge University Press.

Bouras, N. and Holt, G. (eds.) (2007). *Psychiatric and Behavioural Disorders in Intellectual and Developmental Disabilities,* second edition. Cambridge: Cambridge University Press.

Historical and international perspectives of services

Nick Bouras

Introduction

Over the last 25 years we have witnessed remarkable advances in the diagnosis of mental health problems of people with intellectual disabilities (ID) with the use of reliable diagnostic instruments and methods. Our understanding and knowledge on the psychopathology of this population has also improved together with therapeutic interventions. The first and second edition of this book included comprehensive accounts of the historical context for people with ID and mental health problems (Jacobson, 1999; Cumella 2007). This chapter summarizes critically the main points from the above two chapters and adds newly emerged information. Early services for people with ID are briefly presented, while the main historical issues that led to the deinstitutionalization process are discussed. There is a description of the influence of the normalization concept in the development of modern services. Policy initiatives and applied service models for people with ID and mental health problems internationally are highlighted. Perspectives of current and future challenges for people with ID and mental health problems conclude the chapter.

Historical context

Ancient Greeks and Romans believed that ID was a burden on society. Ancient cultures presumed that demon possession caused ID and, similarly, some cultures thought ID was a punishment by God. Early reference to ID dates to the Egyptian Papyrus of Thebes in 1552 B.C. (Harris, 2006). Societies differed in how they conceptualized ID before the 18th century (Harbour and Maulik, 2010). Some early specialist services for people with ID included the founding of an asylum by St. Vincent de Paul in Austria (Barr, 1904/ 1973); the establishment of a hospital in Cairo, Egypt, in the Middle Ages; a form of group care in 13th-century Gheel, Belgium; and residential programs in the early 17th century in Thuringen, Bavaria, and Austria (Meyers and Blacher, 1987).

In the early 19th century there were inspirational innovations for people with mental health problems and disabilities. Philipe Pinel from 1793 reformed asylum care in Paris, to provide a safe environment, characterized by humane vigilance, planned treatment, recreation and vocational preparation, and the elimination of abuse, chains, and indignities (Scheerenberger, 1983). Another one was the publication of *The Wild Boy of Aveyron* by Jean Itard in 1801, which described how the author had worked with a "feral" boy found

Psychiatric and Behavioral Disorders in Intellectual and Developmental Disabilities, ed. Colin Hemmings and Nick Bouras. Published by Cambridge University Press. © Cambridge University Press 2016.

running in the woods. Itard described techniques, which succeeded in engaging the attention of this boy and enabling him to learn some basic skills (Murray, 1988). Edouard Seguin expanded upon Itard's work (Meyers and Blacher, 1987) and developed more extensive instructional methodology. In the following decades the establishment of educational facilities for people with ID was promoted in the USA and some European countries (Meyers and Blacher, 1987).

In the meantime the growth of institutional care gained pace with the rapid development of asylums in the USA, the UK, and other countries. Many countries began building large, publicly funded institutions to accommodate the growing number of people with ID. In the 20th century the theory of eugenics based on an extension of Darwin's theories to societies as a whole, which were conceptualized as "races" in competition for survival, became prominent (Jacobson, 1999; Cumella, 2007).

After the Second World War the new political consensus emphasized the universality of human rights (the United Nations "Universal Declaration of Human Rights" and the European "Convention of Human Rights"), explicitly extended to disabled people in the later "Declaration of Rights of Disabled People" and the "Declaration of Rights of Mentally Retarded Persons." Within democratic societies, politics became increasingly dominated by the demands for full social inclusion for racial and ethnic minorities, women, and people with disabilities (Cumella, 2007)

In 1950, the National Association of Parents and Friends of "Mentally Retarded Children" formed in the USA to advocate for children and families. The organization, now known as Arc, still provides services, coordinates research, and lobbies on behalf of children with ID and their families. By the 1950s social attitudes towards people with ID had developed towards tolerance and compassion, and financial support was made available for programs for them. In the early 1960s, President Kennedy established the "President's Panel on Mental Retardation" (now the "President's Committee for People with Intellectual Disabilities"), thereby setting a national agenda for policy, research, prevention, education, and services. The Education for All Handicapped Children Act in 1975 secured a free public education for children with ID. In 1994, the United Nations passed the "Standard Rules on Equalization of Opportunities for Persons with Disabilities," providing international standards for programs, policies, and laws for those with disabilities (Harbour and Maulik, 2010).

The World Health Organization's atlas on ID (World Health Organization, 2007) reported data on 147 countries who responded to a survey on ID. Institutional settings continued to be the most prevalent type of available services for people with ID in half of the countries. Results also showed that about 70% of countries have legislation related to ID across the world.

Deinstitutionalization

The deinstitutionalization movement's main aim was to replace the asylums with community services. The emerging use of effective new treatments in the 1950s, legislative initiatives, Kennedy's "Administration of New Frontier" program in the 1960s, changes in public opinion about those with mental health problems and or ID, and governments' desire to reduce financial cost gave impetus to the movement of deinstitutionalization (Bouras and Ikkos, 2013). Parallel initiatives and policies appeared in the UK in the 1970s when some disturbing scandals became widely known for some long stay institutions.

The movement gained momentum and spread gradually worldwide when it adopted philosophies from the civil rights movement. Families, professionals, civil rights leaders, and humanitarians saw the shift from institutional confinement to local care as the appropriate approach. Concerns, however, and fears were expressed as well, mostly by psychiatrists but also some patients, carers, and other members of the society. Some historians suggest a combination of social policy, antipsychiatry, and consumer activism contributed to the implementation of deinstitutionalization (Eghigian, 2011).

The last 50 years have seen an increased focus on early intervention, community-based rehabilitation, diagnosis, human rights, and legislation, with particular emphasis on deinstitutionalization (Mansell, 2006; Beadle-Brown et al., 2007). Some of the first clinical effectiveness research in this field found that community-based units had better outcomes in terms of behavior and self-care skills (Raynes and King, 1967). Renewed therapeutic optimism led to the increasing recruitment into services for people with ID of clinical psychologists, educationalists, occupational therapists, and therapists, who had less personal investment in maintaining institutions than medical and nursing staff (Cumella, 2007). Deinstitutionalization of people with ID has been probably the largest social policy experiment of our time. Overall, people with ID and their families have benefited, having a better quality of life and more opportunities.

Normalization

The move from institutional care was also promoted by the "normalization" concept first introduced in Scandinavia (Nirje, 1972). It was Wolfensburger's influential writings emphasizing the need to overcome the social psychology of discrimination of disabled people that influenced the development of services for people with ID (Cumella, 2007). Wolfensburger (1991) noted that disabled people suffer disadvantages not only in the form of overt discrimination but also in an unconscious process of denigration. This confirmed to disabled people their inferior and dependent position in society, which they in turn expressed through their behavior, thereby confirming the initial assumptions of their lower status. He proposed that a key objective of services should, therefore, be to enable disabled people to behave in ways that were socially valued rather than inferior, in order to assert their equal status and achieve acceptance by others in society. This involves living in "normative housing within the valued community with valued people," attending the same schools, and being involved in a valued manner in work, shopping, and leisure activities (Wolfensburger, 1991).

Normalization was implemented in various model services, of which the most influential was that of the Eastern Nebraska Community Office of Retardation (ENCOR), which also became known as the "Core and Cluster" program (Menolascino, 1994). This service was led by the pioneer psychiatrist Frank Menolascino under the inspiration of Wolfensburger who was working with ENCOR at that time. This program carried out the adaptation of ordinary houses to provide staff-supported accommodation for small groups of people with ID. The specialized clinical staff also provided direct teaching to caregivers. The program made use of existing community services, including family support services, and integrated job placements, which had been encouraged through liaison with local industries. In the UK, this model inspired the report *An Ordinary Life* (King's Fund, 1981), which came at the moment when changes in social security regulations inadvertently provided an expansion of public funds for resettling people from long stay hospital care

(Cumella, 2007). Similar policies were adopted gradually around the world, particularly in North America, Europe, and Australasia. The response and attitudes of different societies to people with ID over time has fluctuated in care practices among nations that are consistent with their cultural history and customs.

ID and mental health problems

Until the second half of the 20th century there was little agreement in the professional literature about whether people with ID were susceptible to mental health problems and whether or how treatment should be offered. Research in this field was probably impeded by the eugenic view that mental health problems and antisocial behavior were an inherent characteristic of people with ID. A series of studies in different institutional populations began to estimate prevalence rates for psychiatric disorders and there was recognition that behavioral problems and impoverished institutional environments were very common (Craft, 1959).

Jacobson (1999) noted that instances of coexisting mental health and ID had been described by Seguin as early as 1866. The development, however, of mental health services for people with ID "is largely a phenomenon of the post-modern period. They reflect growth in the financial resources directed via public policy to support and treat people with ID in developed nations during the second half of the 20th century" (Jacobson, 1999).

Service planners and providers assumed that mental health problems for people with ID would substantially diminish when community care programs had been put in place. With the beginnings of deinstitutionalization and the implementation of resettlement programs in the community, the needs of people with ID and mental health problems became evident. Initial longitudinal research indicated the coexistence of ID and mental health problems was a risk factor for reinstitutionalization (Kearney and Smull, 1992). As more and more institutions were closed, people with ID and mental health problems found themselves moving to less restrictive environments, or remaining longer with their families. In such community settings, it became clear that services from both the ID network and the mental health system were required. The provision of the necessary mental health services for people with ID and mental health problems became a major issue in the USA and the UK as community resettlement plans started being implemented.

Strong ideological and political views for services to support people with ID were prevailing in favor of a social care model. However, it became clear that if the plans for community care were going to succeed, a robust clinical mental health service was required. The expectation was that mainstream health services, including mental health, would assume responsibility for the mental health problems of people with ID living in the community. Mainstream psychiatric services were, however, unprepared to respond to the needs of this population, lacking knowledge and expertise on the diagnosis, treatment, and their mental health needs. In addition, the funding for their mental health care from the closure of the institutions was diverted predominately towards social care.

There was a substantial delay before the awareness of the coexistence of ID and mental health problems was converted into public policy. Although mental health clinics for people with ID were established from 1958, in the USA policy-makers were reluctant to accept that people with ID needed more than just a uniform and undifferentiated set of services (Menolascino, 1989).

In the 1960s there were continuing signs of psychiatry's schism with ID services. The American Medical Association (AMA) in 1965 reported that very few psychiatric services were serving people with ID and that these were mostly child psychiatric services (American Medical Association, 1965; Jacobson, 1999). About the same time the American Psychiatric Association (APA) issued a statement on ID (American Psychiatric Association, 1966) advocating for integration of ID with community mental health services. The recommendation was that psychiatry should take the lead in these efforts in collaboration with other organizations to develop standards of care and to avoid establishing duplicative services for people with ID and mental health problems. These recommendations were later to be largely realized in the training sequences for medical and mental health professionals provided by university-affiliated programs (Jacobson, 1999).

Menolascino (1989) recommended that services be provided according to need and be delivered in the context of both ID and coexisting mental health problems, allowing for more appropriate treatment, support, service planning, and development. The result would have been a partnership between the mental health and ID service structures to ensure responsive supports and treatments. The term "dual diagnosis" was first introduced by Menolascino but later became synonymous for people with substance misuse and mental health problems.

Similar issues with the USA were experienced in the UK (Day, 1993). The provision of health services for people with ID should be seen within the context of countries' health systems. The National Health Service (NHS) in the UK is funded by general taxation, while in the USA there are various levels of insurance schemes and state and federal funding systems. Another notable difference between those two countries, and probably from the rest of the world, is that in the UK the Royal College of Psychiatrists has a strong faculty of psychiatrists specializing in people with ID and mental health problems. The Royal College of Psychiatrists in the 1970s debated its involvement with people with ID. The outcome was to focus on the mental health problems of this population with the creation of the subspecialty of "Psychiatry in ID" that has contributed substantially to service developments, training, and research. This development, together with specialization of clinical psychology as well as other professions, has played a decisive role in the development of services in the UK for people with ID.

A government report in 1979 in the UK concluded that people with ID had diverse needs, each requiring an array of specialist services (Department of Health and Social Security, 1979). A series of policy reports in the next two decades (Department of Health and Social Security, 1984; Department of Health, 1993, 2001; Lindsey, 1998) proposed various options for how services could be provided. They identified three overlapping groups of people with ID: those with a mental illness; those with severe antisocial behaviors; and those who have committed offenses against the law. The overall position of governmental policy in the UK has been consistently that people with ID should have access to mainstream health services, but with additional specialist (specifically for people with ID) support when needed (Department of Health, 2001).

The argument for the provision of mental health care for people with ID from mainstream services appeared sound and is supported widely (Bouras and Holt, 2004). Some argued that specialized services leads to stigmatization, labeling, and negative professional attitudes. Others argued that special expertise is required for the diagnosis and treatment of mental health problems in this population, because, although it is theoretically possible to train staff in mainstream settings, the relatively small number of cases gives little opportunity for staff to gain or maintain the necessary skills (Day, 1999). Problems arise particularly when admissions to adult acute inpatient units occur, as people with ID often require longer admissions, and may be vulnerable without additional support on the ward. Furthermore, people with ID represent a very heterogeneous group with a varied range of highly complex mental health needs.

A wide degree of variation in locations, service mix, financing options, and staffing patterns has been reported among service responses to meet the mental health needs of people with ID. Moss et al. (2000) provided a framework to conceptualize the factors that influence service development in this field. They proposed a variant of the matrix model first described for non-disabled people with mental health problems by Thornicroft and Tansella (1999). The model is comprised of two dimensions, one determined by the level within the service system (e.g., national, local, or individual), and the other by the point in the temporal sequence of service provision (e.g., inputs to the service, the process of providing the service, and the resulting outcome). Using this model to characterize various approaches to service, it is possible to observe that national priorities often vary from country to country and from culture to culture. These differences guide and influence inputs to the service system and, ultimately, affect the way a consumer is served and the service products and outcomes. They also emphasize that inputs to every system at all levels are affected by the need for trained personnel to staff and administer the service.

Davidson and O'Hara (2007) suggested that the characteristics of comprehensive mental health services for people with ID should address the conceptualization of the service system model, using techniques to overcome barriers when there are both conceptual and operational gaps between service systems by establishing interagency communication across systems. Additional characteristics should include consensus among providers, interdisciplinary approach by a team of professionals who can address biomedical, behavioral, and environmental interventions, case management, and supports to families and service users. Community-based with tertiary psychiatric links are also required for an acute crisis and may be provided on a supra-district or regional basis. Training and stable funding are also of utmost importance (Davidson and O'Hara, 2007).

The most common model of services for adults with ID and mental health problems that emerged in the UK is an ID community-based, multidisciplinary (interdisciplinary) team offering assessment and specialist services to people with ID. Initially, most of these teams were involved with deinstitutionalization, carrying out tasks such as identifying appropriately adapted and staffed houses, matching people with ID to live together, assessing health and social needs, and so on. Most of them have input from clinical psychologists and usually some input from a psychiatrist specializing in people with ID. There have been some variations of this approach, mostly related to the interface of these teams with mainstream mental health services and or primary care (O'Hara et al., 2013).

Despite the input from a psychiatrist, such teams have been experiencing difficulties in meeting the mental health needs of people, particularly those with mild ID and diagnosable mental illness. The problems are extended to people with ID who may have additional forensic problems, autism spectrum disorders, including Asperger's syndrome, and comorbid conditions, such as those with borderline intellectual functioning. Chaplin et al. (2010) referred to this model as a "one-stop shop," just as it was in the institutions. Bouras and Holt (2010) stated that the provision of mental health services from a specialist Community Intellectual Disability Team was an historical mistake by transferring into community an institutional model of care. This contradiction currently remains and, coupled with ongoing ideological arguments, as to what constitutes challenging behavior versus a diagnosable psychiatric disorder, has led to a fragmentation of services for people with ID in the UK.

The exception to the Community Intellectual Disability Team has been the development of a specialist mental health service for people with ID (MHiID) (also known as mental health services for people with learning disabilities [MHiLD]), fully integrated structurally, organizationally, and operationally with the mainstream (also referred as generic) mental health services. This model is compatible with other specialist mental health services in the UK, e.g., older adults, children and adolescents, drugs misuse, homeless, eating disorders, etc. The MHiID service is one of the longest services in operation, since 1982, based in South East London, providing secondary and tertiary mental health care for people with ID. The evolution of the MHiID service, which first used inpatient beds in a psychiatric unit in a general hospital in the UK, has been well documented. (Holt et al., 1988; Davidson and O'Hara, 2007; Chaplin et al., 2008; Bouras and Holt, 2010; Chaplin et al. 2010; Hemmings, 2010; O'Hara et al., 2013). Other service developments in the UK have also been reviewed in these just-listed publications.

Current research findings on clinical outcomes of different program models for people with mental health problems and ID is presented in Chapter 23. Hemmings et al. (2014) provided an evidence base showing that the way forward is in developing new ways of coworking ID services with mainstream mental health services, including in-community and inpatient settings.

International trends

There has been a growing interest internationally as to how to address the mental health problems of people with ID. Davidson and O'Hara (2007) and Cain et al. (2010) have provided comprehensive reviews of service developments for this population in different countries. The pace and form of change depends on each country's unique historical perspective and national philosophies about care for people with ID. Internationally the trend has been towards the direction of community integration of specialist community ID services with a different degree of inpatient facilities either from mainstream psychiatric services or not. Variation across continents and between services exists on a number of levels. Disparity of service provision also exists between different regions of the same country where local pressures and resources have dictated service developments. These include, service design, care packages, funding streams, commissioning, staffing patterns, and resources (Cain et al., 2010).

Holt et al. (2000) reviewed services for people with ID and mental health problems in five European countries: Austria, England, Greece, Ireland, and Spain. The most common pattern found was a limited number of specialist centers, with the expectation that people with ID and mental health problems will be admitted to mainstream psychiatric services. In some countries, the historical experience of adverse medically dominated institutions led to reluctance among policy-makers to consider any specialist health services for people with ID (Holt et al., 2000). Where emphasis has been on treatment in the community, there was a growing recognition of the need for additional specialist services as well as help to access services. The review concluded that legislation and policy in the five countries tended to separate ID and mental health, resulting in unmet needs remaining largely invisible, to the detriment of people with ID and mental health problems, their families, and carers. Similarly, Weinbach (2004) published a condensed overview of service profiles across Europe (including Belgium, England, Germany, Greece, Spain, Sweden, and the Netherlands) in an attempt to describe the systems of care and support available for people with ID. Dosen has written excessively on services in the Netherlands (Dosen, 1988; Cain et al., 2010) and Salvador-Carulla for Spain (Salvador-Carulla and Martinez-Maroto, 1993; Cain et al., 2010).

Davidson and O'Hara (2007) and Cain et al. (2010) have described several services in the USA that have been providing mental health care for people with mental health problems and ID. Early initiatives for these services in our times were pioneered in the USA by the clinical psychologists Johnny Matson and Steve Reiss and the psychiatrists Frank Menolascino, already mentioned in the development of the ENCOR program in Nebraska, and Ludwik Szymanski in Boston. The development of the National Association for the Dually Diagnosed (NADD) founded in 1983 as a not-for-profit association in the USA by Robert Fletcher acted as a catalyst to promote and exchange ideas, principles, and concepts concerning people having mental health problems and ID. The NADD continues having a strong presence worldwide in the field offering training, publications, and professional, carer, and service user support.

The Rochester Crisis Intervention Model in New York has been one of the well-documented services in North America (Davidson and O'Hara, 2007; Cain et al., 2010). Another well-documented service has been the Greater Boston START Model (Systemic, Therapeutic, Assessment, Respite, and Treatment). The START model was first developed and implemented in Massachusetts in 1989 as a linkage model to overcome disparities in access to mental health care (Charlot and Beasley, 2013). The primary function of START teams is to facilitate collaboration between systems and disciplines in order to improve diagnostic accuracy and treatment outcomes. Service elements include an interdisciplinary clinical consultation team, 24-hour emergency services, planned and emergency therapeutic respite services, and ongoing training in the system of care. There are several START programs in the USA with some state-wide implementation and with more in development. Outcomes associated with START include improved access to appropriate services, reduction in emergency service use, and improvements in the quality of community living (Charlot and Beasley, 2013).

Several other services have been described in the USA over time (Davidson and O'Hara, 2007; Cain et al., 2010) but little is known currently in the literature about their fate. Most of these services appeared in the 1990s led by psychologists, nurses, and social workers, with some involvement from a handful of psychiatrists. There has been a growing interest in recent years to services for people with autism spectrum disorders. One such service is the Autism Speaks Autism Treatment Network (ATN) that has associated a large network of hospitals, physicians, researchers, and families in several locations in the USA and Canada (ATN website: http://www.autismspeaks.org/science/resources-programs/autism-treatment-network). Charlot and Beasley (2013) stated that "In spite of improvements in community systems in the US, change has been sporadic and inconsistent from a national policy perspective. Evidence continues that people with co-occurring ID and mental illness are the last and least served in the community. Recent court decisions with regard to the civil rights of these individuals have helped to motivate states to pay closer attention to the system of care and related outcomes."

In Australia, the term "Dual Disability" was introduced and there have been some specialist mental health services for people with ID that were also reported in some detail by Davidson and O'Hara (2007) and Cain et al. (2010). There are well-established academic units in Australia, e.g., the Centre for Developmental Disability Health Victoria (CDDHV) at Monash University, Queensland Centre for Intellectual and Developmental Disability (QCIDD) at the University of Queensland, and the Intellectual Disability Mental Health at the University of New South Wales. Service provision is also linked with these academic units. Wurth and Brandon (2014) published a 10-year evaluation of the Australian Capital Territory (ACT) Dual Disability Service (DDS) (recently renamed the Mental Health Service for People with Intellectual Disability – MHS-ID), which has been in operation since 2002. Bennett (2014) of the Victorian Dual Disability Service (VDDS) at the Department of Psychiatry at St. Vincent's Hospital in Melbourne has reiterated the need for specialist mental health services for people with ID. Torr (2013) has reviewed the evidence base on mental health for people with ID including services. Trollor, of the academic unit at the University of New South Wales, has reported renewed support from the Royal Australia and New Zealand College of Psychiatrists to reengage in the area of ID, suggesting "Concerted action by government, policymakers, services and practitioners is required if equity of access to mental health services is to be achieved for people with an ID" (Trollor, 2014).

In Hong Kong the Siu Lam Hospital mental health services for people with ID led by Henry Kwok was established in the early 1990s, providing inpatient and outreach services. Within Asia, a survey of 14 countries found a wide variation of services with the type of service relating to wider economic and social considerations (Kwok and Chui, 2008; Kwok et al., 2011). They also reported encouraging developments for children and adults with ID in China. There was, however, a lack of policy to ensure continuity of care or smooth transition from one service to another across the lifespan. Effective implementation of laws and policies remained difficult. They advocated improved coordination, communication, prioritization, and collaboration among government departments, local governments, families, and non-governmental organizations (NGOs) (Kwok and Chui, 2008; Kwok et al., 2011). Similar issues were highlighted by Jeevanandam (2009) for Asian countries, adding the lack of epidemiological studies and evidence-based practices. The lack of policies, poor implementation of plans, low priority, inadequate service provision for people with mental health problems, and ID have been reported by Mercadante et al. (2009) for Latin America, Njenga (2009) for Africa, Adnams (2010) for South Africa, Girimaji and Srinath (2010) for India, Katz et al. (2010) for Mexico, and Ispanovic-Radojkovic and Stancheva-Popkostadinova (2011) for Serbia and Bulgaria.

The issues and dilemmas of the most appropriate services for people with ID and mental health problems have been the focus of important policy documents in recent years. In Canada, in *Moving Forward: National Action on Dual Diagnosis,* the National Coalition on Dual Diagnosis stated that:

> Mainstream mental health services have not welcomed people with a dual diagnosis and have not served their needs well. Further, mental health professionals generally do not have the expertise to diagnose or treat them effectively. Today, mental health and developmental services continue to live in separate worlds with separate cultures (National Coalition on Dual Diagnosis, 2011).

In Ireland, the National Disability Authority made clear in a detailed report that:

> Persons registered with a mainstream ID service provider find it even more difficult or impossible to gain access to appropriate mental health services for assessment, treatment or continuing care. The difference in experience arises mainly because of policy confusion. Service delivery should largely focus on specialist multidisciplinary teams who are dual trained in ID and mental health. Regional units, geographically distributed, must be available to support community teams by providing specialist acute assessment and treatment for the dual diagnosis group. Full consideration to staffing issues is required in order to ensure a stable and sustainable service, supporting the highest standards of care, and providing a rewarding career for those in the services. The need for these services is growing, and provision should be addressed as a matter of urgency (National Disability Authority, 2013).

The Royal College of Psychiatrists (2012, 2013) published documents reiterating that:

> Each organization providing ID and mental health services should have protocols or practices in place to meet the mental health needs of adults with mild ID, jointly agreed between services for people with ID, adult mental health services and Local Authorities. Clinical and non-clinical managers of ID services should ensure that the needs of this group are on the agenda of the local bodies responsible for the development of mental health services.

Conclusions

Service models for people with mental health problems and ID have emerged following successful deinstitutionalization programs. The current trends are geared towards community integration schemes with service users' participation at all levels, including design and implementation, with a person-centered approach. Those commissioning services need to determine what services are needed locally and to decide how they should be provided, monitored, and reviewed. This chapter provides an historical overview of service developments within an international policy context. In spite of some progress, services for people with mental health problems and ID remain underdeveloped. There has been considerable debate as to whether specialist mental health services for people with ID services should be established, or whether mainstream mental health services should serve this population. How specialist mental health services are provided has changed along with key developments, including detection and identification of mental health problems, and a better understanding of therapeutic interventions. The need for specialist services has been recognized as it has become clear that mainstream mental health services, particularly inpatient wards, are unable to cater for all of those with ID. Many reasons have been given for this at a clinical level, including complexity of presentation, the need for more detailed or specialist assessment, and issues of vulnerability. Whatever strategy is undertaken, it should be based on high professional standards and the evidence base.

Over the last two decades, people with ID in many parts of the world live outside of institutions, with families in local communities, and with increased expectations. There is an increasingly diverse population of mild ID, with more complex comorbidity and increased age expectancy. This, along with the issues of ethnicity and gender, has meant the need for services to respond to the needs of ever-changing local communities is now greater than it has ever been. It is the view of the author of this chapter that mental health services for people with ID are due for a major reshape as we have entered the "post-community era."

Key summary points

- Several years into the post-institutional period and the era of community care, meeting the mental health needs of people with ID remains a challenge.
- Provision of community-based interventions is increasing.
- Access to local specialist and mainstream community and inpatient assessment, treatment, forensic, and rehabilitation facilities needs to improve.
- Good interagency communication among health, social, and voluntary sectors should be encouraged.
- Service user and carer participation is essential to ensure that appropriate priorities are set and that services are satisfactorily delivered.
- Resources to meet residential, recreational, and vocational needs of those with enduring needs must be assigned.

References

Adnams, C.M. (2010). Perspectives of intellectual disability in South Africa: epidemiology, policy, services for children and adults. *Current Opinion in Psychiatry*, 23(5), 436–440.

American Medical Association (1965). Mental retardation: a handbook for the primary physician. *Journal of the American Medical Association*, 191, 183–232.

American Psychiatric Association (1966). Psychiatry and mental retardation. *American Journal of Psychiatry*, 122, 1302–1314.

Barr, M.W. (1904/1973). *Mental Defectives, their History, Treatment, and Training*. New York, NY: Arno Press.

Beadle-Brown, J., Mansell, J., Kozma, A. (2007). Deinstitutionalization in intellectual disabilities. *Current Opinion in Psychiatry*, 20, 437–442.

Bennett, C. (2014). Understanding systemic problems in providing mental health services to people with an intellectual disability and co-morbid mental disorders in Victoria. *Australasian Psychiatry*, 22(1), 48–51.

Bouras, N. and Holt, G. (2004). Mental health services for adults with learning disabilities. *British Journal of Psychiatry*, 184, 291–292.

Bouras, N and Holt, G. (eds.) (2010). *Mental Health Services for Adults with Intellectual Disability: Strategies and Solutions*. London: Psychology Press.

Bouras, N. and Ikkos, G. (2013). Ideology, psychiatric practice and professionalism. *Psychiatriki*, 24, 17–27.

Cain, N.N., Davidson, P.W., Dosen, A., et al. (2010). An international perspective of mental health services for people with intellectual disability. In N. Bouras and G. Holt (eds.), *Mental Health Services for Adults with Intellectual Disability: Strategies and Solutions*. London: Psychology Press.

Chaplin, E., O'Hara, J., Holt, G., Hardy, S., Bouras, N. (2008). MHiLD: a model of specialist mental health services for people with learning disabilities. *Advances in Mental Health and Learning Disabilities*, 2(4), 46–50.

Chaplin, E., Paschos, D., O'Hara, J. (2010). The specialist mental health model and other services in a changing environment. In N. Bouras and G. Holt (eds.), *Mental Health Services for Adults with Intellectual Disability: Strategies and Solutions*. London: Psychology Press.

Charlot, L. and Beasley, J.B. (2013). Intellectual disabilities and mental health: United States-based research. *Journal of Mental Health Research in Intellectual Disabilities*, 6(2), 74–105.

Craft, M. (1959). Mental disorder in the defective: a psychiatric survey among in-patients. *American Journal of Mental Deficiency*, 63, 829–834.

Cumella, S. (2007). Mental health and intellectual disabilities: the development of services. In N. Bouras and G. Holt (eds.), *Psychiatric and Behavioural Disorders in Intellectual and Developmental Disabilities*, second edition. Cambridge: Cambridge University Press.

Davidson, P.W. and O'Hara, J. (2007). Clinical services for people with intellectual disabilities and psychiatric or severe behaviour disorders. In N. Bouras and G. Holt (eds.), *Psychiatric and Behavioural Disorders in Intellectual and Developmental Disabilities*, second edition. Cambridge: Cambridge University Press.

Day, K. (1993). Mental health services for people with mental retardation: a framework for the future. *Journal of Intellectual Disability Research*, 37, 7–16.

Day, K. (1999). Professional training in the psychiatry of mental retardation in the United Kingdom. In N. Bouras (ed.), *Psychiatric and Behavioural Disorders in Intellectual and Developmental Disabilities*. Cambridge: Cambridge University Press.

Department of Health (1993). *Services for People with Learning Disabilities and Challenging Behaviours or Mental Health Needs*. London: HMSO.

Department of Health (2001). *Valuing People: A New Strategy for Learning Disabilities in the 21st Century*. London: HMSO.

Department of Health and Social Security (1979). *Report of the Committee of Enquiry into Mental Handicap Nursing and Care*. London: HMSO.

Department of Health and Social Security (1984). *Helping Mentally Handicapped Persons with Special Needs. Report of a DHSS Study Team. A Review of Current Approaches to Meeting the Needs of Mentally Handicapped People with Special Problems*. London: Department of Health and Social Security.

Dosen, A. (1988). Community care for people with mental retardation in the Netherlands. *Australia and New Zealand Journal of Developmental Disabilities*, 14, 15–18.

Eghigian, G. (2011). Deinstitutionalizing the history of contemporary psychiatry. *History of Psychiatry*, 22, 201–214.

Girimaji, S.C. and Srinath, S. (2010). Perspectives of intellectual disability in India: epidemiology, policy, services for children and adults. *Current Opinion in Psychiatry*, 23(5), 441–446.

Harbour, C.K and Maulik, P.K. (2010). History of intellectual disability. In J.H. Stone and M. Blouin (eds.), *International Encyclopedia of Rehabilitation*. At: http://cirrie.buffalo .edu/encyclopedia/en/article/143/

Harris, J.C. (2006). *Intellectual Disability: Understanding its Development, Causes, Classification, Evaluation, and Treatment*. Oxford: Oxford University Press.

Hemmings, C. (2010) Service use and outcomes. In N. Bouras and G. Holt (eds.), *Psychiatric and Behavioural Disorders in Intellectual and Developmental Disabilities*, second edition. Cambridge: Cambridge University Press.

Hemmings, C., Bouras, N., Craig, T. (2014). How should community mental health of intellectual disability services evolve? *International Journal of Environmental Research and Public Health*, 11, 8624–8631.

Holt, G., Bouras, N., Watson, J.P. (1988). Down's syndrome and eating disorders. Mental health services for adults with learning disabilities. *British Journal of Psychiatry*, 152, 847–848.

Holt, G., Costello, H., Bouras, N., et al. (2000). BIOMED–MEROPE project: service provision for adults with intellectual disability: a European comparison. *Journal of Intellectual Disability Research*, 44(6), 685–696.

Ispanovic-Radojkovic, V. and Stancheva-Popkostadinova, V. (2011). Perspectives of intellectual disability in Serbia and Bulgaria: epidemiology, policy and services for children and adults. *Current Opinion in Psychiatry*, 24(5), 419.

Jacobson, J.W. (1999). Dual diagnosis services: history, progress and perspectives. In N. Bouras (ed.), *Psychiatric and Behavioural Disorders in Intellectual and Developmental Disabilities*. Cambridge: Cambridge University Press.

Jeevanandam, L. (2009). Perspectives of intellectual disability in Asia: epidemiology, policy, and services for children and adults. *Current Opinion in Psychiatry*, 22(5), 462–468.

Katz, G., Márquez-Caraveo, M.E., Lazcano-Ponce, E. (2010). Perspectives of intellectual disability in Mexico: epidemiology, policy, and services for children and adults. *Current Opinion in Psychiatry*, 23, 432–435.

Kearney, F.J. and Smull, M.W. (1992). People with mental retardation leaving mental health institutions: evaluating outcomes after five years in the community. In J.W. Jacobson, S.N. Burchard, P.J. Carling (eds.), *Community Living for People with Developmental and Psychiatric Disabilities*. Baltimore, MD: The Johns Hopkins University Press.

King's Fund (1981). *An Ordinary Life. Comprehensive Locally-Based Residential Services for Mentally Handicapped People*. London: King's Fund Centre.

Kwok, H. and Chui, E. (2008). A survey on mental health care for adults with intellectual disabilities in Asia. *Journal of Intellectual Disability Research*, 52, 996–1002.

Kwok, H, Cui, Y., Li, J. (2011). Perspectives of intellectual disability in the People's Republic of China: epidemiology, policy, services for children and adults. *Current Opinion in Psychiatry*, 24, 408–412.

Lindsey, M. (1998). *Signposts for Success in Commissioning and Providing Health Services for People with Learning Disabilities*. London: NHS Executive.

Mansell, J. (2006). Deinstitutionalisation and community living: progress, problems and priorities. *Journal of Intellectual and Developmental Disability*, 31(2), 65–76.

Menolascino, F. (1989). Model services for treatment/management of the mentally retarded-mentally ill. *Community Mental Health Journal*, 25(2), 145–155.

Menolascino, F. (1994). Services for people with dual diagnosis in the USA. In N. Bouras (ed.), *Mental Health in Mental Retardation: Recent Advances and Practices*. Cambridge: Cambridge University Press.

Mercadante, M.T., Evans-Lacko, S., Paula, C.S. (2009). Perspectives of intellectual disability in Latin American countries: epidemiology, policy, and services for children and adults. *Current Opinion in Psychiatry*, 22(5), 469–474.

Meyers, C.E. and Blacher, J. (1987). Historical determinants of residential care. In S. Landesman, P.M. Vietze, M.J. Begab (eds.), *Living Environments and Mental Retardation*. Washington, DC: American Association on Mental Retardation.

Moss, S., Bouras, N., Holt, G. (2000). Mental health services for people with intellectual disability: a conceptual framework. *Journal of Intellectual Disability Research*, 44, 97–107.

Murray, P. (1988). The study of the history of disability services: examining the past to improve the present and future. *Australia and New Zealand Journal of Developmental Disabilities*, 14, 93–102.

National Coalition on Dual Diagnosis (2011). *Moving Forward: National Action on Dual Diagnosis*. At: http://care-id.com/wp-content/uploads/2011/11/moving_forward.pdf

National Disability Authority (2013) *Review of Access to Mental Health Services for People with Intellectual Disabilities*. At: http://www.nda.ie/cntmgmtnew.nsf/0/815EB07591494D9D80256F62005E6964?OpenDocument

Nirje, B. (1972) The right to self-determination. In W. Wolfensburger (ed.), *The Principle of Normalisation in Human Services*. Toronto, ON: National Institute on Mental Retardation.

Njenga, F. (2009) Perspectives of intellectual disability in Africa: epidemiology and policy services for children and adults. *Current Opinion in Psychiatry*, 22(5), 457–461.

O'Hara, J., Chaplin, E., Lockett, J., Bouras, N. (2013). Community mental health services. In E. Tsakanikos and J. McCarthy (eds.), *Handbook of Psychopathology in Intellectual Disability: Research, Practice and Policy*. New York, NY: Springer.

Raynes, N. and King, R. (1967). Residential care for the mentally retarded. In D. Boswell and J. Wingrove (eds.), *The Handicapped Person in the Community*.

A Reader and Sourcebook. London: Tavistock Publications/Open University.

Royal College of Psychiatrists (2012). *CR175. Enabling People with Mild Intellectual Disability and Mental Health Problems to Access Healthcare Services.* At: http://www.rcpsych.ac.uk/usefulresources/publications/collegereports/cr/cr175.aspx

Royal College of Psychiatrists (2013). *People with Learning Disability and Mental Health, Behavioural or Forensic Problems. The Role of Inpatient Services.* At: http://www.rcpsych.ac.uk/pdf/FR%20ID%2003%20for%20website.pdf

Salvador-Carulla, L. and Martinez-Maroto, A. (1993). The European services: Spain. *Journal of Intellectual Disability Research,* 37(Suppl. I), 34–37.

Scheerenberger, R.C. (1983). *A History of Mental Retardation.* Baltimore, MD: Paul H. Brookes.

Thornicroft, G. and Tansella, M. (1999). *The Mental Health Matrix: A Manual to Improve Services.* Cambridge: Cambridge University Press.

Torr, J. (2013). Intellectual disability and mental ill health: a view of Australian research. *Journal of Mental Health Research in Intellectual Disabilities,* 6, 159–178.

Trollor, J. (2014). Australia: making mental health services accessible to people with an intellectual disability. *Australian and New Zealand Journal of Psychiatry,* 48(5), 395–398.

Weinbach, H. (2004). Comparing structure, design and organisation of support of people with learning disabilities in Europe: the work of the Intellectual Disability Research Network (IDRESNET). *Tizard Learning Disability Review,* 9(1), 2–6.

Wolfensberger, W. (1991). Reflections on a lifetime in human services and mental retardation. *Mental Retardation,* 29, 1–16.

World Health Organization (2007). *Atlas: Global Resources for Persons with Intellectual Disabilities.* Geneva: World Health Organization. At: http://www.who.int/mental_health/evidence/atlas_id_2007.pdf

Wurth, P. and Brandon, S.A. (2014). The ACT mental health service for people with intellectual disability, 10 years on. *Australasian Psychiatry,* 22(1), 52–55.

Classification and diagnosis

Marco O. Bertelli, Luis Salvador-Carulla, and
James Harris

Introduction

This chapter is divided in two parts. The first part describes the process of recent developments in the classification of Mental Retardation. It emphasizes the work of the World Health Organization (WHO) International Advisory Group for the revision of classification and diagnostic criteria of Mental Retardation in the *International Classification of Diseases and Related Health Problems, Tenth Revision* (ICD-10; World Health Organization 1992a, 1992b) (WHO-IAGRMR), the Intellectual Disability section of the World Psychiatric Association (WPA-SPID), and the terminology adopted in the *Diagnostic and Statistical Manual of Mental Disorders, Fifth Edition* by the American Psychiatric Association (APA) (DSM-5; American Psychiatric Association, 2013). Though the new *International Classification of Diseases, Eleventh Edition* (ICD-11) is not released at the time this book goes to print, we have described the debate that has taken place and the expected terminology to be finally adopted (World Health Organization, 2011). The second part of this chapter deals with the issue of diagnosis, including arguments for inclusion or not of certain criteria. The importance of taking into consideration the adaptive function in addition to symptoms and behaviors is discussed, as well as the diagnostic challenges for comorbid situations of intellectual disabilities and autism spectrum disorders or different behavioral phenotypes.

Recent developments
Classification

In this chapter we use the term Intellectual Disabilities (ID) instead of Mental Retardation for consistency with the contents throughout the rest of this book, except when referring to DSM-5, which has introduced the term Intellectual Developmental Disorder (IDD). Mental Retardation has a long history within the taxonomy of mental disorders, and its conceptualization has always been controversial. Its recent conceptualization as Intellectual Disabilities (or Intellectual Disability) has proved to be controversial for the forthcoming ICD-11. In fact, Mental Retardation, or ID, is a complex condition implying impairments of mental and personal functions that are difficult to precisely define, such as intelligence, learning, adaptive behavior, and skills, with onset in early life, and that tend to persist life-long. Despite these difficulties in definition, classification and

Psychiatric and Behavioral Disorders in Intellectual and Developmental Disabilities, ed. Colin Hemmings and Nick Bouras. Published by Cambridge University Press. © Cambridge University Press 2016.

diagnostic criteria are crucial issues for ID, having important implications for prevalence, intervention, service provision, and outcomes. ID implies a major impact on functioning and disability throughout the life course, and there is a high co-occurrence of other mental disorders. It is frequently misdiagnosed, is associated with poor access to healthcare services, and is associated with very high costs for the healthcare system and for society as a whole. In spite of this, ID is largely disregarded in the mental health sector, where specific training and specialized services are limited to a few high income countries, primarily in Western Europe and North America.

The question whether ID should be considered a health condition, a disability, or even a life condition is still debated in many contexts. A number of experts in different fields, such as sociology, anthropology, psychology, education, or typology have given different interpretations, which sometimes had – and still have – a considerable impact on classification and choice of diagnostic criteria.

ID has been considered an important topic by the WHO in terms of its complexity relevant to the health construct, and in regards to the definition, categorization, and operationalization of health concepts such as health "condition," "status," and "domain." Apart from the traditional grouping of clinical phenomena into symptoms and signs, syndromes, disorders, discrete entities, and diseases, two other major groupings have been considered by the WHO in recent documents: "other conditions that require specific health care" spectrum disorders and syndrome groupings. ID is also a consideration in the provision of an international definition of "autonomy," "well-being," "deficit," and "limitation in activities" and/or "restriction in participation" (formerly "disabilities and handicaps"; World Health Organization, 2001).

In the WHO classification systems, ID appears in the ICD-10 (World Health Organization, 1992a), with the traditional name Mental Retardation, within the grouping of psychiatric conditions, but also at the same time as impairments in intellectual functions. The latter can also be classified as body functions within WHO's *International Classification of Functioning, Disability and Health (ICF)* (World Health Organization, 2001), and, therefore, can be seen as a part of disability. Genetic syndromes including ID, such as Prader–Willi or Fragile X, can be coded in the ICD independently from associated cognitive impairment.

The APA in the new DSM-5, (American Psychiatric Association, 2013) includes Intellectual Disability (Intellectual Developmental Disorder) as the first disorder of its new meta-structure of neurodevelopmental disorders. Intellectual Developmental Disorder is placed in parenthesis to make clear that the focus of DSM-5 is on brain-based health conditions and not based on the Disability Construct. In contrast, the American Association for Intellectual and Developmental Disorders (AAIDD) explicitly defines ID as a "disability" and not as a "health condition." Based on the disability concept, the AAIDD has assembled a comprehensive definition, classification, and recommended systems of supports. The AAIDD focuses primarily on functioning, adaptive behavior, and support needs; its manual makes clear that it is entirely consistent with the conceptual model proposed by the ICF (World Health Organization, 2001). According to AAIDD, ID is a disability that is characterized by "significant limitations both in intellectual functioning and in adaptive behavior as expressed in conceptual, social, and practical adaptive skills. This disability originates before age 18."

There are serious implications for classification and inclusion in the ICD if ID is defined solely as a disability. If so, ID could be deleted from the ICD because the ICD is a health classification using different codes from the ICF. It is the ICD and not the ICF that is widely used by the 194 WHO member countries to define the responsibilities of governments to provide health care and other services to their citizens. That is, ICD categories, including categories related to ID, are used throughout the world to specify which people are eligible for what health care, educational, and social services, and under what conditions. Therefore, removing ID from the list of health conditions would have a major impact on the visibility of ID, on national and global health statistics, on health policy, and on the services available to this vulnerable population. Interventions related to diet intake (i.e., for disorders such as phenylketonuria), psycho-pharmacotherapy, or education are addressed for attenuation of overall deficits and related activity-functioning and social participation. Conversely, if ID was considered solely as a health condition, then the term "disability" should not be used to refer to it. But this would be at odds with positions already adopted by many governments and international organizations. Such a position might be judged as a reductionist, biomed-ical approach and rejected by many key international stakeholders, users, and experts in the field.

Additionally, there are major unsolved questions in the definition of ID as a health condition, including the large grouping within a health classification regarding where ID should be placed, the age cutoff for onset, and the association between cognitive impairments and behavioral skills. Collective reflections related to ontology and classifi-cation of ID may help to clarify the conceptualization of the disease and disability components in ICD-11 and ICF; that is, where the health condition component of ID can be appropriately classified within a classification of diseases and disorders, and how their functional consequences should be conceptualized using a classification of func-tioning and disability (Salvador-Carulla and Saxena, 2009).

Future perspectives

The discussion and debate regarding these differing conceptualizations of ID was intense in the recent revision of the two major classifications of mental disorders: the ICD-10 and the *Diagnostic and Statistical Manual of Mental Disorders, Fourth Edition, Text Revision* (DSM-IV-TR; American Psychiatric Association, 2000). Important contributions were made by the WPA-SPID and WHO-IAGRMR.

The WPA-SPID considers ID to be a health condition: "a syndromic grouping or meta-syndrome analogous to the construct of dementia, which is characterized by a deficit in cognitive functioning prior to the acquisition of skills through learning. The intensity of the deficit is such to interfere in a significant way with individual normal functioning as expressed in limitations in activities and restriction in participation (disabilities) (Salvador-Carulla et al., 2011).

An important aim for ID in the ICD-11 was to identify and to provide tools to enable more widespread, efficient, and accurate identification and prioritization of service needs for people with ID. In most countries, service eligibility and treatment selection for people with ID are heavily influenced by diagnostic classification. People with ID are more likely to receive the services they need if health workers in the settings where they are most likely to come into contact with the health system have a diagnostic system that is reliable, valid, clinically useful, and feasible. It is highly unlikely that such front-line personnel will be psychiatrists. In low- and middle-income countries, they are unlikely to be specialist mental health professionals of any kind, and often not even physicians. These factors have strongly influenced the conceptualization of the tasks and workflow for the revision of the ICD-10 mental and behavioral disorders classification, as well as the composition of ICD revision Working Groups, including the IAGRMR. The revision process was also influenced by the newly created Content Model for the overall ICD-11, which determines the structure and nature of the information to be provided for each diagnostic category, integrating the category within a much larger informational infrastructure (World Health Organization, 2011).

Because the ICD is used worldwide, it is important that the classification system allows for the use of sophisticated evaluation techniques tailored to local settings taking into account available resources. It is important for the ICD-11 to make clear the prevalence of ID and its functional consequences, because many individuals remain undiagnosed for years in low-income countries. It is also important to consider the proportion of resources available to be used for diagnosis versus treatment and in the development of healthcare programs. However, it must be understood that any marked changes to the ICD may not be incorporated into clinical practice in many countries for some years. It is preferable to keep assessment as user-friendly as possible to encourage its use.

As already mentioned, the APA terminology is now Intellectual Disability (and Intellectual Developmental Disorder). The APA cites the use of the term Intellectual Disability in scientific journals to refer to mental disorder. It refers to the new ICD-11 proposed terminology and refers to the ICD-11 publications justifying the use of the new term Intellectual Developmental Disorder. The WPA-SPID and the WHO-IAGRMR conceptualized ID neither as a disease nor as a disability but as a meta-syndromic group of health conditions (diseases, disorders, and other health conditions), whose clinical entities are parallel to other meta-syndromic conditions such as Dementia, and may be related to a variety of specific etiologies, ranging from genetic (i.e., Fragile X syndrome) to nutritional (e.g., iodine deficiency), infectious (e.g., intrauterine rubella), metabolic (e.g., phenylketonuria), or neurotoxic conditions (e.g., fetal alcohol syndrome and heavy metal intoxications).

The meta-syndrome is characterized by a deficit in cognitive functioning prior to the acquisition of skills through learning. The intensity of the deficit is such that it interferes in a significant way with individual normal functioning as expressed in limitations in activities and restriction in participation (disabilities). The ID spectrum could be incorporated in the meta-construct, after a dimensional approach to early or developmental cognitive impairment. Borderline intellectual functioning may be regarded as "mild cognitive impairment" within the Dementia spectrum. In any case, the nosological dimension should be incorporated into the debate on the concept of ID.

In the DSM-5 the APA did not discuss the rationale for the inclusion of an entity that is labeled as a disability in a classification of mental disorders, other than to cite how this term is used in the scientific literature. However, it made clear that the term "disability" in DSM-5 referred to a mental disorder by categorizing it under the new grouping of Neurodevelopmental Disorders and by placing Intellectual Developmental Disorder in parenthesis. DSM-5 references the rationale for the use of the term Intellectual Developmental Disorder in papers prepared by the ICD study groups. The WPA-SPID and WHO-IAGRMR endorsed a dimensional approach to the classification of ID, which distinguishes between the clinical meta-syndromes and their functioning/disability counterpart having different health, social, and policy applications. The first component should have a place in the ICD, while the second will be included in the ICF. This approach would best support the public health mission of the WHO and the provision of appropriate services and opportunities to people with ID.

Another contribution of the WHO-IAGRMR has been to provide a model of the integration of expert knowledge and empirical evidence in developing consensus related to clinical processes. During the past decade, expert consensus has been much devalued in comparison to experimental evidence, particularly randomized controlled trials, as a basis for developing health procedures and policies. Although this "hierarchy of evidence" has been useful as a basis for the analysis of treatment efficacy, particularly for drugs, it has failed to provide a usable and solid ground for the classification of mental disorders. Efforts to base the classification of mental disorders on brain functions and etiological factors have failed to address serious problems of clinical practice. The issues encountered for the ICD-11, in developing a new classification system for ID and for defining its relationship to mental disorders, have been complex and challenging. In order to transform existing evidence into useful information for taxonomy and classification, the use of techniques that incorporate quantitative data analysis and formal prior expert knowledge should also be explored.

Terminology

The debate for an acceptable term for people with ID from all stakeholders has continued over the last 20 years. The term Intellectual Disability or Intellectual Disabilities has widely replaced the term Mental Retardation in the scientific community and in the scientific literature, and in stakeholders' organizations in many high-income countries and in an increasing number of low- and medium-income countries.

The DSM-5 has chosen ID (IDD) as its terminology based on the usage in recent scientific literature. It chose ID (IDD) using the disorder construct, but recognizes that it is semantically similar (but not the same usage) as the disability term used by the AAIDD (Schalock et al., 2010), other US professional and disability groups (e.g., Division 33 of the American Psychological Association; The Arc), and the US Federal Government (President's Committee for Persons with Intellectual Disabilities, US Social Security Administration, and US PL 111–256 (Rosa's Law)). The DSM-5 terminology includes a parenthesis containing the term Intellectual Developmental Disorder (IDD), which was done to maintain the meaning of a health condition and to be aligned with the first draft version of the ICD-11. However, the WHO has temporarily dropped the use of Intellectual Developmental Disorder in favor of the terminology Disorders of Intellectual Development, making clear its intention to focus on the disorder not the disability construct in its final publication.

The use of ID (IDD) in DSM-5 is unique in the US classification of mental disorders. However, it not expected to cause confusion in healthcare policy (e.g., service eligibility and treatment provision), assessment of treatment outcomes, and legislation because the disability terminology is clearly stated in services law. Services focus on reducing disability by provision of supports. Still, service delivery requires an understanding of the underlying brain disorder as well. In the USA, it is hoped that the DSM-5 definition makes it clear that its focus is on neurodevelopmental disorders of the brain and that greater attention will be paid to neurodevelopmentally focused interventions.

Though the name Intellectual Disability is widely used in the medical literature as preferable to Mental Retardation, it is unsuitable for use in the ICD classification system. If ID is a disability, then it should be coded in the ICF and not the ICD. The ICF defines a disability as "an umbrella term for impairments, activity limitations or participation restriction," and as a result of a dynamic interaction between the "health condition" and the environment (World Health Organization, 2001). The WHO's IAGRMR extensively discussed alternative terms to replace "mental retardation" following a consensus-based approach. Principles considered important for the new name included: a lifespan perspective; persistence; "person first" language; cognition as a key characteristic; and reduced competitiveness in life's struggles.

The WHO-IAGRMR endorsed a multidimensional approach for a new term that distinguishes between Intellectual Developmental Disorder (IDD), the clinical meta-syndrome, and ID, their functioning/disability counterpart. The notion was that these two terms would be regarded as "semantically-proximal" terms describing two different but related aspects of the same construct, to be used in different contexts with different implications, with a socially and policy acceptable term, and a scientific term based on a nosological approach.

For the clinical part, the WHO-IAGRMR Group came to a consensus on the name Intellectual Developmental Disorder (IDD). The word "Intellectual" was chosen with the rationale that it was a well-understood term in most countries, appropriate for public naming and practical use, and more acceptable to families. An alternative considered was the word "cognitive"; though "cognitive" may actually be closer to the phenomenon of this entity, it was decided that this word might cause confusion given its particular use in dementia and schizophrenia. General support was expressed for adopting the term "developmental," in that it refers to a period of time during which the brain and its functions are developing. The term implies a dynamic, long-term process and a lifespan perspective. During the discussion, three words emerged as the main possible descriptors of the entity in question: "impairment," "difficulties," and "disorder." A fourth term, "spectrum," was also considered, but it was discarded due to its low taxonomic value within a categorical classification.

The word "impairment" is a specific term used in the ICF to refer to problems in body functions and body structures that may be associated with a wide variety of health conditions. Although "impairment" would, therefore, capture the meta-syndromic nature of the ID, it has too specific a technical meaning related to single symptoms and functions, and in so doing may minimize the underlying concept of IDD as proposed in ICD-11. The term "difficulties" was proposed to avoid medical connotations and as a term that may be less likely to be rejected by consumers, family groups, and care providers. It may imply that the person can overcome his or her problems with some help or support, but it may also be confusing because for most people these difficulties are long standing and will not be overcome completely.

The ICD-10 Classification of Mental and Behavioural Disorders: Clinical Descriptions and Diagnostic Guidelines (World Health Organization, 1992b) defines a Disorder as a "clinically recognizable set of symptoms or behaviour" that is usually associated with interference with personal functions or with distress. For this reason, the WHO Working Group favored the plural form of the word – that is Disorders – reflecting that ID is not a single condition but multiple disorders. As a result of the above process, the WHO Working Group endorsed the term Intellectual Developmental Disorder as the most accurate and best reflection of underlying concepts. In fact it implies comorbidity and encompasses the variability seen with ID. As underlined by the WHO International Advisory Group, among the concepts considered important in thinking about terminology were: the importance of "person first" language; the importance of cognitive function as the central characteristic; a lifespan perspective; the impact of IDD on development; and the persistence of ID over time (e.g., from birth).

Neurodevelopmental perspective

The WPA-SPID and the WHO-IAGRMR agreed on the relevance of a neurodevelopmental approach and on the lifespan perspective on IDD. Conceptualizing IDD as a neurodevelopmental disorder has implications for the supra-ordinal grouping of IDD with other developmental disorders in the ICD-11. It was suggested that guidance should consider common issues for persons with IDD at different developmental phases. The etiology-specific information may have predictive value in terms of whether functioning is expected to remain relatively stable or deteriorate over time. The incorporation of IDD in the large grouping of neurodevelopmental disorders will have significant implications for this supra-ordinal or parent entity, and it may require a reanalysis of the hierarchy and the conceptual map of neurodevelopmental disorders to avoid double coding (e.g., in the case of Rett syndrome or Fragile X).

The DSM-5 included the adopted term IDD to harmonize with the ICD-11 proposal in a meta-structure named Neurodevelopmental Disorders (NDD), which includes conditions with onset in the developmental age, usually occurring before school age, and characterized by developmental deficits that determine impairment of personal, social, school, and work functioning. Deficits range from very specific difficulties in learning and executive functions to a wide impairment of social skills and intelligence. NDD often co-occur; for example, people with autism spectrum disorders (ASD) often have IDD, and children with attention-deficit/hyperactivity disorder (ADHD) often have an additional specific learning disorder in reading or mathematics.

Diagnosis
Diagnostic criteria

Although general diagnostic criteria are similar in all systems, the WHO classifications underline the IQ level (Criterion A), while the APA, for the first time, includes a definition of intelligence and requires that adaptation functioning (Criterion B) be a consequence of cognitive deficits defined in Criterion A. DSM-5 does not use the term "skills" because of its focus on fluid intelligence and adaptative reasoning. This is a clear distinction from the AAIDD. Moreover, adaptive functioning received greater emphasis than in past definitions. The concept based on IQ and age limit is imprecise and hampers research, needs assessment, and the planning and provision of services for persons with IDD.

To diagnose ID (IDD) in DSM-5 the three following criteria must be met:

A. Deficits in intellectual functions, such as reasoning, problem solving, planning, abstract thinking, judgment, academic learning, and learning from experience, confirmed by both clinical assessment and individualized, standardized intelligence testing.

B. Deficits in adaptive functioning that result in failure to meet developmental and sociocultural standards for personal independence and social responsibility. Without ongoing support, the adaptive deficits limit functioning in one or more activities of daily life, such as communication, social participation, and independent living, across multiple environments, such as home, school, work, and community.

C. Onset of intellectual and adaptive deficits during the developmental period.

A consensus on key aspects related to diagnostic criteria should be reached in the coming years:

1. Criterion A: neural intelligence measurement should be complemented by a grouping of cognitive impairments. Distinctive profiles of cognitive impairments should be considered and looked for.

2. Criterion B: it is necessary to reach international agreement on domains, types, and assessment of adaptive functioning. The assessment of adaptive functioning should be simplified and operationalized.

3. Criterion C: should be defined more clearly.

Intelligence

In the DSM-5 intellectual functioning is defined as cognitive processes that include: reasoning, problem solving, abstract thinking, judgment, learning from instruction, learning from experience, and practical understanding. Subaverage intellectual functioning (Criterion A) is defined based on clinical judgment and standardized testing. In doing so the expectation is that greater attention will be paid to better measures of reasoning, working memory, and cognitive efficacy. Still, in the body of the text it uses the example of an IQ score that is approximately two standard deviations or more below the population mean (i.e., a standard IQ score of 70 on a test with a mean = 100 and standard deviation = 15). However, DSM-5 seeks to reduce reliance on IQ tests and does so by no longer listing IQ scores or standard deviations from the mean in its severity categories that are based on adaptive reasoning and functioning.

The term "approximately" is used purposefully in the DSM-5 because there is a well-documented standard error of measurement and the need to take into consideration clinical judgment in interpreting test scores. All standardized tests of intelligence have a margin of error measurement around the obtained scores. This test error around an obtained score includes the standard error of measurement, which is generally represented by a 95% confidence interval of +5 points. Thus, a person can still obtain an IQ score of between 70 and 75 and still meet criteria for significant subaverage intellectual functioning (American Psychiatric Association, 2013). This is consistent with the AAIDD diagnostic system (Schalock et al., 2010) and a 2014 US Supreme Court decision in Hall v. Florida where it clearly stated that the Florida's stature requiring a bright-line cutoff of IQ 70 was an error. Another source of measurement error cited in the DSM-5 as a potential contributor to artificially inflating the estimate of an individual's true level of intellectual functioning is the obsolescence of the test's normative data or the "Flynn effect" (Flynn, 2009).

It should be noted that there is an effort in DSM-5 to shift over-reliance on the individual's intellectual IQ score in favor of the individual's adaptive behavior. The DSM-5 has abandoned the determination of the levels of severity of intellectual functioning (as noted above) that was previously based on the person's IQ score, in lieu for a severity system that is predicated on the person's level of adaptive functioning across social, conceptual, and practical adaptive functioning.

In the last classification systems, including DSM-5, limited intellectual functioning in the form of standardized IQ reduction has been the shared criterion for defining IDD. This criterion expresses the primacy of mono-component models of intelligence within the international scientific community. Nevertheless, evidence is not definitive on what lies at the core of intelligence, whether it is a general function or if it derives from overlapping component processes. In the last 20 years an increasing number of neuropsychological findings support models of intelligence that consist of distinct, but related, processes. The Cattell–Horn–Carroll, Das–Naglieri's PASS, the Gardner, and the Goleman models are the most renowned examples.

The Cattell–Horn–Carroll model (McGrew, 2005) combines Cattell and Horn's concept of fluidity–crystallization with Carroll's theory of triple stratification (Carroll, 1993) and postulates the existence of nine skills at a general level and over 70 skills at a specific level. The last enhancements of the Planning, Attention, Simultaneous, and Successive (PASS) model (Naglieri and Das, 2002) also describes the existence of interdependent but separate functional systems and, according to the authors, would support clinical and experimental activity precisely in the field of IDD and other neurodevelopmental disorders (Naglieri and Das, 1997). Also, Gardner questioned the validity of IQ and IQ tests as comprehensive indicators of intellectual functioning. According to his theory, IQ and related tools would assess only linguistic and logical–mathematical skills, while the characterization of individual intellectual functioning would require a specific combination of multiple "talents" (Gardner, 1993). Daniel Goleman's theory of emotional intelligence highlighted that people with an under-average IQ can equally achieve relevant levels of adjustment and satisfaction in life, through a harmonious management of their relationship between themselves and with others (Goleman, 1996).

A recent literature mapping indicates that in people with IDD the same IQ score may be associated with very different cognitive profiles, also based on the factors involved in etiopathogenesis (Bertelli et al., 2014). As an example, persons with Down syndrome usually manifest impairments in specific areas of language, long-term memory, and motor performance, while showing relative strengths in visuo-spatial construction (Edgin et al., 2010). In contrast, persons with Williams syndrome show deficits in attention, visuo-spatial construction, short-term memory, and planning (Tiekstra et al., 2009), while showing a distinctive pattern of auditory processing and relative strengths in music and concrete language (Thornton-Wells et al., 2010).

A deficit of a single cognitive function may have a neuropsychological overshadowing effect, and determine low global performance scores. Similarly, erroneous conclusions may be drawn that any anomaly of neuropsychological functioning is explained by a lower than average IQ. In fact, the tools to assess IQ were not originally developed for the evaluation of below-average performance and are not able to describe the complexity of cognitive and behavioral profiles of persons with ID, especially among those with severe degrees, or in the presence of neuropsychiatric comorbidity. Furthermore, IQ ratings may vary as a result of the specific test being used, the testing conditions, and the status of the person being tested, the individual's life course, and even the historical generation. For example, the "Flynn effect" describes a substantial increase in average IQ scores on intelligence tests that may be about three IQ points per decade (Colom et al., 2005), although stagnation has been identified in Scandinavian countries after the 1990s (Flynn, 2009). These variations are especially relevant for the diagnosis of mild IDD and borderline intellectual functioning (BIF), and highlight the need for the periodic standardization of IQ tests. Other evidence suggests that limitations of functioning, behavior problems, and various neurobiopsychological factors that are associated with IDD are more highly correlated with impairments of specific cognitive functions than with reduction in overall IQ (Friedman et al., 2006; Johnson et al., 2008). The functions most frequently studied were associative and working memory, orientation response, and attention switch.

There is still no conceptual map or hierarchy of the cognitive functions and domains important in IDD (Bilder et al., 2009). Different terms are often used for the same functions, and vice versa. However, a series of cognitive domains are significantly impaired in persons with IDD, the most frequently reported in the literature are perceptual reasoning, working memory, processing speed, and verbal comprehension (Deary, 2001; Holdnack et al., 2011).

The current model of intelligence, based on IQ, seems to be of limited utility with respect to the newly envisioned definitions of IDD in the DSM-5 and in the first products of the Working Group for ICD-11 (Salvador-Carulla et al., 2011), given the wide range and variability of cognitive functions in IDD, related to neurobiopsychological factors and range of adaptive capacities (Bertelli et al., 2014).

The ICF (World Health Organization, 2001) already considers intelligence as an umbrella term that includes cognitive functioning, adaptive behavior, and learning, that is age-appropriate and meets the standards of culture-appropriate demands of daily life. Also, the DSM-5 proposed the assessment of intelligence across three domains (conceptual, social, and practical), so as to allow clinicians to base their diagnosis on the impact of the deficit in general mental abilities on functioning needed for everyday life.

The impairment of cognition should be evaluated in the most comprehensive way as possible and tools to investigate specific cognitive functions should, therefore, increasingly become part of standardized assessments for persons with IDD (Bertelli et al., 2014). The assessment of cognition should be aimed at identifying those dysfunctions that have the highest impact on individual behavior, skills, adaptation, autonomy, and quality of life across the lifespan, highlighting personal cognitive strengths and weaknesses that can be useful to understand personal functioning, and to organize intervention. Indication on whether, what, and why some functions should be further investigated can be given by neuropsychological screenings.

Adaptive behavior

In the DSM-5 adaptive functioning is conceptualized as "how well a person meets community standards of personal independence and responsibility, in comparison to others of similar age and social background" (American Psychiatric Association, 2013). The DSM-5 is similar to the tripartite conceptualization of adaptive behavior proposed by the AAIDD, which defines adaptive behavior as "the collection of conceptual, social and practical skills that have been learned and are performed by people in their everyday lives" (Schalock et al., 2010). However the DSM-5 differs from the AAIDD in focusing on adaptive reasoning (not skills) in academic (conceptual), social, and practical situations, and gives examples of each of these in defining severity.

The DSM-5 also acknowledges all the factors that could influence adaptive behavior (e.g., cultural experience, motivation, among others) and highlights the fact that deficits in adaptive functioning should occur across multiple environments, which has important implications for the assessment of adaptive behavior in controlled settings such as prisons or detention centers.

The DSM-5 does not operationalize its definition of deficits in adaptive functioning (Criterion B) using a statistical criterion (e.g., two standard deviations below the mean), as it does for the intellectual functioning criterion. It does, however, recommend the use of psychometrically sound measures of adaptive functioning along with the use of clinical judgment. Criterion B is considered met when at least one domain of adaptive functioning (i.e., conceptual, social, or practical) is "sufficiently impaired that ongoing support is needed" (American Psychiatric Association, 2013). Hence, a deficit (impairment) in one or more of conceptual, social, or practical (adaptive) skills is sufficient to meet Criterion B for a diagnosis of IDD.

These adaptive behavior impairments are defined as mild, moderate, severe, and profound, and replace IQ-based levels of severity, arguing that adaptive functioning is a better predictor of an individual's support needs. Most of the studies have focused on individuals with mild deficits due to their difficulties receiving the services they need. Their support needs may be masked by the fact that these individuals are much more alike than different to the general population. Thus, they may present few difficulties in community use (e.g., communicating with persons outside of the family, instrumental activities of daily living such as shopping or getting around by self) (Fujiura, 2003) and many of them will be able to live independently, get a job, and build their own family (Schalock et al., 2010). Some researchers also highlight that what differentiates individuals with mild deficits from the general population is that they may be especially vulnerable to risks such as social manipulation and maltreatment, due to difficulties in social judgment, social competence, gullibility, and risk awareness (Greenspan, 2006). Other studies propose the existence of different subtypes of mild IDD on the basis of intellectual, adaptive functioning, and behavior problems (Soenen et al., 2009).

Adopting deficits in adaptive functioning as severity-specifiers has important implications. During many years, the results from standardized intelligence tests have solely been used to make a diagnosis of IDD or determine someone's eligibility for IDD services (Greenspan, 2012). As Haydt et al. (2014) point out, this new focus defines IDD much more broadly than IQ scores, and emphasizes what many researchers have reminded us for many years: that it is the deficits in adaptive behavior that constitutes the major impediment to successful inclusion of individuals with IDD (Greenspan, 2006, 2012).

Standardized and psychometrically sound measures should be used for both the assessment of intellectual functioning and adaptive behavior, and should be administered along with clinical assessment or clinical judgment. Schalock and Luckasson (2005) define it as "a special type of judgment rooted in a high level of clinical expertise and experience; it emerges directly from extensive data. Clinical judgment is based on the clinician's explicit training, direct experience with those with whom the clinician is working, and specific knowledge of the person and the person's environment." Clinical judgment is especially important in those situations in which no standardized measures are available and there are no other ways to analyze adaptive behavior or intellectual functioning but direct observation, review of academic reports and psychological assessments, or interviews with those people who know the person very well (Schalock et al., 2010).

The increased role of clinical judgment and adaptive behavior in the new definition of the DSM-5 has been interpreted by some authors (see, for example, Haydt et al., 2014) as an effort to make for greater flexibility, with less emphasis on IQ scores and IQ ceilings. Adaptive behavior refers to the individual's typical ability to cope with and meet environmental demands for personal independence and responsibility (American Psychiatric Association, 2013) according to the expectations of their chronological age and cultural group (Schalock et al., 2010). Thus, adaptive behavior should be assessed in reference to the community settings that are typical for on individual's same-age peer group as well as taking into account factors such as expectations within their cultural group.

Several research studies have described adaptive behavior profiles of individuals with different known etiologies. Knowing adaptive strengths and weaknesses yield important information for diagnostic purposes and may be important with regard to school-based interventions (Reilly, 2012). Down syndrome (Fidler et al., 2006), Angelman syndrome (Brun Gasca et al., 2010), and Williams syndrome (Mervis et al., 2001) are some of the conditions more commonly studied.

Age of onset

One of the most notable changes compared to the DSMs and the AAIDD diagnostic and classification system is the broadened age of onset criteria (Criterion C). Whereas in its revised fourth edition (DSM-IV-TR) the DSM defined IDD as a disorder that occurs before age 18, the current edition does not establish a cutoff age and defines IDD as occurring during the developmental period (American Psychiatric Association, 2013). The previous specific age limit of 18 was considered arbitrary. It was agreed that a developmental perspective would be employed to distinguish IDD as a persistent process that has an impact during early development (and, hence, dynamically influencing further development), as opposed to onset during adult life.

Although IDD is usually a stable diagnosis, there can be significant variability in cognition and functioning across different clinical severity levels throughout the life cycle. Therefore, IDD is considered a dynamic health condition, and it should be reassessed at key developmental phases, life transitions (e.g., at school-entry age, puberty, early and later adulthood), other life events, and traumatic events. No specific temporal qualifier is necessary for the diagnosis.

Adult-onset cognitive impairments are not considered to be neurodevelopmental disorders. While it was agreed by the DSM Working Group that a child who is developing typically and undergoes an acute insult at age 13 has a different experience than a child born with IDD, no consensus was reached about at what point on the developmental trajectory the boundaries of IDD should be defined (i.e., late childhood or adolescence). The DSM Working Group expressed a preference for a narrower focus on IDD, was in favor of limiting the concept of IDD to deficits that begin during childhood, and discussed providing a nuanced explanation of this idea in the diagnostic guidelines for IDD rather than an arbitrary age cutoff.

Subtyping

The WHO-IAGRMR Working Group reached a consensus to maintain the severity levels of mild, moderate, severe, and profound ID, as in the ICD-10 subtyping of Mental

Retardation. A number of important organizations in the field have called for a discontinuation of subtyping based solely on IQ. The AAIDD, for example, proposes a multidimensional system for classification and considers IQ ranges insufficient to be the sole determinant of cognitive functioning or severity level (Schalock et al., 2010). The WHO-IAGRMR Working Group decided that the severity levels for ID will not rely only on IQ but on a clinical description of the characteristics of each subtype.

However, the Working Group decided against discontinuing clinical severity levels altogether because of their diagnostic and clinical utility (Sullivan et al., 2006). For example, increasing severity of IDD has been shown to be associated with lower levels of self-determination in choosing living arrangements, including where and with whom to live (Stancliffe et al., 2011). Those with profound IDD are much more likely to live in a long-term care facility than those with mild IDD, and to less often determine their living arrangement. In addition, severity levels are already in wide use in many public health systems, determining the level of services and benefits provided. They may be helpful for communication between professionals in different disciplines, and can be meaningful labels for families and users.

Subclassifying by clinical severity levels of mild, moderate, severe, and profound may be appropriate in the ICD/health condition context. The classification by clinical severity levels does not contradict use of other subclassifying approaches, including multidimensional approaches aimed at connecting the IDD diagnosis, to needed supports such as intervention and planning (Salvador-Carulla and García-Gutiérrez, 2011). In the future, clinical subtyping based on severity levels should be complemented by function-related subtypings based on personal characteristics and/or supports needed. A number of tools have been developed for classifying support needs and relevant characteristics of persons with IDD (Thompson, 2004; Arnold et al., 2010), but this field is still in its infancy and has not progressed to the point that such measures are available for worldwide use.

Borderline intellectual functioning

Borderline intellectual functioning (BIF) is a mild cognitive-developmental condition not coded in the ICD, which is distinguished from ID by the presence of less extensive and severe impairments in cognitive functioning. The IQ for diagnosis of BIF is usually between 71 and 84. Nevertheless, BIF may not just be understood from a normality approach, as evidence is emerging that there are significant similarities between individuals with BIF and ID; for instance, persons with BIF have higher rates of mental illness, have similar patterns of service response to mental disorders, and have similar communication and support needs (Hassiotis et al., 2008; Emerson et al., 2010).

Development and course

IDD originates during the developmental period and can be caused by prenatal, perinatal, or postnatal risk factors (Schalock et al., 2010), which results in lifelong limitations in intellectual and adaptive functioning. Signs of cognitive impairment can be recognized as early as two years of age (American Psychiatric Association, 2013) and are manifested by difficulties in reaching development milestones (e.g., language, fine and gross motor skills, and social milestones). In up to 60% of cases the etiological factors in IDD are unknown (Rauch et al., 2006) and 80–90% of the population with IDD has mild deficits (Schalock et al., 2010), which could explain why some individuals with IDD are not identified until they reach school age and start having difficulties acquiring and learning new academic skills.

The development and course of this condition may vary depending on different etiological factors. Specific genetic conditions such as Down syndrome or Williams syndrome are associated with different health conditions that have a higher probability of appearing during the life of these persons (e.g., thyroid disorders, cardiovascular disease) than in people with IDD without these syndromes. Other syndromes with known etiology, such as Rett syndrome, present progressive developmental trajectories with periods of worsening (American Psychiatric Association, 2013). Early intervention can contribute to promoting the development of children with IDD (Ramey and Ramey, 1998; Guralnick, 2005), and with appropriate supports across their lifespan and over a sustained period, the life-functioning of individuals with IDD generally will improve (Luckasson et al., 2002; Schalock et al., 2010). Deficits in intellectual functioning tend to remain stable (American Psychiatric Association, 2000), but improvements in adaptive behavior are more likely to occur, in which cases the diagnosis of IDD may no longer be appropriate (American Psychiatric Association, 2013).

Differential diagnosis

About 30–40% of people with IDD have pervasive autistic features (Morgan et al. 2002; Cooper et al., 2007), and about 70% of people with autism have some kind of cognitive impairment (Hoekstra et al., 2009; Matson and Shoemaker, 2009; Noterdaeme and Wriedt, 2010). Although they have many shared features, such as deficits of adaptive skill, stereotypies, or challenging behaviors, IDD and autism spectrum disorders (ASD) have specific core symptoms. IDD is defined by an impairment of logical–deductive skills (IQ under average), while ASD imply a lack of interpersonal skills and relational competences. Onset and age of recognition represent another relevant difference: although there are mild cases identified late (e.g., school entry), IDD is usually diagnosed in the first two years of life, while ASD can be detected at any time, often presenting a normal development till the first or the second year of life. The DSM-5 Working Group also considered that symptoms must be present in early childhood but may not become fully manifest until social demands exceed limited capacities. Anatomic anomalies of the central nervous system have also been reported to be significantly different in IDD and ASD, the former being variable from case to case, the latter mostly presenting diffused gray matter increase (Hazlett et al., 2011) and anomalies in the neuroanatomical networks (Lewis et al., 2014).

Persons with autism who have IDD differ from persons with autism without IDD not only on core symptoms but also on the presence of additional co-occurring comorbid problems. The combination of IDD and ASD presents many challenges and deficits across a range of behaviors and skills that are not seen in IDD or ASD alone (Boucher et al., 2008). In terms of a dual diagnosis (i.e., a developmental disorder such as ASD or IDD and psychiatric disorder), there is increased risk of underestimating ASD in people with IDD when schizophrenia is diagnosed (Palucka et al., 2009; Bradley et al., 2011). About 40% of the items included in diagnostic tools for people with IDD and used to screen for psychosis commonly receive a high score when autism is present (Helverschou et al., 2008; see also Chapter 11). More severe ID was related to higher severity of ASD and higher rates of challenging behaviors (Murphy et al., 2009). High rates of stereotypies tended to be related to severity of autism (Goldmon et al., 2009), but not to severity of ID (Matson and Kozlowski, 2011). ASD may present with specific cognitive impairments or with extensive impairment of verbal comprehension, perceptual reasoning, working memory, and processing speed; in this case the diagnosis of IDD and ASD should both be made. For severe and profound IDD, the identification of autistic features or symptoms is particularly difficult, and the clinician should rely on more in-depth and longitudinal observation.

Several tools are available to assess ASD in ID, including the PDD-MRS scale (a scale of autistic traits in people with ID; Kraijer and de Bildt, 2005) and the recent DIBAS-R (Diagnostic Behavioral Assessment for Autism Spectrum Disorder – Revised; Sappok et al., 2014) for screening, while the GARS-2 (Gilliam Autism Rating Scale–Second Edition; Gilliam, 2006) and the DISCO (Diagnostic Interview for Social and Communication Disorders; Maljaars et al., 2012) can be used to complete the patient evaluation. The DISCO provides a comprehensive assessment of ID and ASD across the range of IQ and functioning ability and subtypes of autism (Wing et al., 2002), it also seems to be useful in differentiating between ASD, IDD, and schizophrenia spectrum disorders (Unenge Hallerbäck et al., 2012).

IDD have also to be differentiated from Specific Learning Disorders (SLD). Although in SLD the cognitive impairment is circumscribed with average or above-average IQ, the learning disability can create considerable gap between ability and performance. Many researchers sustain a significant relationship between SLD and borderline intelligence, while a minority takes a contrary position, stating for a substantial reciprocal independence of the two constructs. A growing number of evidences indicate that the current intelligence model and assessment presents important limits, which can have a significant impact on diagnostic procedures.

IDD are distinguished from cerebral palsy by the presence of abnormal neurological signs and motor delay disproportionate to cognitive functioning. However, cerebral palsy may also be associated with extensive cognitive impairment, in which case diagnosis of both cerebral palsy and IDD are made. In sensory impairment the presence of any impairment in development and skill acquisition is primarily attributable to the underlying sensory impairment and not to early cognitive impairment, like in IDD.

Global Developmental Delay (GDD) and IDD are related, but not synonymous, diagnoses. When the diagnosis of IDD cannot be made reliably in young children, a more global term used in classification systems may be necessary or applicable. IDD requires the presence of significant cognitive impairment but GDD can encompass other developmental problems in childhood not related to cognitive functioning. As the child grows older, a more specific diagnosis should be made (Shevell, 2008).

Neurodegenerative disorders can be distinguished from ID for their late onset in the developmental period, such as mucolipidosis I or Gaucher's disease type III. Extensive brain damage caused by very early birth, multi-infarct, aneurysm, cranial radiotherapy, or brain surgery (e.g., hemispherectomy) shows a complex relationship with IDD that requires careful assessment and extended follow-up. Very early birth and cranial radiotherapy may be associated to mild cognitive impairment and cognitive delays but rarely to IDD. Cranial hemispherectomy for children with intractable epilepsy shows a high individual variability ranging from persistent IDD to cases of cognitive developmental delay with recovery of cognitive functioning in young adulthood. The extension and location of bi-hemispheric damage and the developmental phase at which brain damage occurs play a critical role in recovery.

Conclusions

The classification of IDD involves very complex and challenging conceptual issues that are described in this chapter, including the expert contribution of relevant stakeholders. In recent years, considerable work has been done in the revision of the classification systems, resulting in the APA's DSM-5 and the WHO's ICD-11. In addition, there has been significant contribution by the AAIDD and other American professional and disability groups, e.g., the American Psychological Association and US Federal Government (President's Committee for Persons with Intellectual Disabilities; Social Security Administration). The DSM-5 has adopted the term ID but included a parenthesis with the term Intellectual Developmental Disorder (IDD). It did this in order to maintain the meaning of a health condition and to be aligned with the first draft version of ICD-11. The ICD-11 was not published by the time this book went to print. It seems that the WHO will drop the use of "Intellectual Developmental Disorder" in favor of "Disorders of Intellectual Development." Thus, the construct of disorder will be preserved in ICD-11 in the final version. In this chapter, the importance of taking into consideration the adaptive function of people with ID and the relation to IQ has been reviewed based on the current evidence base as well as the diagnostic challenges for co-occurring diagnoses of ID and ASD.

Key summary points

- The reclassification of mental retardation has been taking place through the ICD-11 and the DSM-5. The DSM-5 has introduced the term Intellectual Developmental Disorder (IDD).
- The classification of ID and IDD involves complex conceptual challenges.
- There is ongoing discussion on terminology by the main US and European professional and stakeholders organizations.
- Health and social parameters should be taken into consideration in the classification systems to give the full benefit of supports and services to people with IDD, their families, and carers.

References

American Psychiatric Association. (2000). *Diagnostic and Statistical Manual of Mental Disorders – Text Revision, Fourth Edition.* Washington, DC: American Psychiatric Association.

American Psychiatric Association. (2013). *Diagnostic and Statistical Manual of Mental Disorders, Fifth Edition.* Washington, DC: American Psychiatric Association.

Arnold, S., Riches, V.C., Stancliffe, R.J. (2010). The I-CAN: developing a bio-psycho-social understanding of support. *Journal of Applied Research in Intellectual Disabilities*, 23(5), 486.

Bertelli, M.O., Salvador-Carulla, L., Scuticchio, D., et al. (2014). Moving beyond intelligence in the revision of ICD-10: specific cognitive functions in intellectual developmental disorders. *World Psychiatry*, 13(1), 93–94.

Bilder, D., Pinborough-Zimmerman, J., Miller, J., McMahon, W (2009). Prenatal, periuatal, and neonatal factors associated with autism spectrum disorders. *Pediatrics*, 123, 1293–1300.

Boucher, J., Bigham, S., Mayes, A., Muskett, T. (2008). Recognition and language in low functioning autism. *Journal of Autism and Developmental Disorders*, 38, 1259–1269.

Bradley, E., Lunsky, Y., Palucka, A. (2011). Recognition of intellectual disabilities and autism in psychiatric inpatients diagnosed with schizophrenia and other psychotic disorders. *Advances in Mental Health and Intellectual Disabilities*, 5, 4–18.

Brun Gasca, C., Obiols, J.E., Bonillo, A., et al. (2010). Adaptive behaviour in Angelman syndrome: its profile and relationship to age. *Journal of Intellectual Disability Research*, 54(11), 1024–1029.

Carroll, J.B. (1993) *Human Cognitive Abilities: A Survey of Factor-Analytic Studies.* Cambridge: Cambridge University Press.

Colom, R., Lluis-Font, J.M., Andrés-Pueyo, A. (2005) The generational intelligence gains are caused by decreasing variance in the lower half of the distribution: supporting evidence for the nutrition hypothesis. *Intelligence*, 33, 83–91.

Cooper, S.A., Smiley, E., Morrison, J., Williamson, A., Allan, L. (2007). Mental ill-health in adults with intellectual disabilities: prevalence and associated factors. *British Journal of Psychiatry*, 190, 27–35.

Deary, I.J. (2001). *Intelligence: A Very Short Introduction.* Oxford: Oxford University Press.

Edgin, J.O., Pennington, B.F., Mervis, C.B. (2010). Neuropsychological components of intellectual disability: the contributions of immediate, working, and associative memory. *Journal of Intellectual Disability Research*, 54(5), 406–417.

Emerson, E., Einfeld, S., Stancliffe, R.J. (2010). The mental health of young children with intellectual disabilities or borderline intellectual functioning. *Social Psychiatry and Psychiatric Epidemiology*, 45(5), 579–587.

Fidler, D.J., Hepburn, S., Rogers, S. (2006). Early learning and adaptive behaviour in toddlers with Down syndrome: evidence for an emerging behavioural phenotype? *Downs Syndrome Research and Practice*, 9(3), 37–44.

Flynn, J.R. (2009). *What is Intelligence? Beyond the Flynn Effect.* Cambridge: Cambridge University Press.

Friedman, N.P., Miyake, A., Corley, R.P., et al. (2006). Not all executive functions are related to intelligence. *Psychological Science*, 17, 172–179.

Fujiura, G.T. (2003). The continuum of intellectual disability: demographic evidence for the "forgotten generation." *Mental Retardation*, 41, 420–429.

Gardner, H. (1993). *Multiple Intelligences: The Theory in Practice.* New York, NY: Basic Books.

Gilliam, J.E. (2006). *Gilliam Autism Rating Scale,* second edition. Austin, TX: PRO-ED.

Goldmon, S., Wang, C., Salgado, M.W., et al. (2009). Motor stereotypies in children with autism and other developmental disorders. *Developmental Medicine and Child Neurology*, 51, 30–38.

Goleman, D. (1996). *Emotional Intelligence: Why it can Matter More than IQ.* New York: Bantam Books.

Greenspan, S. (2006). Functional concepts in mental retardation: finding the natural essence of an artificial category. *Exceptionality*, 14(4), 205–224.

Greenspan, S. (2012). How do we know when it's raining out? Why existing conceptions of intellectual disability are all (or mostly) wet. *Psychology in Intellectual and Developmental Disabilities*, 37, 4–8.

Guralnick, M.J. (2005). Early intervention for children with intellectual disabilities: current knowledge and future prospects. *Journal of Applied Research in Intellectual Disabilities*, 18, 313–324.

Hassiotis, A., Strydom, A., Hall, I., et al. (2008). Psychiatric morbidity and social functioning among adults with borderline intelligence living in private households. *Journal of Intellectual Disability Research*, 52(2), 95–106.

Haydt, N., Greenspan, S., Agharkar, B.S. (2014). Advantages of DSM-5 in the diagnosis of intellectual disability: reduced reliance on IQ Ceilings in Atkins (death penalty) cases. *University of Missouri–Kansas City Law Review*, 82, 2.

Hazlett, H.C., Poe, M.D., Gerig, G., et al. (2011). Early brain overgrowth in autism associated with an increase in cortical surface area before age two years. *Archives of General Psychiatry*, 68, 467–476.

Helverschou S.B., Bakken, T.L., Martinsen, H. (2008). Identifying symptoms of psychiatric disorders in people with autism and intellectual disability: an empirical conceptual analysis. *Mental Health Aspects of Developmental Disabilities*, 11, 105–115.

Hoekstra, R.A., Happé, F., Baron-Cohen, S., Ronald, A. (2009). Association between extreme autistic traits and intellectual disability: insights from a general population twin study. *British Journal of Psychiatry*, 195(6), 531–536.

Holdnack, J.A., Xiaobin, Z., Larrabee, G., Millis, S.R., Salthouse, T.A. (2011). Confirmatory factor analysis of the WAIS-IV/WMS-IV 4. *Assessment*, 18(2), 178–191.

Johnson, W., Nijenhuis, J.T., Bouchard, T.J., Jr. (2008). Still just 1 g: consistent results from five test batteries. *Intelligence*, 36, 81–95.

Kraijer, D. and de Bildt, A. (2005). The PDD-MRS: an instrument for identification of autism spectrum disorders in persons with mental retardation. *Journal of Autism and Development Disorders*, 35(4), 499–513.

Lewis, J.D., Evans, A.C., Pruett, J.R., et al. (2014). Network inefficiencies in autism spectrum disorder at 24 months. *Translational Psychiatry*, 4:e388.

Luckasson, R., Borthwick-Duffy, S., Buntinx, W.H.E., et al. (2002). *Mental Retardation: Definition, Classification, and Systems of Supports*, 10th edition. Washington, DC: American Psychiatric Association.

Maljaars, J., Noens, I., Scholte, E., van Berckelaer-Onnes, I. (2012). Evaluation of the criterion and convergent validity of the Diagnostic Interview for Social and Communication Disorders in young and low-functioning children. *Autism*, 16(5), 487–497.

Matson J.L. and Kozlowski A.M. (2011). The increasing prevalence of autism spectrum disorders. *Research in Autism Spectrum Disorders*, 5, 418–425.

Matson, J.L. and Shoemaker, M. (2009). Intellectual disability and its relationship to autism spectrum disorders. *Research in Developmental Disabilities*, 30(6), 1107–1114.

McGrew, K.S. (2005) The Cattell–Horn–Carroll theory of cognitive abilities: past, present, and future. In D.P. Flanagan, J.L.

Genshaft, P.L. Harrison (eds.), *Contemporary Intellectual Assessment: Theories, Tests, and Issues*. New York, NY: Guilford Press.

Mervis, C.B., Klein-Tasman, B.P., Mastin, M.E. (2001). Adaptive behavior of 4-through 8-year-old children with Williams syndrome. *American Journal on Mental Retardation*, 106(1), 82–93.

Morgan, C.N., Roy, M., Nasr, A., et al. (2002). A community study establishing the prevalence rate of autistic disorder in adults with learning disability. *Psychiatric Bulletin*, 26, 127–129.

Murphy, O., Healy, O., Leader, G. (2009). Risk factors for challenging behaviors among 157 children with autism spectrum disorders in Ireland. *Research in Autism Spectrum Disorders*, 3, 474–482.

Naglieri, J.A. and Das, J.P. (1997). *Das–Naglieri Cognitive Assessment System*. Itasca, IL: Riverside Publishing Co.

Naglieri, J.A. and Das, J.P. (2002). Practical implications of general intelligence and PASS cognitive processes. In R. Sternberg and E. Grigorenko (eds.), *The General Factor of Intelligence. How General is it?* Mahwah, NJ: Lawrence Erlbaum Associates.

Noterdaeme, M.A. and Wriedt, E. (2010). Comorbidity in autism spectrum disorders – I. Mental retardation and psychiatric comorbidity. *Zeitschrift für Kinder-und Jugendpsychiatrie und Psychotherapie*, 38(4), 257–266.

Palucka, A.M., Lunsky, Y., Gofine, T., et al. (2009). Brief report: comparison of referrals of individuals with and without a diagnosis of psychotic disorder to a specialized dual diagnosis program. *Journal on Developmental Disabilities*, 15, 103–109.

Ramey, C.T., and Ramey, S.L. (1998). Early intervention and early experience. *American Psychologist*, 53, 109–120.

Rauch, A., Hoyer, J., Guth, S., et al. (2006). Diagnostic yield of various genetic approaches in patients with unexplained developmental delay or mental retardation. *American Journal of Medical Genetics Part A*, 140(19), 2063.

Reilly, C. (2012). Behavioural phenotypes and special educational needs: is aetiology important in the classroom? *Journal of Intellectual Disability Research*, 56, 929–946.

Salvador-Carulla, L. and García-Gutiérrez, J.C. (2011). The WHO construct of Health-related Functioning (HrF) and its implications for health policy. *BMC Public Health*, 11(4), S9.

Salvador-Carulla, L. and Saxena, S. (2009). Intellectual disability: between disability and clinical nosology. *Lancet*, 374(9704), 1798–1799.

Salvador-Carulla, L., Reed, G.M., Vaez-Azizi, L.M., et al. (2011). Intellectual developmental disorders: towards a new name, definition and framework for "mental retardation/ intellectual disability" in ICD-11. *World Psychiatry*, 10(3), 175–180.

Sappok, T., Gaul, I., Bergmann, T., et al. (2014) The Diagnostic Behavioral Assessment for Autism Spectrum Disorder – Revised: a screening instrument for adults with intellectual disability suspected of autism spectrum disorders. *Research in Autism Spectrum Disorders*, 8(4), 362–375.

Schalock, R.L. and Luckasson, R. (2005). *Clinical Judgment*. Washington, DC: American Association on Intellectual and Developmental Disabilities.

Schalock, R.L., Borthwick-Duffy, S.A., Bradley, M., et al. (2010). *Intellectual Disability: Definition, Classification, and Systems of Supports*, 11th edition. Washington, DC: American Association on Intellectual and Developmental Disabilities.

Shevell, M. (2008). Global developmental delay and mental retardation or intellectual disability: conceptualization, evaluation, and etiology. *Pediatric Clinics of North America*, 55, 1071–1084.

Soenen, S., Van Berckelaer-Onnes, I., Scholte, E. (2009). Patterns of intellectual, adaptive and behavioral functioning in individuals with mild mental retardation. *Research in Developmental Disabilities*, 30(3), 433–444.

Stancliffe, R.J., Lakin, K.C., Larson, S., et al. (2011). Choice of living arrangements.

Journal of Intellectual Disability Research, 55(8), 746–762.

Sullivan, W.F., Heng, J., Cameron, D., et al. (2006). Consensus guidelines for primary health care of adults with developmental disabilities. *Canadian Family Physician*, 52(11), 1410–1418.

Thompson, J.R. (2004). *Supports Intensity Scale: User's Manual*. Washington, DC: American Association on Mental Retardation.

Thornton-Wells, T.A., Cannistraci, C.J., Anderson, A.W., et al. (2010). Auditory attraction: activation of visual cortex by music and sound in Williams syndrome. *American Journal on Intellectual and Developmental Disabilites*, 115(2), 172–189.

Tiekstra, M., Hessels, M.G., Minnaert, A.E. (2009). Learning capacity in adolescents with mild intellectual disabilities. *Psychological Reports*, 105(3 Pt 1), 804–814.

Unenge Hallerbäck, M., Lugnegård, T., Gillberg, C. (2012). Is autism spectrum disorder common in schizophrenia? *Psychiatry Research*, 198(1), 12–17.

Wing, L., Leekam, S.R., Libby, S.J., Gould, J., Larcombe, M. (2002). The diagnostic interview for social and communication disorders: background, inter-rater reliability and clinical use. *Journal of Child Psychology and Psychiatry, and Allied Disciplines*, 43, 307–325.

World Health Organization. (1992a). *International Statistical Classification of Diseases and Related Health Problems, 10th Revision*, Vol. 1. Geneva: World Health Organization.

World Health Organization. (1992b). *The ICD-10 Classification of Mental and Behavioural Disorders: Clinical Descriptions and Diagnostic Guidelines*. Geneva: World Health Organization.

World Health Organization (2001). *International Classification of Functioning, Disability and Health (ICF)*. Geneva: World Health Organization.

World Health Organization. (2011). *ICD-11 Alpha. Content Model Reference Guide, 11th Revision*. Geneva: World Health Organization.

The epidemiology of psychiatric disorders in adults with intellectual disabilities

Jason Buckles

Introduction

Obtaining accurate data regarding the prevalence of psychiatric disorders in adults with intellectual disabilities (ID) is a necessary aspect in the path toward achieving functional distribution and allocation of services (Kerker et al., 2004; Smiley, 2005). Without such data it may be difficult to create or maintain the complex networks necessary for targeted, effective, and sustainable systems of treatment and support. Over the past several decades, research in this domain has been affected by changing notions of the abilities of people with ID, inconsistency of definition and classification of both ID and psychiatric disorder, and variation in assessment procedures (Moss et al., 1997; Yoo et al., 2011). There appears to be movement toward research methods and foci that may attenuate some of these concerns (Bouras, 2013). This chapter critically reviews recent studies regarding the epidemiology of co-occurring psychiatric disorder(s) in adults with ID in order to elucidate recent developments and suggest areas for improvement. The means by which prevalence data may continue to be complicated by sampling methodology, differences in definition, classification, and measurement of ID and psychiatric disorder, and geographical distribution of studies are addressed. Examples of promising practice, areas in need of examination, and developing concerns are provided.

Review

Reviews of the research by Kerker et al. (2004) and Whitaker and Read (2006) form the starting point for the current analysis. The studies analyzed in these previous reviews evidenced wide variation (0–74%) in reported prevalence rates of psychiatric disorder in people with ID. Both reviews suggested that sampling methodologies (i.e., administrative or population-based) as well as diagnostic criteria and assessment methods might have played significant roles in this variation.

Twelve articles were identified for this chapter using a combination of electronic search and citation review. In order to meet inclusion criteria articles must have: (i) been published in peer-reviewed English language journals between January 2004 and July 2014; and (ii) included data on the prevalence of ID and co-occurring psychiatric disorder in an adult (i.e., 16 years and older) sample. The cutoff age of 16 was established

Psychiatric and Behavioral Disorders in Intellectual and Developmental Disabilities, ed. Colin Hemmings and Nick Bouras. Published by Cambridge University Press. © Cambridge University Press 2016.

in line with the method utilized in certain studies from the UK (e.g., Cooper et al., 2007b) that defined "adult" as age 16 and above. Exclusion criteria included: (i) any article reviewed by Whitaker and Read (2006) or Kerker et al. (2004); (ii) articles that addressed "problem behavior" or like terms without data regarding assessment of psychiatric disorder; and (iii) articles that focused solely on individuals identified as having border-line intelligence but not ID (e.g., Hassiotis et al., 2008). In addition, articles were excluded if they were secondary analyses of previously published, larger datasets. This criterion applied mainly to the series of articles (i.e., Cooper et al., 2007a, 2007c, 2007d; Mantry et al., 2008; Melville et al., 2008) that stemmed from the work represented in Cooper, et al. (2007b). Comprehensive reviews of each of these non-included articles may be found in Buckles et al. (2013).

Searches of PsychINFO, ERIC, PubMed, and MEDLINE were conducted using the following terms: "comorbid" OR "mental-ill health" OR "dual-diagnosis" OR "mental disorder" OR "psychiatric disorder" OR "psychopathology" AND "mental retardation" OR "intellectual disability" OR "learning disability" AND "prevalence" OR "epidemiology." Searches revealed 305 articles. A brief review of titles and abstracts left 99 as potentially relevant. Of these 99, 34 articles were identified as candidates for review. Full-text versions of the 34 identified articles were obtained and read by the author. Following this initial read-through, 12 articles were identified as fulfilling inclusion criteria.

Reviewed articles were grouped according to sampling methodology (i.e., adminis-trative or population-based). Studies were identified as utilizing administrative sampling if participants were entirely identified/recruited from services specific to individuals with ID. Also, studies were identified as utilizing population-based sampling if participants were recruited from the population as a whole regardless of enrollment in specialized services.

Prevalence data

Estimates of prevalence of psychiatric disorders in population-based samples of adults with ID were found to range from 13.9% (Cooper et al., 2007b) when using criteria from the *Diagnostic and Statistical Manual of Mental Disorders, Fourth Edition, Text Revision* (DSM-IV-TR; American Psychiatric Association, 2000) and not including autism spec-trum disorders or challenging behavior, to 74% (Strydom et al., 2005). In the group of studies that utilized administrative samples, prevalence estimates ranged from 13.2% (Bailey, 2007; when using DSM-IV criteria) to 72.3% (Turygin et al., 2014). The highest reported rates appear to have been influenced by inclusion of less stringent definitions of disorder, age or administrative status of study sample, and differences in manner of assessment.

Due to rigorous protocols, the work presented in Cooper et al. (2007b) was of particular note. Specifically, this team's methodology included: (a) a large sample size ($N = 1023$; representing ~70.6% of the population with ID in the study area); (b) clear and current medical/physiological assessment; (c) clear definition and standardized tools to assess/report intellectual status; and (d) the use and comparison of multiple psychiatric assessment tools and criteria sets as applied by specially trained physicians. Prevalence estimates in this study ranged from 13.9% (DSM-IV criteria not including autism or challenging behaviors) to 40.9% ("clinical criteria" and including autism and challenging behavior). Kerker et al.'s (2004) review reported prevalence rates varied from 0% to 45% depending on similar variables. When the data from Cooper et al. (2007b) were distinguished by level of ID and based upon clinical criteria not including autism and challenging behavior, prevalence rates for all groups (i.e., mild, moderate, and profound ID) were reported at 22.4%. In short, it appears that the inclusion of challenging behavior in the definition of mental disorder may account for much of the perceived increased risk of co-occurring mental disorder in the population of persons with ID. Figure 3.1 provides a visual perspective on this variation in the data that is perhaps due to inclusion/exclusion criteria and sampling methods.

Consistently higher prevalence rates were reported in the studies that utilized administrative sampling. Of the examined studies in this group, Bailey (2007) appeared to utilize the most robust protocol (i.e., medical screening, multiple diagnostic methods conducted by a specialist psychiatrist, and reported on how the rate is affected by inclusion/exclusion of certain conditions) and also reported the highest rate of co-occurrence (61.2% – "clinical criteria" and including "behavior disorder"). This rate appeared to be markedly influenced by the applied diagnostic classification system. Specifically, the reported prevalence of psychiatric disorder, in the same individuals, reduced respectively to 57.0%, 24.8%, and 13.2% when the *Diagnostic Criteria for Psychiatric Disorders for Use with Adults with Learning Disabilities/Mental Retardation* (DC-LD; Royal College of Psychiatrists, 2001), *ICD-10 Diagnostic Criteria for Research* (DCR-10; World Health Organization, 1993), and DSM-IV criteria were applied.

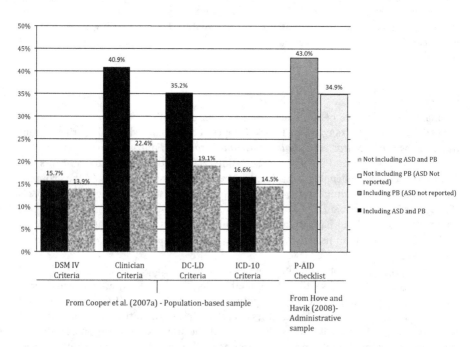

Figure 3.1 Variation of point prevalence of mental disorder in adults with ID. Effect of diagnostic criteria, inclusion/exclusion of autism spectrum disorders (ASD) and/or problem behavior (PB), and sampling method. From Buckles et al. (2013). Used with permission.

Sampling methodology

Since the reviews by Kerker et al. (2004) and Whitaker and Read (2006) there has been a modest increase in the use of population-based sampling methods. Four of the 12 studies identified for review utilized such methods As described above, these advances have provided models for how such endeavors may be undertaken in a focused, thorough manner that addresses several of the limitations which have historically affected this type of research. Administrative sampling methods, however, remain dominant. This is perhaps due to the financial and organizational demands of carrying out large-scale, multisite investigations. Reviewed studies that utilized administrative sampling methods added to the literature base in several areas including: (a) examination of the role of challenging behavior (Myrbakk and von Tetzchner, 2008); (b) co-occurring psychiatric conditions in persons with ID involved in criminal justice systems (Vanny et al., 2009; Dias et al., 2013); (c) comparison of urban/rural differences (Kiani et al., 2013); and (d) examination of prevalence in a sample from institutional settings in the USA (Turygin et al., 2014). In short, utilization of administrative sampling may reveal specific areas of concern and potential intervention for individuals in particular residential or specialized service systems. Caution must be used, however, in applying these data to estimates of overall prevalence in the population of people with ID.

Diversity in definition, measurement, and assessment processes

The reviewed studies evidenced a wide array of definitions and interpretations of what constitutes a psychiatric condition. In short, there continues to be little to "no consensus about which problems should be included in the term 'mental health problem'" (Costello and Bouras, 2006). As there is also considerable, potentially irreconcilable, variability in cross-cultural definitions of psychopathology, problem behavior, and deviance (Tanaka-Matsumi, 2001; Fabrega, 2004), this is more than just a matter of standardizing professional nomenclature. In order to supply meaningful data that may be compared across studies, research in this domain must continue to increase consistency and clarity of diagnostic inclusion and exclusion criteria while remaining sensitive to cultural, linguistic, and geographic differences. Likewise, there is the distinct concern of applying existing definitional systems of mental disorder with persons identified as ID. The most widely used diagnostic manuals in this research area (e.g., DSM-IV-TR; *International Classification of Disease, Tenth Edition, Classification of Mental and Behavioural Disorders* (ICD-10; World Health Organization, 1993)) often rely on self-report of internal experiences for key symptom criteria. It may, therefore, be exceedingly difficult to accurately apply these criteria to individuals with ID, who have difficulty with nuanced verbal expression (Moss et al., 1996; Costello and Bouras, 2006) or identification of emotional states. In this manner, concern about diagnostic overshadowing (Reiss and Syszko, 1993; White, M.J., et al., 1995) remains present. Conversely, the possibility of *over*diagnosis may emerge when certain psychiatric disorders are assessed for the purpose of clinical treatment rather than empirical research (Berardi et al., 2005; Mojtabi, 2013). This issue is particularly germane in estimates of prevalence that have utilized data from medical charts in healthcare systems, such as the USA, where approval for treatment may be contingent upon application of a qualifying diagnosis.

Perhaps stemming from the above, the reviewed studies revealed significant variation in the particular tools used to assess psychiatric symptoms. Methods ranged from questionnaires or checklists completed by support persons or carers (e.g., Hove and Havik, 2008) to multimodal integration of face-to-face professional interview and assessment with structured tools applied by trained specialists (e.g., Cooper et al., 2007b). Similar limitations have been noted in the previous reviews of this topic (Kerker et al., 2004; Whitaker and Read, 2006). Tailored tools, such as the *Psychiatric Assessment Schedule for Adults with Developmental Disabilities* (PAS-ADD; Moss et al., 1998), were utilized in several studies and findings suggested promising crossover with estimates based on clinical criteria (e.g., Bailey, 2007; Cooper et al., 2007b).

Complicating this matter further, there appears to be ongoing variation and inconsistency regarding the terminology, assessment, and classification of ID (Luckasson and Reeve, 2001). Reviewed projects utilized a litany of methods for determining the label of ID, including but not limited to: (i) review of registry records (e.g., Morgan et al., 2008); (ii) self-report and/or report of close others (e.g., White, P., et al., 2005); and (iii) use of multiple normed measures applied by trained healthcare professionals (e.g., Cooper et al., 2007c). In essence, while studies may utilize similar terminology regarding ID, the methods of defining or measuring what is meant by these terms may, at times, be quite disparate and affected by historical and functional variation.

The above issues regarding methods of definition, classification, and assessment are cumulative. Collectively, these aspects compound the difficulty of arriving at any consensus regarding the prevalence of co-occurring disorders in people with ID. At each turn in the process – from sampling method, to definition of disorder or disability, to inclusion or exclusion of specific disorders or symptoms, to choice of tool and assessment method – there are multiple points of potential divergence. Such variation of methods may result in a relative kaleidoscope of findings, which will remain difficult to compare in a valid fashion either to each other or to general population data. As certain regions begin to integrate use of the fifth edition of the *Diagnostic and Statistical Manual of Mental Disorders* (DSM-5; American Psychiatric Association, 2013), these matters, as discussed below, may increase in complexity.

Inclusion of physiological assessment

It is essential to note that only two of the 12 reviewed studies (Bailey, 2007; Cooper et al. 2007b) included protocols that integrated medical/physiological evaluation in an attempt to identify potentially confounding health variables. When utilizing certain psychiatric manuals (e.g., DSM-IV-TR), practitioners are cautioned to determine (i.e., "rule-out") if the examined set of symptoms are attributable to the effects of a general medical condition. If a medical condition is found to be etiologically connected, the behavioral or psychiatric diagnosis may be coded as "due to" said condition. As so few of the reviewed studies examined these issues, it is unclear if such conditions were intentionally or unintentionally included in the base definition of psychiatric disorder and resultant prevalence estimates. Delineating between what conditions may be defined as a psychiatric disorder versus a neurological condition may be difficult (Wakefield and First, 2003). In addition, many physical conditions may influence presentation or interpretation of psychiatric symptoms in people with ID (Lennox, 2007; King et al., 2014). There is also convincing evidence that while progress has been made, people with ID overall may continue to encounter inadequate attention to medical health (Anderson et al., 2013). Thus, historical or chart-based data sources may lack an adequate examination of potentially confounding medical conditions. Incorporation of these types of data must increase if we hope to arrive at valid prevalence estimates.

Geographical, cultural, and linguistic representation

Only one of the 12 reviewed studies (Turygin et al., 2014) examined a sample of individuals from North America. Other represented regions included: (i) the UK ($N = 4$); (ii) Australia ($N = 4$); (iii) Sweden ($N = 1$); and (iv) Norway ($N = 2$). No studies that matched inclusion/exclusion criteria were found from Central or South America, Asia, Eastern Europe, or Africa. Reviewed studies were overwhelmingly conducted in culturally and linguistically homogenous areas. In order to ensure robust prevalence estimates there is clearly a need to expand the diversity of sampled populations both geographically and culturally.

Emergent concerns: changes and developments in diagnostic manuals

In its most recent iteration, the DSM-5 (American Psychiatric Association, 2013) introduced several areas of adjustment to manners of classifying and defining certain psychiatric disorders. There are also data which indicate that certain changes may effect measurement of conditions such as autism spectrum disorders (Matson et al., 2012; Wilson et al., 2013; Kim et al., 2014; Maenner et al. 2014), post-traumatic stress disorder (Weathers et al., 2014), certain presentations of major depression (Koukpoulos and Sani, 2014), negative symptoms of schizophrenia (Malaspina et al., 2014), and the role of chronic pain in symptom presentation (Young, 2013). Similar questions have been posed regarding pending revisions in ICD-11 (Reed et al., 2013; Goldberg, 2014). Studies that compare prevalence estimates, via previous, current, and emergent diagnostic sets, must continue if we hope to better understand how definitional differences and adjustments may affect epidemiological estimates and resultant system development (Goldman et al., 2012).

In relation to the above, promising advances have been made toward tailoring diagnostic manuals for potential expressive differences in people with ID. The DC-LD was utilized in several of the reviewed studies and results were comparable to clinical criteria (e.g., Bailey, 2007; Cooper et al., 2007b). Additionally, there is early evidence that the *Diagnostic Manual – Intellectual Disability* (DM-ID; Fletcher et al., 2007), which is based upon DSM-IV criteria, may provide improved clinical utility while reducing the use of not-otherwise-specified diagnostic labels (Fletcher et al., 2009). Questions remain, however, regarding: (a) how application of DM-ID criteria may affect prevalence estimates; (b) how future editions of the DC-LD and DM-ID may accommodate and be affected by respective changes in the ICD-11 and DSM-5; and (c) potential development or modification of specialized assessment tools based upon these emergent criteria.

Conclusions

This chapter provided a critical review of research regarding the prevalence of psychiatric disorders in people with ID published from 2004 to 2014. The findings suggest that there have been improvements in methodological considerations of sampling techniques and use/comparison of varying assessment tools and diagnostic criteria. Specifically, there has been marked increase in the use of adjusted criteria sets for assessing psychiatric disorders in this population. In particular, both the DC-LD manual and the PAS-ADD Checklist appear to have promising correlation with clinically derived assessment data (e.g., Cooper et al., 2007b). Unfortunately, limitations of this research base continue to prevent confidence in statements of overall prevalence of co-occurring psychiatric conditions in people with ID. Similar to findings of previous reviews (Kerker et al., 2004; Whitaker and Read, 2006, Yoo, et al., 2011) and position papers (Costello and Bouras, 2006), there remains ongoing disparity in definition of what is meant by the term psychiatric disorder, including decisions to include or exclude certain conditions (for example, behavioral problems, autism spectrum disorders, diagnoses secondary to general medical conditions). Additional variation was found to be present in the tools and methods of assessment, as well as the use of physiological screening. When viewed in conjunction with similar issues regarding terminology and measurement of ID – the concerns are additive and continue to hamper comparison/aggregation of findings. The introduction and potential effect of revised and adjusted diagnostic manuals (e.g., DSM-5, ICD-11) is a potential further confound and must be addressed in the upcoming literature. Lastly, there is a clear need for an expanded physical and cultural geography of prevalence research regarding psychiatric disorders in people with ID. Efforts in this arena will be best informed by use of population-based sampling, clearly stated definitions and consistent measurement of both psychiatric disorder and ID, use/comparison of multiple diagnostic sets and assessment methods, and inclusion of medical screening.

Key summary points

- Clear consensus regarding the prevalence of mental health conditions in people with ID remains elusive.
- There has been an increase in the use of population-based sampling over the past 10 years.
- Variation in prevalence data may stem from a multitude of factors including but not limited to:
  - The nature of the study sample (i.e., administrative or population based);
  - The nature of the definition/classification system(s) used to identify psychiatric disorders and ID;
  - The particular tool(s) used for assessment of potential psychiatric disorders;
  - The inclusion or exclusion of 'challenging behavior' and/or autism spectrum disorders under the general mantle of psychiatric disorders;
  - The inclusion or exclusion of biomedical conditions as a potential contributing/ etiological factor in presentation of behavioral or affective symptoms;
  - The training and experience of the individual(s) applying assessment tools.
- In order to address shortcomings in the literature base, further research in this area must focus on:
  - Continued utilization of population-based sampling; and
  - Inclusion of non-ID comparison groups; and
  - Utilization and comparison of multiple assessment tools and methods including medical screening; and
  - Expanded geographic, cultural, and linguistic representation (e.g., studies from the Americas, Asia, Eastern Europe).

References

American Psychiatric Association. (2000). *Diagnostic and Statistical Manual of Mental Disorders – Text Revision, Fourth Edition.* Washington, DC: American Psychiatric Association.

American Psychiatric Association. (2013). *Diagnostic and Statistical Manual of Mental Disorders, Fifth Edition.* Washington, DC: American Psychiatric Association.

Anderson, L.L., Humphries, K., McDermott, S., et al. (2013). The state of the science of health and wellness for adults with intellectual and developmental disabilities. *Intellectual and Developmental Disabilities*, 51, 385–398.

Bailey, N.M. (2007). Prevalence of psychiatric disorders in adults with moderate to profound learning disabilities. *Advances in Mental Health and Learning Disabilities*, 1, 36–44.

Berardi, D., Menchetti, M., Cevenini, N., et al.. (2005). Increased recognition of depression in primary care: comparison between primary care physician and ICD-10 diagnosis of depression. *Psychotherapy and Psychosomatics*, 74, 225–230.

Bouras, N. (2013). Reviewing research of mental health problems for people with intellectual disabilities. *Journal of Mental Health Research in Intellectual Disabilties*, 6, 71–73.

Buckles, J., Luckasson, R., Keefe, E. (2013). A systematic review of the prevalence of psychiatric disorders in adults with intellectual disability, 2003-2010. *Journal of Mental Health Research in Intellectual Disabilities*, 6, 181–207.

Cooper, S.A., Smiley, E., Finlayson, J., et al. (2007a). The prevalence, incidence, and factors predictive of mental ill-health in adults with profound intellectual disabilities. *Journal of Applied Research in Intellectual Disabilities*, 20, 493–501.

Cooper, S.A., Smiley, E., Morrison, J., Williamson, A., Allan, L. (2007b). Mental ill-health in adults with intellectual disabilities: prevalence and associated factors. Mental health services for adults with learning disabilities. *British Journal of Psychiatry*, 190, 27–35.

Cooper, S.A., Smiley, E., Morrison, J., Williamson, A., Allan, L. (2007c). An epidemiological investigation of affective disorders with a population-based cohort of 1023 adults with intellectual disabilities. *Psychological Medicine*, 37, 873–882.

Cooper, S.A., Smiley, E., Morrison, J., et al. (2007d). Psychosis and adults with intellectual disabilities: prevalence, incidence, and related factors. *Social Psychiatry and Psychiatric Epidemiology*, 42, 530–536.

Costello, H. and Bouras, N. (2006). Assessment of mental health problems in people with intellectual disabilities. *Israeli Journal of Psychiatry and Related Sciences*, 43, 241–251.

Dias, S., Ware, R.S., Kinner, S.A., Lennox, N.G. (2013). Co-occurring mental disorder and intellectual disability in a large sample of Australian prisoners. *Australia and New Zealand Journal of Psychiatry*, 47, 938–944.

Fabrega, H., Jr. (2004). Culture and the origins of psychopathology. In U.P. Gielen, J.M. Fish, J.G. Draguns (eds.), *Handbook of Culture, Therapy, and Healing.* Mawah, NJ: Lawrence Earlbaum Associates.

Fletcher, R., Loschen, E., Stavrakaki, C., et al. (eds.) (2007). *Diagnostic Manual – Intellectual Disability: A Textbook of Diagnosis of Mental Disorders in Persons with Intellectual Disability.* Kingston, NY: NADD Press.

Fletcher, R., Havercamp, S.M., Ruedrich, S.L., et al. (2009). Clinical usefulness of the Diagnostic Manual – Intellectual Disability for mental disorders in persons with intellectual disability: results from a brief field survey. *Journal of Clinical Psychiatry*, 70, 967–974.

Goldberg, J.F. (2014). What should ICD-11 do that DSM-5 did not? *Australia and New Zealand Journal of Psychiatry*, 48, 87–88.

Goldman, H.H., Horvitz-Lennon, M.V., Hu, T-W., et al. (2012). Economic consequences of revising the diagnostic nomenclature for mental disorders. In S. Saxena, P. Esparza, D.A. Regier, B. Saraceno, N. Satorius (eds.),

Public Health Aspects of Diagnosis and
Classification of Mental and Behavioral
Disorders: Refining the Research Agenda for
DSM-5 and ICD-11. Arlington, VA:
American Psychiatric Association.

Hassiotis, A., Strydom, A., Hall, I., et al.
(2008). Psychiatric morbidity and social
functioning among adults with borderline
intelligence living in private households.
Journal of Intellectual Disability Research,
52, 95–106.

Hove, O. and Havik, O.E. (2008). Mental
disorders and problem behavior in a
community sample of adults with
intellectual disability: three-month
prevalence and comorbidity. *Journal of
Mental Health Research in Intellectual
Disabilities*, 1, 223–237.

Kerker, B.D., Owens, P.L., Zigler, P.I., et al.
(2004). Mental health disorders among
individuals with mental retardation:
challenges to accurate prevalence estimates.
Public Health Reports, 119, 409–417.

Kiani, R., Tyrer, F., Hodgson, A., et al. (2013).
Urban–rural differences in the nature and
prevalence of mental ill-health in adults
with intellectual disabilities. *Journal
of Intellectual Disability Research*,
57, 119–127.

Kim, Y.S., Fombonne, E., Koh, Y.-J., et al.
(2014). A comparison of DSM-IV pervasive
developmental disorder and DSM-5 autism
spectrum disorder prevalence in an
epidemiologic sample. *Journal of the
American Academy of Child and Adolescent
Psychiatry*, 53, 500–508.

King, B.H., de Lacy, N., Siegel, M. (2014).
Psychiatric assessment of severe
presentations in autism spectrum disorders
and intellectual disability. *Child and
Adolescent Psychiatric Clinics of North
America*, 23, 1–14.

Koukpoulos, A. and Sani, G. (2014).
DSM-5 criteria for depression with
mixed features: a farewell to mixed
depression. *Acta Psychiatrica Scandinavia*,
129, 4–16.

Lennox, N. (2007). The interface between
medical and psychiatric disorders in people
with intellectual disabilities. In N. Bouras

and G. Holt (eds.), *Psychiatric and
Behavioural Disorders in Intellectual and
Developmental Disabilities*, second edition.
Cambridge: Cambridge University Press.

Luckasson, R. and Reeve, A. (2001). Naming,
defining, and classifying in mental
retardation. *Mental Retardation*, 39, 47–52.

Maenner, M.J., Rice, C.E., Arneson, C.L., et al.
(2014). Potential impact of DSM-5 criteria
on autism spectrum disorder prevalence
estimates. *Journal of the American Medical
Association – Psychiatry*, 71, 292–300.

Malaspina, D., Walsh-Messinger, J., Gaebel,
W., et al. (2014). Negative symptoms, past
and present: a historical perspective and
moving to DSM-5. *European
Neuropsychopharmacology*, 24, 710–724.

Mantry, D., Cooper, S.A., Smiley, E., et al.
(2008). The prevalence and incidence of
mental ill-health in adults with Down
syndrome. *Journal of Intellectual Disability
Research*, 52, 141–155.

Matson, J.L., Belva, B.C., Horovitz, M.,
Kozlowski, A.M., Bamburg, J.W. (2012).
Comparing symptoms of autism spectrum
disorders in a developmentally disabled
adult population using the current DSM-
IV-TR diagnostic criteria and the proposed
DSM-5 diagnostic criteria. *Journal of
Developmental and Physical Disabilities*,
24, 403–414.

Melville, C.A., Cooper, S.A., Morrison, J., et al.
(2008). The prevalence and incidence of
mental ill-health in adults with autism and
intellectual disabilities. *Journal of Autism
and Developmental Disorders*, 38, 1676–1688.

Mojtabi, R. (2013). Clinician-identified
depression in community settings:
concordance with structured-interview
diagnoses. *Psychotherapy and
Psychosomatics*, 82, 161–169.

Morgan, V.A., Leonard, H., Bourke, J.,
Jablensky, A. (2008). Intellectual disability
co-occurring with schizophrenia and other
psychiatric illness: population-based study.
Mental health services for adults with
learning disabilities. *British Journal of
Psychiatry*, 193, 364–372.

Moss, S., Prosser, H., Ibbotson, B., et al. (1996).
Respondent and informant accounts of

psychiatric symptoms in a sample of patients with learning disability. *Journal of Intellectual Disability Research*, 40, 457–465.

Moss, S., Emerson, E., Bouras, N., et al. (1997). Mental disorders and problematic behaviours in people with intellectual disability: future directions for research. *Journal of Intellectual Disability Research*, 41, 440–447.

Moss, S., Prosser, H., Costello, H., et al. (1998). Reliability and validity of the PAS-ADD checklist for detecting psychiatric disorders in adults with intellectual disability. *Journal of Intellectual Disability Research*, 42, 173–183.

Myrbakk, E. and von Tetzchner, S. (2008). Psychiatric disorders and behavior problems in people with intellectual disability. *Research in Developmental Disabilities*, 29, 316–332.

Reed, G.M., Roberts, M.C., Keeley, J., et al. (2013). Mental health professionals' natural taxonomies of mental disorders: implications for the clinical utility of the ICD-11 and the DSM-5. *Journal of Clinical Psychology*, 69, 1191–1212.

Reiss, S. and Syszko, J. (1993). Diagnostic overshadowing and professional experience with mentally retarded persons. *American Journal of Mental Deficiency*, 87, 396–402.

Royal College of Psychiatrists (2001). *Diagnostic Criteria for Psychiatric Disorders for Use with Adults with Learning Disabilities/Mental Retardation (DC-LD)*. Occasional Paper OP 48. London: Royal College of Psychiatrists.

Smiley, E. (2005). Epidemiology of mental health problems in adults with learning disabilities: an update. *Advances in Psychiatric Treatment*, 18, 214–222.

Strydom, A., Hassiotis, A., Livingston, G. (2005). Mental health and social care needs of older people with intellectual disabilities. *Journal of Applied Research in Intellectual Disabilities*, 18, 229–235.

Tanaka-Matsumi, J. (2001). Abnormal psychology and culture. In D. Matsumoto (ed.), *Handbook of Culture and Psychology*. New York, NY: Oxford University Press.

Turygin, N., Matson, J.L., Adams, H. (2014). Prevalence of co-occurring disorders in a sample of adults with mild and moderate intellectual disabilities who reside in a residential treatment setting. *Research in Developmental Disabilities*, 35, 1802–1808.

Vanny, K.A., Levy, M.H., Greenberg, D.M., Hayes, S.C. (2009). Mental illness and intellectual disability in Magistrates Courts in New South Wales, Australia. *Journal of Intellectual Disability Research*, 53, 289–297.

Wakefield, J.C. and First, M.B. (2003). Clarifying the distinction between disorder and nondisorder: confronting the overdiagnosis (false-positives) problem in DSM-V. In K.A. Phillips, M.B. First, H.A. Pincus (eds.), *Advancing DSM: Dilemmas in psychiatric diagnosis*. Washington, DC: American Psychiatric Association.

Weathers, F.W., Marx, B.P., Friedman, M.J., Schnurr, P.P. (2014). Posttraumatic stress disorder in DSM-5: new criteria, new measures, and implications for assessment. *Psychological Injury and Law*, 7, 93–107.

Whitaker, S. and Read, S. (2006). The prevalence of psychiatric disorders among peoples with intellectual disabilities: an analysis of the literature. *Journal of Applied Research in Intellectual Disabilities*, 19, 330–345.

White, M.J., Nichols, C.N., Cook, R.S., et al. (1995). Diagnostic overshadowing and mental retardation: a meta-analysis. *American Journal on Mental Retardation*, 100, 293–298.

White, P., Chant, D., Edwards, N., et al. (2005). Prevalence of intellectual disability and comorbid mental illness in an Australian community sample. *Australian and New Zealand Journal of Psychiatry*, 39, 395–400.

Wilson, C.E., Gillan, N., Spain, D., et al. (2013). Comparison of ICD-10R, DSM-IV-TR, and DSM-5 in an adult autism spectrum disorder diagnostic clinic. *Journal of Autism and Developmental Disorders*, 43, 2515–2525.

World Health Organization (1993) *ICD-10 Classification of Mental and Behavioural*

Disorders: Diagnostic Criteria for Research. Geneva: World Health Organization.

Yoo, J.H., Valdovinos, M.G., Schroeder, S.R. (2011). The epidemiology of psychopathology in people with intellectual disability: a 40-year review. In R.M. Hodapp (ed.), *International Review of Research in Developmental Disabilities,* Vol. 42. New York, NY: Academic Press.

Young, G. (2013). Ill-treatment of pain in the DSM-5. *Psychological Injury and Law,* 6, 299–306.

Assessment instruments and rating scales

Heidi Hermans

Introduction

Assessment instruments and rating scales are a vital part in evaluating mental health and identifying mental health problems in people with intellectual disabilities (ID). An advantage of adding rating scales to clinical assessments is that it allows objective comparison over time. Consequently, it gives insight into the effectiveness of treatments or interventions. It also allows for comparison over persons and over groups, e.g., the suitability of a particular treatment can be compared for different patient-groups. Standardized measurement of complaints is especially important for people with more severe ID who live in residential care, in which healthcare workers often change. Rating scale outcomes give an overview of functioning across changing healthcare workers. Therefore, using rating scales improves the quality of care.

Self-report versus informant-report

In the general population, assessment of psychiatric disorders is regularly done by means of self-report. In the population with ID, psychiatric assessment using self-report is only possible for people with sufficient cognitive and verbal skills, whereas informant-report is used for people with insufficient cognitive or verbal skills. It has been established that people with mild or moderate ID are able to report reliably about their feelings and thoughts (Lindsay et al., 1994; Costello and Bouras, 2006; Hartley and MacLean, 2006; Hurley, 2006). However, it is important that the content and wording of the questions are concrete (Finlay and Lyons, 2001). Furthermore, comprehension of the questions' content needs to be checked, as acquiescence may mask a lack of comprehension. Self-report enables questions about thoughts and feelings, whereas informant-report only allows questions about observable behavior. Therefore, self-report, if possible, is preferable. A combination of self-report and informant-report is even more desirable.

Screening instruments versus diagnostic instruments

Psychiatric and behavioral disorders can only be diagnosed with a diagnostic assessment performed by a skilled diagnostic investigator. In a diagnostic assessment, the criteria listed in diagnostic systems are used as a guideline. A structured diagnostic interview, in which the diagnostic criteria of a particular disorder are systematically questioned, can be part of the assessment. Even if a structured interview is used, diagnostic assessment still requires particular expertise in people with ID. Consequently, it is rather time-consuming and expensive. Therefore, it is common to screen with questionnaires first, to guide the decision for further diagnostic assessment.

Screening instruments

Screening instruments contain questions about symptoms or complaints of one or more disorders. In general, each question is scored with a standardized scoring system containing three to five answering categories. The score on the total questionnaire or its subscales reflects the number or severity of the symptoms. Some questionnaires have been provided with a cutoff score or norms, representing the clinical significance of the symptoms. A score above the cutoff score indicates that the presence of a psychiatric disorder is plausible. Hence, further diagnostic assessment is necessary.

Psychopathology

Quite a few instruments contain questions about symptoms of multiple psychiatric disorders. An advantage is that you are able to collect information on several disorders using only one instrument. Considering the comorbidity of psychiatric disorders, it seems convenient to assess multiple disorders with one instrument. A disadvantage is that most disorders are questioned rather briefly to limit the length of the instrument. Considering the complexity of mental health problems, one should be cautious with using instruments which are too non-specific. A risk of broad questions is that they do not discriminate between disorders or between people with and without mental health problems.

Self-report instruments assessing multiple disorders which are developed for adults with ID are scarce. Instruments developed for the general population are often used, but their applicability, reliability, and validity in people with ID have hardly been studied. The *Brief Symptom Inventory* (BSI) (Derogatis, 1975) is such an instrument used in the general population and also applied in adults with ID. The BSI is a shortened version of the widely used Symptom Checklist-90-R and consists of 53 items covering symptoms about somatization, interpersonal sensitivity, obsession–compulsion, interpersonal sensitivity, depression, anxiety, phobic anxiety, hostility, paranoid ideation, and psychoticism. Its utility and validity for adults with borderline or mild ID seems to be good, except for people with autism spectrum disorders (Kellett et al., 2003, Wieland et al., 2011). An advantage of the BSI is its broad scope.

Informant-report instruments assessing psychopathology that are especially developed for people with ID are more numerous. The *Psychiatric Assessment Schedule for Adults with Developmental Disabilities Checklist* (PAS-ADD Checklist) (Moss et al., 1993) and the *Mini Psychiatric Assessment Schedule for Adults with Developmental Disabilities* (Mini PAS-ADD) (Prosser et al., 1997) were developed for people with mild to profound ID. They are both based on the PAS-ADD Interview and cover a broad range of mental health problems. The reliability and validity of the PAS-ADD Checklist are good (Sturmey et al., 2005), whereas those of the Mini PAS-ADD are moderate for most subscales. Although the Mini PAS-ADD has weaker psychometric properties, caregivers are actively involved in the assessment of mental health, whereas the PAS-ADD Checklist is a regular questionnaire requiring no active input.

The *Anxiety, Depression And Mood Scale* (ADAMS) (Esbensen et al., 2003) consists of 28 items and focuses on depression, anxiety, mania, social avoidance, and obsessive-compulsive behavior. The ADAMS has been developed for adolescents and adults with mild to profound ID, and the reliability and validity of the total scale and its subscales are good in all levels of ID. The short length and its focus on two very common mental disorders (depression and anxiety) make this a suitable questionnaire for quick screening and monitoring of treatment effects.

The *Psychopathology Instrument for Mentally Retarded Adults* (PIMRA) consists of a self-report and an informant-report version and is suitable for all levels of ID. The PIMRA consists of 56 items assessing psychopathology on basis of DSM-III criteria. The PIMRA covers affective disorders, anxiety disorders, schizophrenia, psychosexual disorders, adjustment disorders, somatoform disorders, personality disorders, and inappropriate adjustment (Kazdin et al., 1983). In general, the PIMRA is able to distinguish between people with and without psychopathology. However, further differentiation between different disorders seems to be rather poor (Senatore et al., 1985; Ramirez and Lukenbill, 2007). The *Reiss Screen for Maladaptive Behaviour* (RSMB) (Reiss, 1988) is shorter and consists of 38 items covering aggressive behavior, autism, psychosis, paranoia, depression (both behavioral and physical signs), dependent personality disorder, and avoidant disorder. The RSMB is applicable for all levels of ID. The total RSMB has good reliability and validity results, but the psychometric quality of the separate subscales varies (Sturmey et al., 1995). *The Assessment of Dual Diagnosis* (ADD) (Matson and Bamburg, 1998) consists of 79 items covering mania, depression, anxiety, post-traumatic stress disorder, substance abuse, somatoform disorders, dementia, conduct disorder, pervasive developmental disorder, schizophrenia, personality disorders, sexual disorders, and eating disorders. The ADD was developed for people with mild or moderate ID, whereas the *Diagnostic Assessment for the Severely Handicapped–II* (DASH-II) (Matson, 1995) was developed for people with severe or profound ID. The DASH-II consists of 84 symptoms covering impulse control, organic syndromes, anxiety, mood, mania, autism, schizophrenia, stereotypies, self-injurious behavior, eliminating disorders, eating disorders, sleep disorders, and sexual disorders. Both instruments are quite lengthy to apply in clinical practice, and the reliability and validity results of both scales have varied among studies. Therefore, it is recommended to further study these instruments before they can be adopted in clinical practice. The *Psychopathology in Autism Checklist* (PAC) (Helverschou et al., 2009) has been especially developed for people with ID and autism. It consists of 42 items covering psychosis, depression, anxiety, and obsessive-compulsive disorder. This instrument has been developed to overcome the urgent problem of autistic features overshadowing other psychiatric symptoms. However, not all subscales differentiate well enough between the several included psychiatric diagnoses. Though potentially a very useful instrument, improvement of its differentiating ability, especially for anxiety disorders, is necessary.

In conclusion, most psychopathology instruments are suitable to screen for psychopathology in general, but are not first-choice instruments to examine specific disorders. The PAS-ADD questionnaires and the ADAMS seem currently the most applicable and valid (Matson et al., 2012) instruments for use in clinical practice.

Mood disorders

Mood disorders include mania and depression, but most instruments focus on depression (Hermans and Evenhuis, 2010). For depression, there are several self-report instruments available; both instruments developed for the general population and instruments especially developed for people with ID. Instruments developed for the general population which are often used in adults with borderline, mild, or moderate ID are the *Beck Depression Inventory* (BDI) (Beck, 1996), the *Zung Self-Rating Depression Scale* (Zung, 1965), and the *Hamilton Depression Rating Scale* (Hamilton, 1960). Although these instruments are applicable, the psychometric quality of instruments specifically developed for people with ID has been studied more often and seems to be better. Therefore, instruments developed for people with ID are preferable. The *Glasgow Depression Scale for people with a Learning Disability* (GDS-LD) (Cuthill et al., 2003) has been developed for people with mild or moderate ID, and is currently the most promising self-report instrument for this population. It contains 20 items and has an additional Carer Supplement of 16 items. The combination of self-report and informant-report allows for a broader, more thorough, assessment. The reliability and validity of the GDS-LD are good. Another self-report instrument for people with borderline, mild, or moderate ID is the *Self-report Depression Questionnaire* (SRDQ) (Reynolds and Baker, 1988), which is a structured interview of 32 items. The reliability is good, but the results for the validity are inconsistent. An informant-report instrument focusing on depression is the *Mood, Interest, and Pleasure Questionnaire* (MIPQ) (Ross and Oliver, 2003). The MIPQ consists of 25 items and has been developed for people with severe or profound ID. It has good reliability, but the validity has not been studied yet. The narrow target population may be a disadvantage for use in clinical practice or research, but it also improves the applicability of the items for this particular population.

Anxiety disorders

Most instruments focusing on anxiety are self-report (Hermans et al., 2011). This is not surprising, because most symptoms of anxiety (e.g., racing thoughts, heart pounding, and dizziness) are hard or impossible to observe by a third party. Two well-known instruments for anxiety in adults with ID are the *Glasgow Anxiety Scale for people with an Intellectual Disability* (GAS-ID) (Mindham and Espie, 2003) and the *Fear Survey for Adults with Mental Retardation* (FSAMR) (Ramirez and Lukenbill, 2007). The GAS-ID consists of 27 items and covers physical symptoms, worrying, and specific fears. The FSAMR consists of 85 items, including six items to check for acquiescence. Both instruments are applicable in adults with borderline, mild, or moderate ID and have good reliability and validity. An advantage of the GAS-ID over the FSAMR is the lower number of questions, requiring a shorter attention span and, therefore, broadening its applicability.

Instruments developed for children without ID are also often used for adults with ID. These instruments contain simple language and are, therefore, specifically suitable for this group. However, some topics questioned in these instruments (e.g., about school or play-dates) are not applicable for adults with ID. Therefore, it is better not to use such instruments solely because of their suitable language.

Dementia

Dementia or pathological cognitive decline is mostly assessed using neuropsychological tests or informant-report instruments (Zeilinger et al., 2013). Two well-known instruments for dementia in people with ID, which have been thoroughly studied for their psychometric qualities, are the Dementia Scale for Down Syndrome (DSDS) (Gedye, 1995) and the Dementia Questionnaire for Learning Disabilities (DMR), formally known as the Dementia Questionnaire for Mentally Retarded Persons (Evenhuis et al., 1995). The DSDS consists of 60 items that are divided in three categories, which reflect the three stages of dementia. The DMR consists of 50 items covering eight subscales, which can be divided in two main categories: cognitive subscales (short-term memory, long-term memory, orientation) and social subscales (mood, activities and interests, speech, practical skills, and behaviors). Although the DMR has been developed to use in all levels of ID, its suitability in people with profound ID is rather poor, because of their premorbid limited level of skills. Consequently they have a premorbid high score and further functional decline cannot be measured. Nevertheless both instruments are able to discriminate between most people with dementia and those without dementia (Shultz et al., 2004). However, periodic recordings seem to significantly improve the accuracy of both instruments. Periodic recordings enable comparison of functioning over time and they objectify cognitive or physical decline. Two other measures which are broadly used in the general population and which have been adapted for people with ID are the Cambridge Examination for Mental Disorders of Older People with Down's Syndrome and Others with Intellectual Disabilities (CAMDEX-DS) (Holland and Huppert, 2006) and the *Shultz Mini-Mental State Exam* (Shultz et al., 2004). Both instruments require participation from the person with ID, which adds valuable information about functional decline, but which limits the number of people for whom these instruments are valid. If possible, it is advisable to combine periodic recordings of functioning collected through rating scales with functional tests for memory and orientation.

Behavioral problems

Behavioral problems are often assessed with observation schemes and not with a standardized instrument. Consequently, only few standardized instruments are more or less studied for their psychometric properties. The *Aberrant Behavior Checklist* (ABC) (Aman et al., 1985) seems to be the most studied instrument. The ABC is an informant-rated instrument and consists of 58 items containing all kinds of behavioral problems. Its items are divided over five subscales: irritability, lethargy, stereotypies, hyperactivity, and inappropriate speech. The ABC is applicable for all levels of ID and specifically suitable to measure treatment effects (Shedlack et al., 2005). Its psychometric properties seem to be sufficient (Aman et al., 1985).

Other frequently used informant-report instruments are the *Adult Behavior Checklist* (ABCL) (Achenbach and Rescorla, 2003), the *Behavior Problems Inventory* (BPI) (Rojahn et al., 2001), and the *Developmental Behavior Checklist* (DBC) (Einfeld and Tonge, 1995). The ABCL was originally developed for the general population, but seems to have sound psychometric properties in people with mild ID (Tenneij and Koot, 2007). It has to be noted that it is a long rating scale containing more than 100 items. The BPI has been developed for people with ID and is also available in a short-form version. Both versions seem to be applicable and reliable in children and adults with mild to profound ID (Van Ingen et al., 2010; Rojahn et al., 2012). The DBC has been developed for children, adolescents, and adults with mild to profound ID, and its reliability and validity seems to be sufficient (Einfeld and Tonge, 1995).

Standardized diagnostic interviews

Probably the best-known standardized diagnostic interview developed for people with ID is the *Psychiatric Assessment Schedule for Adults with Developmental Disabilities* (PAS-ADD) (Moss et al., 1994, Moss, 2011). The PAS-ADD is a semi-structured, diagnostic interview that is based on the *Schedules for Clinical Assessment in Neuropsychiatry* (SCAN). With the latest version of the PAS-ADD, the *PAS-ADD Clinical Interview*, diagnoses of major depressive disorder, manic disorder, general anxiety disorder, panic disorder, agoraphobia, social phobia, specific phobia, obsessive-compulsive disorder, and schizophrenia based on ICD-10 or DSM-IV criteria can be made. The questions of the *PAS-ADD Clinical Interview* can be answered by people with ID, their caregivers, or both. The *PAS-ADD Clinical Interview* is slightly different from the former version, and its psychometric properties have not been studied yet. The former version of the *PAS-ADD Clinical Interview* has been validated in people with ID against expert psychiatric diagnosis and showed satisfactory psychometric properties (Costello et al., 1997; Moss et al., 1997).

Two other, more recently developed instruments are the *Mood and Anxiety Semi-Structured* (MASS) interview (Charlot et al., 2007) and the *Psychopathology checklists for Adults with Intellectual Disability* (P-AID) (Hove and Havik, 2008). The MASS interview has been developed for assessment with caregivers of people with ID. "Presence" or "absence" in the last month is assessed for 35 symptoms that are based on behavioral descriptions of DSM-IV criteria. The validity of the MASS interview is good (Charlot et al., 2007). The P-AID has also been developed for completion by informants and consists of 18 different checklists: 8 for problem behaviors and 10 for psychiatric disorders. The items are based on the diagnostic criteria of the Diagnostic Criteria for Psychiatric Disorders for Use with Adults with Learning Disabilities/Mental Retardation (DC-LD) (Royal College of Psychiatrists, 2001). The reliability of the P-AID was fair to good (Hove and Havik, 2008). An advantage of the *PAS-ADD Clinical Interview* is that it allows for self-report and informant-report, whereas an advantage of the P-AID is the inclusion of problem behavior. All three interviews require knowledge of psychiatric disorders and some training in how to use the instrument.

Choosing an instrument

There are a few steps in choosing the most suitable instrument for your assessment in clinical practice. Assuming that you start with a screening, you first have to decide what the scope of the instrument should be; e.g., if you want to screen for psychopathology in general or for one particular disorder. Second, you have to evaluate if self-report is possible. If relevant questions can only be partly answered reliably, maybe a caregiver is able to add information. If reliable self-report is not possible at all, you should select an informant-report instrument. Also for individuals who are capable of self-report, additional information from caregivers or a spouse can be valuable. Third, you need to consider the target group of the instrument. A self-report instrument developed for people with mild ID is not suitable for someone with a severe ID. Fourth, you need to consider the psychometric properties of the instrument. Even if an instrument has passed your earlier selection steps, an instrument with invalid results barely adds to your assessment.

New developments

New developments focus mainly on empowerment and digitalization. One innovative development, linked to self-report, is the SAINT. This is a guided self-help pack for people with ID (Chaplin et al., 2012; Chaplin et al., 2013). It helps people to recognize their mental health problems and adopt fitting coping strategies. An initiative such as SAINT empowers people with ID to recognize and deal with mental health problems. Another promising development is the use of e-health devices for people with ID. Preventive strategies and contacts with the social and medical network are offered, with applications accessible through a smartphone or tablet (Verdonschot and Soest, 2011). Adding information about key symptoms to applications improves timely recognition of mental health problems. Furthermore, outcomes of rating sales should be discussed with clients (if possible) and their caregivers or significant others. Periodic recordings should be visualized in graphics to clarify improvement after intervention or functional decline with aging. Moreover, professionals may need training or instruction on how particular outcomes can be translated to daily care and how these outcomes can add value to clinical practice.

Conclusions

In the last three decades many instruments have been developed specifically for people with ID. However, the number of instruments is quite variable per psychiatric disorder. Furthermore, the level of knowledge about reliability and validity is varying across instruments and for most instruments this knowledge is still scarce. Using these instruments, both in clinical practice and in research, leads to more knowledge on the utility of these instruments. It is more valuable to further develop existing instruments than to keep developing new instruments. To improve mental health care for people with ID it is important to embed the use of rating scales in clinical practice. Systematic use of standardized instruments improves the quality of assessment by objectifying symptoms and supporting the formation of clear intervention goals. It also enables comparison within a person over time, which makes it possible to evaluate the effect of treatment. To encourage the use of rating scales in clinical practice, it is essential that their content is complementary to regular care. In the last decade, researchers and clinicians have increasingly collaborated in the development of instruments. Also people with ID seem to be involved more often.

Although the "image" of assessment instruments and rating scales is rather dull, adding them to your clinical work can be real fun. Using different instruments will give you insight into the advantages and disadvantages of several instruments for particular disorders or particular target groups. They improve understanding of symptoms of psychiatric disorders and objectify the treatment effect. In summary, if you choose your instrument carefully, you will experience benefits in clinical practice.

Key summary points

- Using assessment instruments and rating scales improves quality of care.
- Results from instruments and scales should be embedded in daily care.
- To evaluate the suitability of an instrument not only applicability but also psychometric quality is of importance.
- Effects of treatment or intervention can be demonstrated by using standardized instruments and rating scales.

References

Achenbach, T.M. and Rescorla, L.A. (2003). *Manual for the ASEBA Adult Forms and Profiles*.Burlington, VT: University of Vermont, Research Center for Children, Youth, and Families.

Aman, M.G., Singh, N.N., Stewart, A.W., Field, C.J. (1985). The aberrant behavior checklist: a behavior rating scale for the assessment of treatment effects. *American Journal of Mental Deficiency*, 89, 485–491.

Beck, A. (1996). *Beck Depression Inventory-II (BDI-II)*. San Antonio, TX: The Psychological Corporation, San Antonia Harcourt Brace and Company.

Chaplin, E., Craig, T., Bouras, N. (2012). Using service user and clinical opinion to develop the SAINT: a guided self-help pack for adults with intellectual disability. *Advances in Mental Health and Intellectual Disabilities*, 6, 17–25.

Chaplin, E., Chester, R., Tsakanikos, E., et al. (2013). Reliability and validity of the SAINT: a guided self-help tool for people with intellectual disabilities. *Journal of Mental Health Research in Intellectual Disabilities*, 6, 245–253.

Charlot, L., Deutsch, C., Hunt, A., Fletcher, K., McLlvane, W. (2007). Validation of the Mood and Anxiety Semi-Structured (MASS) interview for patients with intellectual disabilities. *Journal of Intellectual Disability Research: JIDR*, 51, 821–834.

Costello, H. and Bouras, N. (2006). Assessment of mental health problems in people with intellectual disabilities. *Israel Journal of Psychiatry and Related Sciences*, 43, 241–251.

Costello, H., Moss, S., Prosser, H., Hatton, C. (1997). Reliability of the ICD-10 version of the Psychiatric Assessment Schedule for Adults with Developmental Disability (PAS-ADD). *Social Psychiatry and Psychiatric Epidemiology*, 32, 339–343.

Cuthill, F.M., Espie, C.A., Cooper, S.A. (2003). Development and psychometric properties of the Glasgow Depression Scale for people with a learning disability. Individual and carer supplement versions. Mental health services for adults with learning disabilities. *British Journal of Psychiatry*, 182, 347–353.

Derogatis, L.R. (1975). *Brief Symptom Inventory*. Baltimore, MD: Clinical Psychometric Research.

Einfeld, S.L. and Tonge, B.J. (1995). The Developmental Behavior Checklist: the development and validation of an instrument to assess behavioral and emotional disturbance in children and adolescents with mental retardation. *Journal of Autism and Developmental Disorders*, 25, 81–104.

Esbensen, A.J., Rojahn, J., Aman, M.G., Ruedrich, S. (2003). Reliability and validity of an assessment instrument for anxiety, depression, and mood among individuals with mental retardation. *Journal of Autism and Developmental Disorders*, 33, 617–629.

Evenhuis, H.M., Kengen, M.M.F., Eurlings, H.A.L. (1995). *Manual of the Dementia Questionnaire for Persons with Mental Retardation (DMR)*. Amsterdam: Harcourt Assessment B.V.

Finlay, W.M. and Lyons, E. (2001). Methodological issues in interviewing and using self-report questionnaires with people with mental retardation. *Psychological Assessment*, 13, 319–335.

Gedye, A. (1995). *Dementia Scale for Down Syndrome Manual*. Vancouver, BC: Gedye Research and Consulting.

Hamilton, M. (1960). A rating scale for depression. *Journal of Neurology, Neurosurgery, and Psychiatry*, 23, 56–62.

Hartley, S.L. and MacLean, W.E., Jr. (2006). A review of the reliability and validity of Likert-type scales for people with intellectual disability. *Journal of Intellectual Disability Research: JIDR*, 50, 813–827.

Helverschou, S.B., Bakken, T.L., Martinsen, H. (2009). The Psychopathology in Autism Checklist (PAC): a pilot study. *Research in Autism Spectrum Disorders*, 3, 179–195.

Hermans, H. and Evenhuis, H.M. (2010). Characteristics of instruments screening for depression in adults with intellectual disabilities: systematic review. *Research in Developmental Disabilities*, 31, 1109–1120.

Hermans, H., van der Pas, F.H., Evenhuis, H.M. (2011). Instruments assessing anxiety in adults with intellectual disabilities: a systematic review. *Research in Developmental Disabilities*, 32, 861–870.

Holland, T. and Huppert, F.A. (2006). *CAMDEX-DS: The Cambridge examination for mental disorders of older people with Down's syndrome and others with intellectual disabilities.* Cambridge: Cambridge University Press.

Hove, O. and Havik, O.E. (2008). Psychometric properties of Psychopathology checklists for Adults with Intellectual Disability (P-AID) on a community sample of adults with intellectual disability. *Research in Developmental Disabilities*, 29, 467–482.

Hurley, A.D. (2006). Mood disorders in intellectual disability. *Current Opinion in Psychiatry*, 19, 465–469.

Kazdin, A.E., Matson, J.L., Senatore, V. (1983). Assessment of depression in mentally retarded adults. *American Journal of Psychiatry*, 140, 1040–1043.

Kellett, S.C., Beail, N., Newman, D.W., Frankish, P. (2003). Utility of the Brief Symptom Inventory (BSI) in the assessment of psychological distress. *Journal of Applied Research in Intellectual Disabilities: JARID*, 16, 127–135.

Lindsay, W.R., Michie, A.M., Baty, F.J., Smith, A.H., Miller, S. (1994). The consistency of reports about feelings and emotions from people with intellectual disability. *Journal of Intellectual Disability Research: JIDR*, 38(1), 61–66.

Matson, J.L. (1995). *Diagnostic Assessment for the Severely Handicapped – II.* Baton Rouge, LA: Scientific Publishers.

Matson, J.L. and Bamburg, J.W. (1998). Reliability of the Assessment of Dual Diagnosis (ADD). *Research in Developmental Disabilities*, 19, 89–95.

Matson, J.L., Belva, B.C., Hattier, M.A., Matson, M.L. (2012). Scaling methods to measure psychopathology in persons with intellectual disabilities. *Research in Developmental Disabilities*, 33, 549–562.

Mindham, J. and Espie, C.A. (2003). Glasgow Anxiety Scale for people with an Intellectual Disability (GAS-ID): development and psychometric properties of a new measure for use with people with mild intellectual disability. *Journal of Intellectual Disability Research: JIDR*, 47, 22–30.

Moss, S. (2011). *The PAS-ADD Clinical Interview.* Brighton, UK: Pavilion.

Moss, S., Patel, P., Prosser, H., et al. (1993). Psychiatric morbidity in older people with moderate and severe learning disability. I: development and reliability of the patient interview (PAS-ADD). Mental health services for adults with learning disabilities. *British Journal of Psychiatry*, 163, 471–480.

Moss, S.C., Ibbotson, B., Prosser, H. (1994). *The Psychiatric Assessment Schedule for Adults with a Developmental Disability (the PAS-ADD): Interview Development and Compilation of the Clinical Glossary.* Manchester, UK: Hester Adrian Research Centre, University of Manchester.

Moss, S., Ibbotson, B., Prosser, H., et al. (1997). Validity of the PAS-ADD for detecting psychiatric symptoms in adults with learning disability (mental retardation). *Social Psychiatry and Psychiatric Epidemiology*, 32, 344–354.

Prosser, H., Moss, S., Costello, H., Simpson, N., Patel, P. (1997). *The Mini PAS-ADD: An Assessment Schedule for the Detection of Mental Health Needs in Adults with Learning Disability (Mental Retardation).* Manchester, UK: Hester Adrian Research Centre, University of Manchester.

Ramirez, S.Z. and Lukenbill, J.F. (2007). Development of the fear survey for adults with mental retardation. *Research in Developmental Disabilities*, 28, 225–237.

Reiss, S. (1988). *The Reiss Screen Test Manual.* Orland Park, IL: International Diagnostic Systems.

Reynolds, W.M. and Baker, J.A. (1988). Assessment of depression in persons with mental retardation. *American Journal on Mental Retardation*, 93, 93–103.

Rojahn, J., Matson, J.L., Lott, D., Esbensen, A.J., Smalls, Y. (2001). The Behavior Problems Inventory: an instrument for the assessment of self-injury, stereotyped behavior, and aggression/destruction in individuals with developmental disabilities. *Journal of Autism and Developmental Disorders*, 31, 577–588.

Rojahn, J., Rowe, E.W., Sharber, A.C., et al. (2012). The Behavior Problems Inventory – Short Form for individuals with intellectual disabilities. Part II: reliability and validity. *Journal of Intellectual Disability Research: JIDR*, 56, 546–565.

Ross, E. and Oliver, C. (2003). Preliminary analysis of the psychometric properties of the Mood, Interest and Pleasure Questionnaire (MIPQ) for adults with severe and profound learning disabilities. *British Journal of Clinical Psychology*, 42, 81–93.

Royal College of Psychiatrists (2001). *Diagnostic Criteria for Psychiatric Disorders for Use with Adults with Learning Disabilities/Mental Retardation (DC-LD)*. London: Royal College of Psychiatrists.

Senatore, V., Matson, J.L., Kazdin, A.E. (1985). An inventory to assess psychopathology of mentally retarded adults. *American Journal of Mental Deficiency*, 89, 459–466.

Shedlack, K.J., Hennen, J., Magee, C., Cheron, D.M. (2005). A comparison of the Aberrant Behavior Checklist and the GAF among adults with mental retardation and mental illness. *Psychiatric Services (Washington, D.C.)*, 56, 484–486.

Shultz, J., Aman, M., Kelbley, T., et al. (2004). Evaluation of screening tools for dementia in older adults with mental retardation. *American Journal on Mental Retardation*, 109, 98–110.

Sturmey, P., Burcham, K.J., Perkins, T.S. (1995). The Reiss Screen for Maladaptive Behaviour: its reliability and internal consistencies. *Journal of Intellectual Disability Research: JIDR*, 39(Pt 3), 191–195.

Sturmey, P., Newton, J.T., Cowley, A., Bouras, N., Holt, G. (2005). The PAS-ADD Checklist: independent replication of its psychometric properties in a community sample. *British Journal of Psychiatry*, 186, 319–323.

Tenneij, N.H. and Koot, H.M. (2007). A preliminary investigation into the utility of the Adult Behavior Checklist in the assessment of psychopathology in people with low IQ. *Journal of Applied Research in Intellectual Disabilities*, 20, 391–400.

Van Ingen, D.J., Moore, L.L., Zaja, R.H., Rojahn, J. (2010). The Behavior Problems Inventory (BPI-01) in community-based adults with intellectual disabilities: reliability and concurrent validity vis-a-vis the Inventory for Client and Agency Planning (ICAP). *Research in Developmental Disabilities*, 31, 97–107.

Verdonschot, M. and Soest, V.K. (2011). *Technology in Care for People with Intellectual Disabilities*. Utrecht: Vilans.

Wieland, J., Wardenaar, K.J., Fontein, E., Zitman, F.G. (2011). Utility of the Brief Symptom Inventory (BSI) in psychiatric outpatients with intellectual disabilities. *Journal of Intellectual Disability Research*, 55, 843–853.

Zeilinger, E.L., Stiehl, K.A., Weber, G. (2013). A systematic review on assessment instruments for dementia in persons with intellectual disabilities. *Research in Developmental Disabilities*, 34, 3962–3977.

Zung, W.W. (1965). A self-rating depression scale. *Archives of General Psychiatry*, 12, 63–70.

Dementias

Jennifer Torr

Introduction

Unprecedented numbers of people with intellectual disabilities (ID) are now living into middle and old age, with a concurrent increase in prevalence of general age-related health conditions (Haveman et al., 2009) and dementias (Strydom et al., 2010b) associated with increased morbidity and mortality (Coppus et al., 2008; Strydom et al., 2013b). A review of care of people with ID and dementia highlights concerns regarding pathways to assessment, changing care needs, transitions, end-of-life care, training, and support of care staff and families. Pharmacological and non-pharmacological management of behavioral and psychological symptoms of dementia (BPSD) is extrapolated from the general population (Courtenay et al., 2010). Whilst the cost of care increases with age, especially for those in residential services, dementia per se does not necessarily increase the overall care costs (Strydom et al., 2010a).

Diagnosing dementias in people with ID

The dementias are a meta-syndrome of acquired cognitive deficits across multiple domains, secondary to a range of brain disorders, resulting in loss of independence in daily functioning. The dementias encompass neurodegenerative disorders, vascular dementias, traumatic brain injury, alcohol-related dementia, and other brain insults. Historically, memory loss has been a fundamental of dementia diagnosis regardless of the severity of deficits in other cognitive domains. The *Diagnostic and Statistical Manual of Mental Disorders, Fifth Edition* (DSM-5), whilst accommodating the continuing use of the term "dementia," has introduced the category of Neurocognitive Disorder, with two levels of severity of acquired cognitive impairment (mild and major) across multiple domains, with or without memory impairment (American Psychiatric Association, 2013).

People with ID are a heterogeneous population with a multiplicity of neurodevelopmental disorders, severity and profile of pre-existing impairments in cognitive and adaptive functioning, and confounding multi-comorbidity, rendering the assessment and diagnosis of dementias a complex task (Torr, 2009). Standard diagnostic criteria for dementia have acceptable expert inter-rater reliability (0.68) and high specificity (95%); however, there is a risk for false-positive diagnoses, especially in those who are

Psychiatric and Behavioral Disorders in Intellectual and Developmental Disabilities, ed. Colin Hemmings and Nick Bouras. Published by Cambridge University Press. © Cambridge University Press 2016.

young, or have more severe ID and sensory impairments (Strydom et al., 2007, 2013a). Demonstrating decline in cognition and functioning from baseline is essential to a diagnosis of dementia. Furthermore, what degree of functional change warrants a diagnosis of dementia? Perhaps it is the increases in support needs requiring changes in the supports provided. The diagnosis of dementia also depends upon which criteria are used. Use of the *Diagnostic and Statistical Manual of Mental Disorders, Fourth Edition, Text Revision* (DSM-IV-TR) (American Psychiatric Association, 2000) criteria for dementia diagnosis is comparable with use of the *Diagnostic Criteria for Psychiatric Disorders for Use with Adults with Learning Disabilities/Mental Retardation* (DC-LD) (Royal College of Psychiatrists, 2001). However, dementia, even to a moderate degree, may be missed by the *ICD-10 Diagnostic Criteria for Research (DCR-10)* (World Health Organization, 1993; Strydom et al., 2007).

Lack of general and disorder-specific normative cognitive data requires the demonstration of changes from individual rather than group baselines. Baseline assessments in early adulthood are recommended for people with Down syndrome and longitudinal assessments for people with other ID when changes in cognition and/or functioning are noted. There is currently no standard protocol for the assessment of dementias in people with ID. A recent review identified 114 instruments; 35 informant-based, 79 direct assessments, and 4 test batteries (Zeilinger et al., 2013). For more detailed reviews of selected neuropsychological assessments, see Prasher (2009). Selected instruments should assess memory, executive functioning, visual spatial skills and language, attention, and speed of processing, if possible, as well as daily functioning. For people with severe cognitive impairment, instruments such as the Severe Impairment Battery (Saxton et al., 1993) have utility (Witts and Elders, 1998).

Deterioration in self-care and other activities of daily living are often reported by carers to precede memory and other cognitive impairments. Both retrospective carer report and prospective monitoring for functional decline have potential in the screening for dementia, especially for people with moderate and severe ID. Reports of memory change are better predictors of dementia than functional change for people with mild ID. Although emotional and behavioral changes also occur early on, these changes are nonspecific and not predictive of dementia (Jamieson-Craig et al., 2010).

Sensory and motor impairments, medical and mental illnesses may mimic or be comorbid with dementia. The risk for delirium is high in people with ID given the higher rates of neurodevelopmental brain abnormalities, epilepsy, chest and urinary infections, and polypharmacy. Yet delirium is often overlooked. In a community cohort of 187 adults with Down syndrome, only one case of delirium was identified over two years (Mantry et al., 2008). Persistent subacute delirium can be mistaken for dementia. Long-term psychotropic medications, especially medications with anticholinergic effects, can result in persistent cognitive impairment (Gedye, 1998). Many people with ID do not have access to specialist clinical services (Torr et al., 2010a), and in practice there are real risks of false-positive and false-negative diagnoses of dementia.

Dementia in people with ID not due to Down syndrome
The Becoming Older with Learning Disability (BOLD) study is a community population longitudinal study of dementias in people with ID, excluding Down syndrome, aged 60 years plus (Strydom et al., 2007). Following screening, standardized clinical assessments

were conducted, and diagnosis of dementias made by expert consensus according to DC-LD (Royal College of Psychiatrists, 2001), DSM-IV-TR (American Psychiatric Association, 2000), and DCR-10 (World Health Organization, 1993). Prevalence of any dementia was 13% for 60 years plus; 18% for 65 years plus; and 33% for 75 years plus (Strydom et al., 2007, 2009). This is consistent with a similar community-population study reporting overall prevalence of dementia of 22% for people with ID over the age of 65 years, whereby prevalence increased across age cohorts: 15% at 65–74 years; 24% at 65–84 years; and 70% at 85–94 years (Cooper, 1997) Although prevalence is related to age, when compared with the general population the Standardized Morbidity Ratio (SMR) for dementia is 2.77 for those aged ≥65 years. However the SMR diminishes with age from 7.7 for those aged 65–74 years to 2.7 for those ≥85 years, indicating differential risk for earlier onset of dementia in people with ID. (Strydom et al., 2009). Overall, there was no association between gender or severity of ID and prevalence of dementia (Strydom et al., 2007). The incidence of dementia was up to five times that of the general population, and estimated to be 55/1000 person-years in those over 60 years of age and 98/1000 person-years in the 70–74-year age group (Strydom et al., 2013b).

The most common subtype of dementia was Alzheimer's disease (≥60 years, 8.6%; ≥65 years, 12%), followed by Lewy body dementia (≥60 years, 5.9%; ≥65 years, 7.7%), frontal type dementia (≥60 years, 3.2%; ≥65 years, 4.2%) and vascular dementia (≥60 years, 2.7%; ≥65 years, 3.5%; Strydom et al., 2007). Frontal type dementia was over-represented and vascular dementia is not as common as might have been expected. Lewy body dementia was "possible" rather than "probable" in the majority of cases, raising questions about delirium, which has common clinical features, as well as possible extra-pyramidal side effects from antipsychotic medications. The stability of diagnostic sub-type was not reported at follow-up (Strydom et al., 2009). Very early-onset dementias have been described for some rare genetic intellectual and developmental disorders (Strydom et al., 2010b).

The minimal research into the risk factors for dementia in people with ID focuses on associations such as age, multiple physical problems, and poorly controlled epilepsy (Cooper, 1997). There are more hypotheses than evidence. For example, vitamin D deficiency is more common in people with ID (Frighi et al., 2014), and vitamin D deficiency is a risk factor for Alzheimer's disease in the general population (Littlejohns et al., 2014). Repeated head trauma and head banging are associated with taupathy, atrophy, and cognitive impairment/dementia (Carlock et al., 1997). The big questions relate to the interplay between the complexities of neurodevelopment and neurodegeneration at the cellular level, and the impacts of environmental factors, and how a life is lived, upon these processes. In the absence of evidence to the contrary, it might be prudent to foster healthy lifestyles, with good nutrition, management of weight and vascular risk, regular exercise, educational and occupational endeavors, social engagement, and inclusion.

Down syndrome and Alzheimer's disease

People with Down syndrome account for 15% plus of the identified population with ID. Life expectancy is now about 60 years. Reported prevalence varies, but overall about 50% of people with Down syndrome will develop the dementia of Alzheimer's disease in the 6th decade, with an average age of diagnosis of Alzheimer's disease in the mid 50s

(Torr et al., 2010b). The reported incidence is 4.88 per 100 person–years during the 6th decade, increasing to 13.3 per 100 person-years in the 7th decade. Nonetheless, not all people with Down syndrome have dementia in older age and the prevalence falls to 25% in the over-60-year-old age group (Coppus et al., 2006). Emotional and behavioral changes precede frank cognitive decline, beginning with emerging executive dysfunction (Ball et al., 2006, 2008) before the development of impairments in memory, language, visual, spatial, and learnt motor skills.

Down syndrome is caused by trisomy 21 in 95% of cases, the remainder being due to mosaic or partial trisomy 21 and various translocations (Mulcahy, 1979; Stoll et al., 1998). Triplication of the amyloid precursor protein (APP) gene on chromosome 21 is a primary risk factor for the high rates of early-onset dementia of Alzheimer's disease. Indeed, a 78-year-old woman, with partial trisomy 21, not involving the APP gene, showed no clinical or neuropathological evidence of Alzheimer's disease (Prasher et al., 1998), and two women with Down syndrome and partial disomy for chromosome 21 living into their 70s and 80s showed no signs of dementia (Schupf and Sergievsky, 2002). Triplication of chromosome 21 results in complex whole of genome and epigenetic effects. Expression of the APP gene is 3–4 times higher than the expected 1.5-fold gene dosage effect. Moderate overexpression of ETS2, a transcription factor located on chromosome 21, increases transcription of both APP and presenelin-1 and β-amyloid production (Wolvetang et al., 2003) The gene for DYRK1A is also located on chromosome 21 and expression is increased further by β-amyloid. DYRK1A phosphorylates the tau protein, helping to drive the development of neurofibrillary tangles (Jones et al., 2008; Wegiel et al., 2008).

There is an age-related continuum from precocious and excessive cerebral amyloid deposition to the progressive development of amyloid plaques, followed by intracellular accumulation of neurofibrillary tangles, proceeding to neurodegeneration and dementia. Deposition of amyloid plaques may occur in the 2nd and 3rd decades, and the number of number of plaques and tangles increases greatly from the age of 30 years. By 40 years of age the concentration of plaques and tangle meet the neuropathological criteria for Alzheimer's disease (Wisniewski et al., 1985). Positron emission tomographic (PET) methodologies also demonstrate increasing amyloid and tau concentration with age (Nelson et al., 2011). Amyloid plaques alone are not associated with significant cognitive change (Jones et al., 2009; Hartley et al., 2014). The development of neurofibrillary tangles occurs later, and behavioral and early cognitive changes begin with increasing concentration of neurofibrillary tangles (Nelson et al., 2011; Koran et al., 2014). Neurodegeneration progresses with age, with loss of total brain volume as well as orbitofrontal, parietal, and hippocampal atrophy, and increase in ventricular volume, and is associated with ongoing cognitive decline and dementia (Strydom et al., 2002; Koran et al., 2014). Clinically, serial neuroimaging may be required to delineate atrophy from pre-existing brain differences (Prasher et al., 1996; Strydom et al., 2002).

A number of factors modulate individual risk for the age of onset of dementia in people with Down syndrome. Increased risk is associated with the apolipoprotein E4 allele (Apo E4) whilst the apolipoprotein E2 allele is protective (Schupf and Sergievsky, 2002). Increased risk is also associated with female gender, lower age of menopause, lower weight, certain polymorphisms of CYP17 and CYP19, which are involved in synthesis of estrogen, and reduced bioavailability of estradial (Chace et al., 2012) and high total cholesterol, although statins reduced this risk (Zigman et al., 2007). In one study, serum levels of both amyloid peptides Aβ1–42 β1–40 were increased in adults with Down syndrome. The apolipoprotein E4 allele is associated with increased levels of Aβ1–42, and levels of Aβ1–42 are selectively increased in those with dementia (Schupf et al., 2001). Other studies have found no relationship between Aβ1–42, Apo E4, or the age of dementia (Jones et al., 2009). However, earlier age of onset of dementia is associated with the extended tau haplotype (Jones et al., 2008). Randomized controlled trials with antioxidants (Tyrrell et al., 2001) and memantine (Hanney et al., 2012) have not been of preventive benefit. The trial numbers are small and participants are older adults, including those with dementia. It is likely that preventive interventions will need to begin in early adulthood if not before.

Cholinesterase inhibitors and memantine

People with Down syndrome are of smaller stature and have differences in brain structure, cardiac conduction, and drug metabolism; hence, caution is required in extrapolating evidence from general population research into clinical practice. *Cochrane Systematic Reviews* report insufficient research into the treatment of Alzheimer's disease in Down syndrome with acetylcholinesterase inhibitors, donepezil, rivastigmine and galantamine, and memantine, a glutamate *N*-methyl-D-aspartate (NMDA)-receptor antagonist (Mohan et al., 2009a, 2009b, 2009c, 2009d). Only one study met the inclusion criteria – a 24-week randomized double-blind placebo-controlled trial of donepezil 5–10 mg in 30 patients with Down syndrome and Alzheimer's disease (Prasher et al., 2002). Improvements were not statically significant; however, significant benefits were found in the treatment group in an open-label extension study (Prasher et al., 2003). Improvements, or less rapid deterioration in cognition and functioning, have also been reported in small case series and non-randomized trials for donepezil (Lott et al., 2002; Boada-Rovira et al., 2005; Kondoh et al., 2005a) and rivastigmine (Prasher et al., 2005). In the absence of brady-cardia and cardiac abnormalities, that are common in Down syndrome, cholinesterase inhibitors seem to be safe but not well tolerated. For equal doses of donepezil, people with Down syndrome have higher serum levels, which are associated with more adverse effects (Kondoh et al., 2005b), including fatigue, anorexia, nausea, vomiting, abdominal discomfort, diarrhoea, incontinence, insomnia, agitation, and muscle weakness (Prasher, 2004). Commencing at lower doses, with slow titration and dose adjustments, is recommended (Prasher, 2004). Memantine in adults with Down syndrome aged 40 years plus, with and without dementia, found memantine to be safe but of no benefit (Hanney et al., 2012). However, benefits have only been demonstrated for moderate to severe Alzheimer's disease in the general population (McShane et al., 2006).

Complications of Alzheimer's disease in Down syndrome

Behavioral and psychological symptoms of dementia in people with Down syndrome include social disengagement, amotivation and apathy, slowness, resistiveness, aggressive behaviors, restlessness, wandering, and neuropsychiatric symptoms such as depression, delusions, and hallucinations (Urv et al., 2010). Medical complications include incontinence, gait disturbance, falls and injury including fractures and head injury, eating and swallowing problems with malnutrition, episodes of choking and recurrent aspiration pneumonia, myoclonus, and generalized seizures. Loss of mobility, feeding problems, pneumonia, and seizures increase with progression from early- to middle- to end-stage dementia. Prevalence of seizures increases from 40% at mid-stage to 85% by end-stage. The onset of seizures is a poor prognostic indicator, with death occurring within two years (Tyrrell et al., 2001; McCarron et al., 2005).

Conclusions

As ever-increasing numbers of people with ID are living well into middle and old age, the prevalence of age-related dementias is also increasing. The dementias are associated with increased morbidity and earlier death. Epidemiological studies are finding that, in comparison with the general population, dementias in people with ID other than Down syndrome, are of earlier onset, with higher incidences and greater age-related prevalence. The reasons for this much greater risk for dementia in people with ID are yet to be determined. The diagnosis of dementia is a complex task; however, it has been demonstrated that the diagnosis of dementia, including dementia subtype, is possible through rigorous clinical assessment. Longitudinal assessment is recommended to validate diagnosis.

It is well established that people with Down syndrome are at very high risk of early-onset dementia of Alzheimer's, conferred by triplication of the *APP* and other genes on chromosome 21. The average age of onset is the mid 50s, and, whilst not all people with Down syndrome will develop dementia even in much older age, the majority will be affected. There is evidence for the use of cholinesterase inhibitors, at lower doses due to poor tolerability.

The overall quality of dementia research in people with ID has been improving with the application of methodologically sound protocols, including the establishment of epidemiological cohorts, standardized assessments, and randomized controlled trials, as well as studies of the genetic, cellular, and molecular aspects of neurodegenerative disorders, most notably Alzheimer's disease in Down syndrome.

Key summary points

- Dementias in people with ID other than Down syndrome are earlier in onset, and of higher incidence and age-related prevalence than the general population. Dementia is associated with an increased risk of death.
- There is limited research into risk factors and prevention.
- People with Down syndrome have very high rates of early-onset dementia of Alzheimer's disease with an average age of onset in the mid 50s. Most, but not all, older adults will be affected. There is evidence to support careful treatment with low-dose cholinesterase inhibitors. The progression of dementia is associated with increasing behavioral and psychological symptoms, medical complications, and early death.
- There is increasing research into the pathological mechanisms of Alzheimer's disease in Down syndrome.
- Randomized controlled treatment trials are possible in people with ID and are essential in establishing an evidence base to guide clinical practice.

References

American Psychiatric Association (2000). *Diagnostic and Statistical Manual of Mental Disorders – Text Revision, Fourth Edition.* Washington, DC: American Psychiatric Association.

American Psychiatric Association (2013). *Diagnostic and Statistical Manual of Mental Disorders, Fifth Edition.* Washington, DC: American Psychiatric Association.

Ball, S.L., Holland, A.J., Hon, J., et al. (2006). Personality and behaviour changes mark the early stages of Alzheimer's disease in adults with Down's syndrome: findings from a prospective population-based study. *International Journal of Geriatric Psychiatry*, 21(7), 661–673.

Ball, S.L., Holland, A.J., Treppner, P., Watson, P.C., Huppert, F.A. (2008). Executive dysfunction and its association with personality and behaviour changes in the development of Alzheimer's disease in adults with Down syndrome and mild to moderate learning disabilities. *British Journal of Clinical Psychology*, 47(1), 1–29.

Boada-Rovira, M., Hernandez-Ruiz, I., Badenas-Homiar, S., Buendia-Torras, M., Tarraga-Mestre, L. (2005). Clinical-therapeutic study of dementia in people with Down syndrome and the effectiveness of donepezil in this population. *Revista de Neurologia*, 41(3), 129–136.

Carlock, K.S., Williams, J.P., Graves, G.C. (1997). MRI findings in headbangers. *Clinical Imaging*, 21(6), 411–413.

Chace, C., Pang, D., Weng, C., et al. (2012). Variants in CYP17 and CYP19 cytochrome P450 genes are associated with onset of Alzheimer's disease in women with Down syndrome. *Journal of Alzheimer's Disease*, 28(3), 601–612.

Cooper, S.A. (1997). High prevalence of dementia among people with learning disabilities not attributable to Down's syndrome. *Psychological Medicine*, 27(3), 609–616.

Coppus, A., Evenhuis, H., Verberne, G.-J., et al. (2006). Dementia and mortality in persons with Down's syndrome. *Journal of Intellectual Disability Research*, 50(10), 768–777.

Coppus, A., Evenhuis, H., Verberne, G.-J., et al. (2008). Survival in elderly persons with Down syndrome. *Journal of the American Geriatrics Society*, 56(12), 2311–2316.

Courtenay, K., Jokinen, N.S., Strydom, A. (2010). Caregiving and adults with intellectual disabilities affected by dementia. *Journal of Policy and Practice in Intellectual Disabilities*, 7(1), 26–33.

Frighi, V., Morovat, A., Stephenson, M.T., et al. (2014). Vitamin D deficiency in patients with intellectual disabilities: prevalence, risk factors and management strategies. *British Journal of Psychiatry*, 205(6), 458–464.

Gedye, A. (1998). Neuroleptic-induced dementia documented in four adults with mental retardation. *Mental Retardation*, 36(3), 182–186.

Hanney, M., Prasher, V., Williams, N., et al. (2012). Memantine for dementia in adults older than 40 years with Down's syndrome (MEADOWS): a randomised, double-blind, placebo-controlled trial. *Lancet*, 379(9815), 528–536.

Hartley, S.L., Handen, B.L., Devenny, D.A., et al. (2014). Cognitive functioning in relation to brain amyloid-β in healthy adults with Down syndrome. *Brain*, 137(9), 2556–2563.

Haveman, M.J., Heller, T., Lee, L.A., et al. (2009). *Report on the State of Science on Health Risks and Ageing in People with Intellectual Disabilities.* Dortmund, Germany: IASSID Special Interest Research Group on Ageing and Intellectual Disabilities/Faculty Rehabilitation Sciences, University of Dortmund.

Jamieson-Craig, R., Scior, K., Chan, T., Fenton, C., Strydom, A. (2010). Reliance on carer reports of early symptoms of dementia among adults with intellectual disabilities. *Journal of Policy and Practice in Intellectual Disabilities*, 7(1), 34–41.

Jones, E.L., Margallo-Lana, M., Prasher, V.P., Ballard, C.G. (2008). The extended tau haplotype and the age of onset of dementia in Down syndrome. *Dementia and Geriatric Cognitive Disorders*, 26(3), 199–202.

Jones, E.L., Hanney, M., Francis, P.T., Ballard, C.G. (2009). Amyloid β concentrations in older people with Down syndrome and dementia. *Neuroscience Letters*, 451(2), 162–164.

Kondoh, T., Amamoto, N., Doi, T., et al. (2005a). Dramatic improvement in Down syndrome-associated cognitive impairment with donepezil. *Annals of Pharmacotherapy*, 39(3), 563–566.

Kondoh, T., Nakashima, M., Sasaki, H., Moriuchi, H. (2005b). Pharmacokinetics of donepezil in Down syndrome. *Annals of Pharmacotherapy*, 39(3), 572–573.

Koran, M.E., Hohman, T., Edwards, C., et al. (2014). Differences in age-related effects on brain volume in Down syndrome as compared to Williams syndrome and typical development. *Journal of Neurodevelopmental Disorders*, 6(1), 8.

Littlejohns, T.J., Henley, W.E., Lang, I.A., et al. (2014). Vitamin D and the risk of dementia and Alzheimer disease. *Neurology*, 83(10), 920–928.

Lott, I.T., Osann, K., Doran, E., Nelson, L. (2002). Down syndrome and Alzheimer disease: response to donepezil. *Archives of Neurology*, 59(7), 1133–1136.

Mantry, D., Cooper, S.A., Smiley, E., et al. (2008). The prevalence and incidence of mental ill-health in adults with Down syndrome. *Journal of Intellectual Disability Research*, 52(2), 141–155.

McCarron, M., Gill, M., McCallion, P., Begley, C. (2005). Health co-morbidities in ageing persons with Down syndrome and Alzheimer's dementia. *Journal of Intellectual Disability Research*, 49(7), 560–566.

McShane, R., Areosa, S.A., Minakaran, N. (2006). Memantine for dementia (review). *Cochrane Database of Systemic Review*, 2, CD003154.

Mohan, M., Bennett, C., Carpenter, P.K. (2009a). Galantamine for dementia in people with Down syndrome. *Cochrane Database of Systematic Reviews*, 1, CD007657.

Mohan, M., Bennett, C., Carpenter, P.K. (2009b). Memantine for dementia in people with Down syndrome. *Cochrane Database of Systematic Reviews*, 1, CD007657.

Mohan, M., Bennett, C., Carpenter, P.K. (2009c). Rivastigmine for dementia in people with Down syndrome. *Cochrane Database of Systematic Reviews*, 1, CD007658.

Mohan, M., Carpenter, P.K., Bennett, C. (2009d). Donepezil for dementia in people with Down syndrome. *Cochrane Database of Systematic Reviews*, 1, CD007178.

Mulcahy, M.T. (1979). Down's syndrome in Western Australia: cytogenetics and incidence. *Human Genetics*, 48(1), 67–72.

Nelson, L.D., Siddarth, P., Kepe, V., et al. (2011). Positron emission tomography of brain β-amyloid and tau levels in adults with Down syndrome. *Archives of Neurology* 68, 768–774.

Prasher, V. (2004). Review of donepezil, rivastigmine, galantamine and memantine for the treatment of dementia in Alzheimer's disease in adults with Down syndrome: implications for the intellectual disability population. *International Journal of Geriatric Psychiatry*, 19(6), 505–515.

Prasher, V. (ed.) (2009). *Neuropsychological Assessments of Dementia in Down Syndrome and Intellectual Disabilities*. London: Springer-Verlag.

Prasher, V.P., Barber, P.C., West, R., Glenholmes, P. (1996). The role of magnetic resonance imaging in the diagnosis of Alzheimer disease in adults with Down syndrome. *Archives of Neurology*, 53(12), 1310–1313.

Prasher, V.P., Farrer, M.J., Kessling, A.M., et al. (1998). Molecular mapping of Alzheimer-type dementia in Down's syndrome. *Annals of Neurology*, 43(3), 380–383.

Prasher, V.P., Huxley, A., Haque, M.S., Down Syndrome Ageing Study Group (2002). A 24-week, double-blind, placebo-controlled trial of donepezil in patients with Down syndrome and Alzheimer's disease – pilot study. *International Journal of Geriatric Psychiatry*, 17(3), 270–278.

Prasher, V.P., Adams, C., Holder, R. (2003). Long term safety and efficacy of donepezil in the treatment of dementia in Alzheimer's disease in adults with Down syndrome: open label study. *International Journal of Geriatric Psychiatry*, 18(6), 549–551.

Prasher, V.P., Fung, N., Adams, C. (2005). Rivastigmine in the treatment of dementia in Alzheimer's disease in adults with Down syndrome. *International Journal of Geriatric Psychiatry*, 20(5), 496–497.

Royal College of Psychiatrists (2001). *Diagnostic Criteria for Psychiatric Disorders for Use with Adults with Learning Disabilities/Mental Retardation (DC-LD)*. London: Royal College of Psychiatrists.

Saxton, J., McGonigle, K.L., Swihart, A.A., Boller, F. (1993). *The Severe Impairment Battery*. Bury St. Edmunds, Norfolk, UK: Thames Valley Test Company.

Schupf, N. and Sergievsky, G.H. (2002). Genetic and host factors for dementia in Down's syndrome. *British Journal of Psychiatry*, 180, 405–410.

Schupf, N., Patel, B., Silverman, W., et al. (2001). Elevated plasma amyloid beta-peptide 1–42 and onset of dementia in adults with Down syndrome. *Neuroscience Letters*, 301(3), 199–203.

Stoll, C., Alembik, Y., Dott, B., Roth, M.P. (1998). Study of Down syndrome in 238,942 consecutive births. *Annales de Genetique*, 41(1), 44–51.

Strydom, A., Hassiosis, A., Walker, Z. (2002). Clinical use of structural magnetic resonance imaging in the diagnosis of dementia in adults with Down's syndrome. *Irish Journal of Psychological Medicine*, 19(2), 60–63.

Strydom, A., Livingston, G., King, M., Hassiotis, A. (2007). Prevalence of dementia in intellectual disability using different diagnostic criteria. *British Journal of Psychiatry*, 191, 150–157.

Strydom, A., Hassiotis, A., King, M., Livingston, G. (2009). The relationship of dementia prevalence in older adults with intellectual disability (ID) to age and severity of ID. *Psychological Medicine*, 39(1), 13–21.

Strydom, A., Romeo, R., Perez-Achiaga, N., et al. (2010a). Service use and cost of mental disorder in older adults with intellectual disability. *British Journal of Psychiatry*, 196(2), 133–138.

Strydom, A., Shooshtari, S., Lee, L.A., et al. (2010b). Dementia in older adults with intellectual disabilities – epidemiology, presentation and diagnosis. *Journal of Policy and Practice in Intellectual Disabilities*, 7(2), 96–110.

Strydom, A., Chan, T., Fenton, C., et al. (2013a). Validity of criteria for dementia in older people with intellectual disability. *American Journal of Geriatric Psychiatry*, 21(3), 279–288.

Strydom, A., Chan, T., King, M., et al. (2013b). Incidence of dementia in older adults with intellectual disabilities. *Research in Developmental Disabilities*, 34(6), 1881–1885.

Torr, J. (2009). Assessment of dementia in people with learning disabilities. *Advances in Mental Health and Learning Disabilities*, 3(3), 3–9.

Torr, J., Carling-Jenkins, R., Iacono, T., Bigby, C. (2010a). Pathways to assessment and diagnosis of dementia in adults with Down syndrome. *Journal of Applied Research in Intellectual Disabilities*, 23(5), 408–418.

Torr, J., Strydom, A., Patti, P., Jokinen, N. (2010b). Ageing in Down syndrome: morbidity and mortality. *Journal of Policy and Practice in Intellectual Disabilities*, 7(1), 70–81.

Tyrrell, J., Cosgrave, M., McCarron, M., et al. (2001). Dementia in people with Down's syndrome. *International Journal of Geriatric Psychiatry*, 16(12), 1168–1174.

Urv, T., Zigman, W.B., Silverman, W. (2010). Psychiatric symptoms in adults with Down syndrome and Alzheimer's disease. *American Journal on Intellectual and Developmental Disabilities*, 115(4), 265–276.

Wegiel, J., Dowjat, K., Kaczmarski, W., et al. (2008). The role of overexpressed DYRK1A protein in the early onset of neurofibrillary degeneration in Down syndrome. *Acta Neuropathologica*, 116(4), 391–407.

Wisniewski, K.E., Wisniewski, H.M., Wen, G.Y. (1985). Occurrence of neuropathological changes and dementia of Alzheimer's disease in Down's syndrome. *Annals of Neurology*, 17(3), 278–282.

Witts, P. and Elders, S. (1998). The "Severe Impairment Battery": assessing cognitive ability in adults with Down syndrome. *British Journal of Clinical Psychology*, 37(2), 213–216.

Wolvetang, E.W., Bradfield, O.M., Tymms, M., et al. (2003). The chromosome 21 transcription factor ETS2 transactivates the beta-APP promoter: implications for Down syndrome. *Biochimica et Biophysica Acta*, 1628(2), 105–10.

World Health Organization (1993) *ICD-10 Classification of Mental and Behavioural Disorders: Diagnostic Criteria for Research*. Geneva: World Health Organization.

Zeilinger, E.L., Stiehl, K.A.M., Weber, G. (2013). A systematic review on assessment instruments for dementia in persons with intellectual disabilities. *Research in Developmental Disabilities*, 34(11), 3962–3977.

Zigman, W.B., Schupf, N., Jenkins, E.C., et al. (2007). Cholesterol level, statin use and Alzheimer's disease in adults with Down syndrome. *Neuroscience Letters*, 416(3), 279–284.

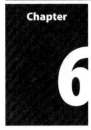

Schizophrenia spectrum disorders

Rory Sheehan, Lucy Fodor-Wynne, and Angela Hassiotis

Introduction

Schizophrenia spectrum disorders (SSD) comprise of a cluster of mental disorders in which the most prominent feature is psychosis. They are more common in people with intellectual disabilities (ID) than in the general population. Operationalized criteria used to diagnose mental disorders in the general population may not be generalizable to people with ID, particularly in those with the greatest degree of disability (Clarke et al., 1994). The *Diagnostic Manual – Intellectual Disability* (DM-ID) (Fletcher et al., 2007) and *Diagnostic Criteria for Psychiatric Disorders for Use with Adults with Learning Disabilities/Mental Retardation* (DC-LD)(Royal College of Psychiatrists, 2001) have been developed from the *Diagnostic and Statistical Manual* (DSM) and *International Classification of Diseases* (ICD) criteria respectively, to better serve this population, although there remains debate about their utility in improving ascertainment of SSD, especially in people with more severe ID (Melville, 2003).

Prevalence

Studies investigating the prevalence rates of SSD in people with ID report varying results. Reasons for such variation include: diversity in sampling frames; inconsistent definitions of both ID and psychosis; and differences in case ascertainment and assessment (Buckles et al., 2013). As a general estimate, schizophrenia prevalence is often quoted as 3% in people with ID, compared with an approximately 1% lifetime risk in the general population (Perälä et al., 2007).

Cooper et al. conducted a population-based cohort study of over 1000 adults with ID who were followed up for two years (Cooper et al., 2007). The point prevalence of psychotic disorders was reported as 2.6–4.4%, depending on the diagnostic criteria used, and the two-year incidence of a psychotic episode was 1.4%. Findings of this study are in agreement with an earlier work that reported a prevalence rate of schizophrenia of 4.4% in a Welsh cohort of adults with ID (Deb et al., 2001).

Morgan et al. report the results of a large study based on a population register in Western Australia. They found that between 3.7% and 5.2% of the study population had an ICD-9 diagnosis of schizophrenia, with the lifetime risk of experiencing at least one episode of non-organic psychosis to be just over 10% (Morgan et al., 2008). These

Psychiatric and Behavioral Disorders in Intellectual and Developmental Disabilities, ed. Colin Hemmings and Nick Bouras. Published by Cambridge University Press. © Cambridge University Press 2016.

results contrast with a previous Australian study, which found a lower point prevalence of 1.3% for the broader diagnosis of "psychosis" (White et al., 2005).

In a study of over 3000 inmates of British prisons, Hassiotis and colleagues not only found that people with ID were over-represented in the prison system, but also that those with ID were twice as likely as inmates of normal intelligence to have probable psychosis (Hassiotis et al., 2011). Although the time of onset of the psychosis was not recorded, it was speculated that the stressful and complex prison environment might precipitate the development of psychotic illness in those already at risk.

Risk factors

Risk factors for schizophrenia have traditionally been considered as genetic and environmental, but there is increasing evidence in support of interaction of the two in the genesis of the disorder (Van Os et al., 2008). Owing to the lack of investigation, not all risk factors have been established in the population with ID, but it might be reasonable to assume that exposures that place individuals in the general population at a higher risk of developing schizophrenia have similar effects in those with ID. However, the association of certain factors with increased rates of schizophrenia does not prove evidence of causation, and the mechanisms by which risk factors influence the development of such complex psychopathology are generally not well understood. Specific risk factors that have been investigated in people with ID include:

- Pregnancy and birth complications – pregnancy and birth complications are more common in people with ID, and may be causative in some instances (Sussmann et al., 2009). Prenatal and perinatal complications have also been associated with the later development of schizophrenia. There is evidence that pregnancy and birth complications are more common in people with ID who develop schizophrenia than in a matched cohort of people with ID who do not (O'Dwyer, 1997).
- Ethnic minority status – people from an ethnic minority group in the UK who have ID are more likely to develop SSD than their White counterparts (Tsakanikos et al., 2010).
- The use of cannabis increases the incidence of psychosis in the general population, and the response appears to be dose-dependent (Moore et al., 2007). The role of cannabis in the risk of developing SSD in people with ID has not been thoroughly studied; one study demonstrated that cannabis use is prevalent amongst people with ID presenting to specialist psychiatric services and is particularly associated with those suffering SSD (Chaplin et al., 2011).
- Negative life events – events such as moving house, death of a relative, and victimization are common in people with ID and have been associated with the subsequent development of a range of psychiatric problems, including psychotic illness (Hulbert-Williams et al., 2014).

The nature of the link between ID and SSD

The association between SSD and intellectual functioning has prompted research in people with ID and SSD with the aim of gaining a broader understanding of the pathophysiology of schizophrenia itself (Moorhead et al., 2009). Such work has challenged the traditional view of schizophrenia as a neurodegenerative condition with onset in early adulthood (indeed, the Kraeplinian term "dementia praecox" implies a slow progressive decline arising after normal development), and a neurodevelopmental model of schizophrenia is increasingly dominant (Fatemi and Folsom, 2009; Owen et al., 2011).

Proponents of a social causative theory of schizophrenia might argue that the increased rates of social and economic disadvantage, exclusion, bullying, and adverse life events that people with ID suffer cause additional stress, which underlies the observation of increased rates of SSD (and mental illness in general) in this group (Tsakanikos et al., 2007). That is, the effects of a hostile environment are borne out by increased rates of psychopathology in vulnerable individuals. Alternatively, it may be the case that cognitive impairment in itself increases susceptibility to developing an SSD, mediated by an "overload" of an individual's cognitive and adaptive capacity resulting from multiple episodes of only partly understood stimuli (Doody et al., 1998).

Results from imaging studies, although relatively sparse in people with ID and SSD, support a neurodevelopmental model, which maintains that SSD arise as a result of disturbed early development of the nervous system. A number of structural brain abnormalities have been described in individuals with schizophrenia, including enlargement of the ventricles, dilatation of cortical sulci, and a reduction in brain volume with proportionately greater loss in the amygdala and hippocampus, particularly on the left side. Many of the changes in gross brain morphology demonstrated in people with schizophrenia are also seen in people with ID without schizophrenia; however, imaging studies have shown the brains of people with comorbid ID and schizophrenia to show greater similarity to the brains of people of normal intelligence with schizophrenia than to a control group with ID alone (Sanderson et al., 1999). This observation leads to the suggestion that a common pathophysiological process is at work in both comorbid schizophrenia and ID and in schizophrenia alone. Therefore, the association of ID and schizophrenia may be a function of a severe and early-onset form of schizophrenia (of which the global intellectual impairment is part of the natural history of the disease), rather than the pre-existing ID itself acting as a risk factor for the development of schizophrenia (Sanderson et al., 1999; Bonnici et al., 2007). Further advocating a neurodevelopmental theory of schizophrenia is the finding that both functional decline (Fuller et al., 2002) and morphological brain changes are evident at the onset of the disease or may even predate the clinical disorder, rather than developing after the disease becomes manifest (Steen et al., 2006). Moreover, people with ID tend to develop schizophrenia at a younger age than those of normal intellectual functioning. Such findings suggest a biological underpinning to SSD, the expression of which may be influenced by later environmental exposures.

Genetic conditions and SSD

See also Chapter 18.

Several genetic conditions that cause ID are also associated with increased rates of SSD, although the mechanisms mediating the links have not been defined.

22q11.2 deletion syndrome, also known as velocardiofacial or DiGeorge syndrome, is caused by the deletion of a small region of DNA on the long arm of chromosome 22. It occurs at a population frequency of approximately 1 in 4000 live births (Botto et al. 2003). Features include facial dysmorphia, cleft palate, structural heart defects, and immune disorders in addition to mild–moderate ID. The syndrome is one of the strongest known risk factors for psychosis – 1% of people with schizophrenia are estimated to have the mutation (Horowitz et al., 2005; Bassett et al., 2010) and SSD develop in up to 41% people with the syndrome (Shprintzen, 2008; Ousley et al., 2013; Schneider et al., 2014).

Prader–Willi syndrome results from failure of expression of paternally inherited genes on the long arm of chromosome 15. Psychiatric illness is highly prevalent, particularly in the subtype caused by maternal disomy, and usually manifests as an affective psychosis (Boer et al., 2002; Soni et al., 2008; Sinnema et al., 2011).

Usher syndrome is an autosomal-recessive condition that results from defects in one of several genes. The syndrome involves ID and varying degrees of deafness, blindness, and vestibular dysfunction. The lifetime incidence of psychosis is increased, though the mechanisms underlying this association have yet to be explained (Hess-Röver et al., 1999; Waldeck et al., 2001).

There is evidence that people with *Down syndrome* are less likely to be diagnosed with schizophrenia than people with ID not due to Down syndrome (Collacott et al., 1992; Mantry et al., 2008). However, whether this represents a true differential in rates of the illness is not clear.

Differential diagnosis

Several illnesses or disorders can present in a similar way to SSD and must be excluded before diagnosis, for example *autism spectrum disorders (ASD)* (Starling and Dossetor, 2009; Raja and Azzoni, 2010). People with ASD have impaired social interactions, commonly talk to themselves, may hold unconventional beliefs or peculiar ideas, have a high likelihood of sensory abnormalities, and often display stereotypies of speech and movement, all of which could be misinterpreted as psychosis. Poor social judgment and theory-of-mind skills may suggest paranoid delusions (Deprey and Ozonoff, 2008). However, true delusions and hallucinations are not among the symptoms of ASD (Cochran et al., 2013) (see also Chapter 11).

Difficulties in recognizing and diagnosing psychotic disorders in people with ID

Accurate diagnosis is essential to direct the correct treatment and supportive interventions.

There are no laboratory, radiological, or psychometric tests that confirm diagnosis, which is, therefore, based on clinical interview and observation. Diagnosis of SSD in people with ID can be difficult for several reasons:

- Deficits in communication skills and limitations in verbal ability can make it difficult for people with ID to describe their symptoms. This is especially pertinent in psychotic disorders where symptoms include complex and subjective mental phenomena.
- People with ID may express their thoughts in a muddled or disjointed manner resembling thought disorder, or may seem overly concerned about the motives of others in a way resembling paranoid thinking, but which could be normal when viewed in the context of past experiences of abuse or victimization.
- Distinguishing developmentally appropriate behaviors from psychotic experiences can be difficult. Magical thinking and imaginary friends are two such examples

that could be misinterpreted as evidence of delusions, or hallucinations (Pickard and Paschos, 2005).

• People with ID may lack insight into their illness and, thus, not report symptoms, quite before barriers to accessing health care are considered.

There is some evidence that people with ID experience a different pattern of psychotic symptoms to people of average intelligence. In people with mild ID, the symptoms and clinical features of schizophrenia are thought to be broadly the same as the population with normal intelligence (Doody et al., 1998). The content of delusions and hallucinations will be commensurate with an individual's developmental level, and people with ID are less likely to hold complex systematized delusional beliefs or to report conceptually complex symptoms such as passivity delusions (Meadows et al., 1991; Moss et al., 1996). Auditory hallucinations have been shown to be the most reliable and consistently reported psychotic symptom in those with mild ID (Meadows et al., 1991; Moss et al., 1996).

Bouras et al. (2004) compared people diagnosed with SSD with and without mild ID. The study found that, although the groups did not differ in terms of reported psychopathology, the group with ID showed greater levels of observable psychopathology and more negative symptoms (Bouras et al., 2004). This finding was corroborated by a meta-analysis of studies comparing the presentation of schizophrenia in people with mild ID or borderline intellectual functioning with those with average–high IQ, which demonstrated that those with lower IQ experience substantially greater negative symptoms (Welch et al., 2011). This contrasts with evidence from people with severe–profound ID in whom negative symptoms seem to be under-represented (Cherry et al., 2000), although there is, of course, inherent difficulty in diagnosing functional decline in people who may never have attained basic adaptive skills, and some authors have questioned the validity of the construct of negative symptoms when applied to people with ID (Melville, 2003; Hatton et al., 2005). In recognition of this, the DC-LD gives less significance to negative symptoms than diagnostic criteria developed for use in the general population.

In the absence of detailed self-report, observable signs of psychiatric illness that might manifest as changes in behavior and functioning are important. Maladaptive behaviors such as unexplained screaming, aggression, and self-injury, can suggest psychotic illness, particularly in those with greater degrees of impairment. Change in presentation is a particularly important indicator of the development of a psychotic illness. Collateral information is vital to establish a baseline premorbid state and family and carers should be engaged at all stages, although reliance on third-party information is not without its own complications (Costello and Bouras, 2006).

The *Psychiatric Assessment Schedule for Adults with Developmental Disabilities* (PAS-ADD) is a diagnostic interview suitable for direct use with people with ID and separately with informants (Moss et al., 1993). Psychotic symptoms are covered in detail, and the outcome is a specific diagnosis aligned to diagnostic criteria specified in the ICD or DSM. The Clinical Interview has been validated in the diagnosis of schizophrenia (Moss et al., 1996). The Diagnostic Assessment for the Severely Handicapped–Revised (DASH-II) is an alternative scale for use in people with severe and profound ID, and has been demonstrated to be useful in screening for schizophrenia in this group (Bamburg et al., 2001).

Management

Treatment approaches can be broadly divided into pharmacological and non-pharmacological. The evidence base for such interventions in people with ID is generally lacking and management is guided by research in the non-ID population and clinical experience.

Pharmacological treatment

See also Chapter 13.

The mainstay of pharmacological management in SSD in people with ID is antipsychotic medication. However, there is a lack of high-quality evidence for their use in people with ID (Duggan and Brylewski, 2004), and studies suggest that a significant proportion of prescribed antipsychotics are used to treat behavioral, rather than psychotic symptoms (De Kuijper et al., 2010).

Atypical antipsychotics have largely replaced older antipsychotics as first-line treatment and seem to be better tolerated (Connor and Posever, 1998; Advokat et al., 2000). Choice is determined by individual factors and the presence of comorbid conditions, and should be made jointly by practitioners and patients where possible (National Institute for Health and Care Excellence, 2014). An important side effect of atypical antipsychotics is the "metabolic syndrome" comprising of obesity, insulin resistance, impaired glucose tolerance, and dyslipidaemia (Newcomer, 2007). However, an observational study found that there were no clinical or statistically significant differences in metabolic indices between people with ID treated with antipsychotics and those who were antipsychotic naïve, although there was a trend towards increased rates of type 2 diabetes in the treated group (Frighi et al., 2011). Guidelines recommend regular monitoring of blood glucose, lipids, and weight for people taking antipsychotic medication (American Diabetes Association, 2004), although there are indications that people with ID frequently do not receive such investigations (Devapriam et al., 2009; Teeluck-dharry et al., 2013).

Extra-pyramidal side effects (EPSEs) of antipsychotic medication comprise of drug-induced Parkinsonism, akathisia, acute dystonic reactions, and tardive dyskinesia. Such side effects can be persistent, impair quality of life, and may be mistaken for core symptoms or features of ID. Although the newer, atypical antipsychotics have been promoted as having less propensity to cause EPSEs than older drugs, there is evidence that those with ID who take atypical antipsychotic drugs remain at increased risk of developing abnormal movement disorders (Fodstad et al., 2010). The Matson Evaluation of Drug Side effects (MEDS) has been developed as a comprehensive informant-based measure that can be used to assess side effects of psychotropic medication in people with ID (Matson et al., 1998).

The atypical antipsychotic clozapine is effective in improving symptoms in treatment-resistant schizophrenia (Kane, 1992). It is licensed where two adequate trials of alternative antipsychotics have failed. Studies suggest that clozapine is safe and efficacious in people with ID (Antonacci and De Groot, 2000; Thalayasingam et al., 2004). Clozapine has also been used to treat aggression in people with ID with some success in small trials (Cohen and Underwood 1994), but a more recent review concluded that "research on the use of clozapine to manage behavior among individuals with ID is inconclusive at best" (Singh et al., 2010). In addition, the risk of serious side effects, including potentially fatal agranulocytosis, and necessity of regular blood tests may deter clinicians from using the drug.

Non-pharmacological treatment

See also Chapter 15.

Psychosocial interventions are often used in combination with medication and require input from the wider multidisciplinary team. A broad range of psychosocial interventions has been used, including cognitive-behavioral therapy (CBT), psychoeducation programs, and family-based interventions (Chien et al., 2013). The focus may be on managing or reducing symptoms, psychoeducation and improving insight, or maximizing functional ability. Delivery of therapies needs to be adapted to reflect a person's developmental level, which may involve incorporating flexibility in the location and structure of sessions, and supporting the individual with prompts or accessible written information.

Case reports detailing successful group and individual interventions for people with ID and SSD have been published (Crowley et al. 2008; Hurley 2012; Allott et al. 2013), but interventions have not been systematically evaluated and robust evidence of their effectiveness and acceptability is lacking.

Psychosis co-occurring with ID confers additional carer burden (Irazábal et al., 2012) and efforts should be made to involve and support family carers (National Institute for Health and Care Excellence, 2014). Research in the mainstream population has consistently demonstrated the effectiveness of family therapy in improving several aspects of the condition, including frequency of relapse and number of admissions to hospital (Pharoah et al., 2010). Although further research is required, adapted family therapy shows signs of being a promising treatment in people with ID (Marshall and Ferris, 2012).

Service provision

The majority of people with ID and psychosis will be managed in the community and their usual home. People with ID and SSD are likely to be heavy consumers of psychiatric resources (Spiller et al., 2007). Amongst people with ID suffering mental illness, those with schizophrenia have been shown to use psychiatric services more than those with any other diagnosis (Morgan et al., 2008). Despite this, there has been little research to inform the most effective models of community care (Balogh et al., 2008; Hemmings, 2008). A consultation exercise involving a large multidisciplinary group identified the "need for a focused approach on the service user and their illness" and "working within the wider context of the service user" as essential components of services managing people with ID and psychosis (Hemmings et al., 2009).

Assertive community treatment (ACT) teams are a feature of many mainstream psychiatric services and work with people with severe and chronic mental illness who engage poorly with services (Stein and Test, 1980). Evaluation of such services for people with ID have failed to show evidence of improvement in any outcome measure (Oliver et al., 2002; Martin et al., 2005).

At times of symptom exacerbation or where the risk associated with the illness is too great, facilities for hospital admission must be available. Being diagnosed with a schizophrenia spectrum condition increases the likelihood of having a psychiatric admission over people with other psychiatric diagnoses (Cowley et al., 2005). Moreover, a study conducted in Taiwan found that hospital admissions for people with ID and co-occurring schizophrenia cost more than admissions for people with ID and other mental illnesses (Lai et al., 2011).

Whether psychiatric services for people with ID who develop serious mental illness, including SSD, are provided within specialist ID teams or by generic mental health services is the focus of a, as yet unanswered, debate (Hemmings et al., 2014).

Outcome/prognosis

The "recovery model" of rehabilitation from serious mental illness has gained currency in the general population. Advocates from within both professional and service user and carer populations uphold that principles of hope, healing, and empowerment should drive the development of positive, person-centered services that work collaboratively with, and are acceptable to, users of those services (Warner, 2009). Under this model, recovery is not merely remission from symptoms but implies broader gains in social and functional outcome. Respect for the individual's experience and their priorities are at the heart of the model. Although the concept of "recovery" from SSD in this sense has sparsely been covered in people with ID, certain aspects of the model, such as supported employment, social skills training, and promotion of community inclusion, will be familiar to those working in ID services.

Despite the optimism inherent in the recovery model, SSD tend to run a chronic course and can impair relationships, functioning, and quality of life (Morgan et al., 2008; Jääskeläinen et al., 2013). A study by Cooper and colleagues reported a full remission rate of just under 15% over a two-year period (Cooper et al., 2009).

When comparing people with SSD with and without co-occurring ID, studies have shown people with borderline intellectual functioning or diagnosed ID have a more severe illness, greater functional disability, and lower quality of life (Bouras et al., 2004; Chaplin et al., 2006).

Conclusions

Schizophrenia spectrum disorders are not uncommon in people with ID and confer an additional degree of impairment. The presentation of these disorders in people with ID is often atypical and, as such, they can be difficult to recognize and might be overlooked. Treatment guidelines are extrapolated from those used in the general population, as research addressing interventions specifically tailored to people with ID is relatively sparse.

Key summary points

- Schizophrenia spectrum disorders are more common in people with ID than the general population.
- The nature of the link between SSD and ID is not clear and the development of pathology is likely to be multifactorial. There is increasing evidence in support of aberrant early development of the nervous system in predisposing individuals to developing SSD.

- The clinical manifestations of SSD are diverse and are likely to be different to those in the general population. The disorders can be difficult to recognize in people with ID, leading to underdiagnosis and treatment, and continuing distress and disturbance.
- Treatment methods are extrapolated from research in the general population, but there are issues unique to people with ID that must also be considered.

References

Advokat, C.D., Mayville, E.A., Matson, J.L. (2000). Side effect profiles of atypical antipsychotics, typical antipsychotics, or no psychotropic medications in persons with mental retardation. *Research in Developmental Disabilities*, 21(1), 75–84.

Allott, K.A., Francey, S.M., Velligan, D.I. (2013). Improving functional outcome using compensatory strategies in comorbid intellectual disability and psychosis: a case study. *American Journal of Psychiatric Rehabilitation*, 16(1), 50–65.

American Diabetes Association. (2004). Consensus development conference on antipsychotic drugs and obesity and diabetes. *Diabetes Care*, 27(2), 596–601.

Antonacci, D.J. and De Groot, C.M. (2000). Clozapine treatment in a population of adults with mental retardation. *Journal of Clinical Psychiatry*, 61(1), 22–25.

Balogh, R., Ouellette-Kuntz, H., Bourne L., Lunsky, Y., Colantonio, A. (2008). Organising health care services for persons with an intellectual disability. *Cochrane Database of Systematic Review*, 4, CD007492.

Bamburg, J.W., Cherry, K.E., Matson, J.L., Penn, D. (2001). Assessment of schizophrenia in persons with severe and profound mental retardation using the Diagnostic Assessment for the Severely Handicapped-II (DASH-II). *Journal of Developmental and Physical Disabilities*, 13(4), 319–331.

Bassett, A.S., Costaina, G., Funga, W.L.A., et al. (2010). Clinically detectable copy number variations in a Canadian catchment population of schizophrenia. *Journal of Psychiatric Research*, 44(15), 1005–1009.

Boer, H., Holland, A., Whittington, J., et al. (2002). Psychotic illness in people with Prader Willi syndrome due to chromosome 15 maternal uniparental disomy. *Lancet*, 359(9301), 135–136.

Bonnici, H.M., William, T., Moorhead, J., et al. (2007). Pre-frontal lobe gyrification index in schizophrenia, mental retardation and comorbid groups: an automated study. *Neuroimage*, 35(2), 648–654.

Botto, L.D., May, K., Fernhoff, P.M., et al. (2003). A population-based study of the 22q11. 2 deletion: phenotype, incidence, and contribution to major birth defects in the population. *Pediatrics*, 112(1), 101–107.

Bouras, N., Martin, G., Leese, M., et al. (2004). Schizophrenia-spectrum psychoses in people with and without intellectual disability. *Journal of Intellectual Disability Research*, 48(6), 548–555.

Buckles, J., Luckasson, R., Keefe, E. (2013). A systematic review of the prevalence of psychiatric disorders in adults with intellectual disability, 2003–2010. *Journal of Mental Health Research in Intellectual Disabilities*, 6(3), 181–207.

Chaplin, R., Barley, M., Cooper, S.J., et al. (2006). The impact of intellectual functioning on symptoms and service use in schizophrenia. *Journal of Intellectual Disability Research*, 50(4), 288–294.

Chaplin, E., Gilvarry, C., Tsakanikos, E. (2011). Recreational substance use patterns and co-morbid psychopathology in adults with intellectual disability. *Research in Developmental Disabilities*, 32(6), 2981–2986.

Cherry, K.E., Penn, D., Matson, J.L., et al. (2000). Characteristics of schizophrenia among persons with severe or profound mental retardation. *Psychiatric Services*, 51(7), 922–924.

Chien, W.T, Leung, S.F., Yeung, F.K.K., et al. (2013). Current approaches to treatments for schizophrenia spectrum disorders, Part

II: psychosocial interventions and patient-focused perspectives in psychiatric care. *Neuropsychiatric Disease and Treatment*, 9, 1463.

Clarke, D.J., Cumella, S., Corbett, J., et al. (1994). Use of ICD-10 research diagnostic criteria to categorise psychiatric and behavioural abnormalities among people with learning disabilities: the West Midlands field trial. *Mental Handicap Research*, 7(4), 273–285.

Cochran, D.M., Dvir, Y., Frazier, J.A. (2013). "Autism-plus" spectrum disorders: intersection with psychosis and the schizophrenia spectrum. *Child and Adolescent Psychiatric Clinics of North America*, 22(4), 609–627.

Cohen, S.A. and Underwood, M.T. (1994). The use of clozapine in a mentally retarded and aggressive population. *Journal of Clinical Psychiatry*, 55(10), 440–444.

Collacott, R.A., Cooper, S.-A., McGrother, C. (1992). Differential rates of psychiatric disorders in adults with Down's syndrome compared with other mentally handicapped adults. *British Journal of Psychiatry*, 161(5), 671–674.

Connor, D.F. and Posever, T.A. (1998). A brief review of atypical antipsychotics in individuals with developmental disability. *Mental Health Aspects of Developmental Disabilities*, 1, 93–101.

Cooper, S-A., Smiley, E., Morrison, J., et al. (2007). Psychosis and adults with intellectual disabilities. *Social Psychiatry and Psychiatric Epidemiology*, 42(7), 530–536.

Cooper, S-A., Smiley, E., Jackson, A., et al. (2009). Adults with intellectual disabilities: prevalence, incidence and remission of aggressive behaviour and related factors. *Journal of Intellectual Disability Research*, 53(3), 217–232.

Costello, H. and Bouras, N. (2006). Assessment of mental health problems in people with intellectual disabilities. *Israel Journal of Psychiatry and Related Sciences*, 43(4), 241.

Cowley, A., Newton, J., Sturmey, P., et al. (2005). Psychiatric inpatient admissions of adults with intellectual disabilities:

predictive factors. *American Journal on Mental Retardation*, 110(3), 216–225.

Crowley, V., Rose, J., Smith, J., et al. (2008). Psycho-educational groups for people with a dual diagnosis of psychosis and mild intellectual disability: a preliminary study. *Journal of Intellectual Disabilities*, 12(1), 25–39.

De Kuijper, G., Hoekstra, P., Visser F., et al. (2010). Use of antipsychotic drugs in individuals with intellectual disability (ID) in the Netherlands: prevalence and reasons for prescription. *Journal of Intellectual Disability Research*, 54(7), 659–667.

Deb, S., Thomas, M., Bright, C. (2001). Mental disorder in adults with intellectual disability. 1: prevalence of functional psychiatric illness among a community-based population aged between 16 and 64 years. *Journal of Intellectual Disability Research*, 45(6), 495–505.

Deprey, L. and Ozonoff, S. (2008). Assessment of comorbid psychiatric conditions in autism spectrum disorders. In G. Sam and S. Ozonoff (eds.), *Assessment of Autism Spectrum Disorders*. New York, NY: Guilford Press.

Devapriam, J., Anand, A., Raju, L.B., et al. (2009). Monitoring for metabolic syndrome in adults with intellectual disability on atypical antipsychotic drugs. *British Journal of Development Disabilities*, 55(108), 3–13.

Doody, G.A., Johnstone, E.C., Sanderson, T.L., et al. (1998). "Pfropfschizophrenie"revisited. Schizophrenia in people with mild learning disability. *British Journal of Psychiatry*, 173(2), 145–153.

Duggan, L. and Brylewski, J. (2004). Antipsychotic medication versus placebo for people with both schizophrenia and learning disability. *Cochrane Database Syst Rev*, 4, CD000030.

Fatemi, S.H. and Folsom, T.D. (2009). The neurodevelopmental hypothesis of schizophrenia, revisited. *Schizophrenia Bulletin*, 35(3), 528–548.

Fletcher, R., Loschen, E., Stavrakaki, C., et al. (eds.) (2007). *Diagnostic Manual – Intellectual Disability: A Textbook of*

Diagnosis of Mental Disorders in Persons with Intellectual Disability. Kingston, NY: NADD Press.

Fodstad, J.C., Bamburg, J.W., Matson, J.L., et al. (2010). Tardive dyskinesia and intellectual disability: an examination of demographics and topography in adults with dual diagnosis and atypical antipsychotic use. *Research in Developmental Disabilities*, 31(3), 750–759.

Frighi, V., Stephenson, M.T., Morovat, A., et al. (2011). Safety of antipsychotics in people with intellectual disability. *British Journal of Psychiatry*, 199(4), 289–295.

Fuller, R., Nopoulos, P., Arndt, S., et al. (2002). Longitudinal assessment of premorbid cognitive functioning in patients with schizophrenia through examination of standardized scholastic test performance. *American Journal of Psychiatry*, 159(7), 1183–1189.

Hassiotis, A., Gazizova, A., Akinlonu, L., et al. (2011). Psychiatric morbidity in prisoners with intellectual disabilities: analysis of prison survey data for England and Wales. *British Journal of Psychiatry*, 199(2), 156–157.

Hatton, C., Haddock, G., Taylor, J.L., et al. (2005). The reliability and validity of general psychotic rating scales with people with mild and moderate intellectual disabilities: an empirical investigation. *Journal of Intellectual Disability Research*, 49(7), 490–500.

Hemmings, C.P. (2008). Community services for people with intellectual disabilities and mental health problems. *Current Opinion in Psychiatry*, 21(5), 459–462.

Hemmings, C.P., Underwood, L.A., Bouras, N. (2009). Services in the community for adults with psychosis and intellectual disabilities: a Delphi consultation of professionals' views. *Journal of Intellectual Disability Research*, 53(7), 677–684.

Hemmings, C.P., Bouras, N., Craig, T. (2014). How should community mental health of intellectual disability services evolve? *International Journal of Environmental Research and Public Health*, 11(9), 8624–8631.

Hess-Röver, J., Critchton, J., Byrne, K., et al. (1999). Case report: diagnosis and treatment of a severe psychotic illness in a man with dual severe sensory impairments caused by the presence of Usher syndrome. *Journal of Intellectual Disability Research*, 43(5), 428–434.

Horowitz, A., Shifman, S., Rivlin, N., et al. (2005). A survey of the 22q11 microdeletion in a large cohort of schizophrenia patients. *Schizophrenia Research*, 73(2), 263–267.

Hulbert-Williams, L., Hastings, R., Owen, D.M., et al. (2014). Exposure to life events as a risk factor for psychological problems in adults with intellectual disabilities: a longitudinal design. *Journal of Intellectual Disability Research*, 58(1), 48–60.

Hurley, A.D. (2012). Treatment of erotomania using cognitive behavioural psychotherapy approaches. *Advances in Mental Health and Intellectual Disabilities*, 6(2), 76–81.

Irazábal, M., Marsà, F., García, M., et al. (2012). Family burden related to clinical and functional variables of people with intellectual disability with and without a mental disorder. *Research in Developmental Disabilities*, 33(3), 796–803.

Jääskeläinen, E., Juola, P., Hirvonen N., et al. (2013). A systematic review and meta-analysis of recovery in schizophrenia. *Schizophrenia Bulletin*, 39, 1363–1372.

Kane, J.M. (1992). Clinical efficacy of clozapine in treatment-refractory schizophrenia: an overview. *British Journal of Psychiatry*, 160(17), 41–45.

Lai, C.-I., Hung, W.J., Lin, L.P., et al. (2011). A retrospective population-based data analyses of inpatient care use and medical expenditure in people with intellectual disability co-occurring schizophrenia. *Research in Developmental Disabilities*, 32(3), 1226–1231.

Mantry, D., Cooper, S-A., Smiley, E., et al. (2008). The prevalence and incidence of mental ill-health in adults with Down syndrome. *Journal of Intellectual Disability Research*, 52(2), 141–155.

Marshall, K. and Ferris, J. (2012). Utilising behavioural family therapy (BFT) to help support the system around a person with intellectual disability and complex mental health needs: a case study. *Journal of Intellectual Disabilities*, 16(2), 109–118.

Martin, G., Costello, H., Leese M., et al. (2005). An exploratory study of assertive community treatment for people with intellectual disability and psychiatric disorders: conceptual, clinical, and service issues. *Journal of Intellectual Disability Research*, 49(7), 516–524.

Matson, J.L., Mayville, E.A., Bielecki, J.A., et al. (1998). Reliability of the Matson evaluation of drug side effects scale (MEDS). *Research in Developmental Disabilities*, 19(6), 501–506.

Meadows, G., Turner, T., Campbell, L., et al. (1991). Assessing schizophrenia in adults with mental retardation. A comparative study. *British Journal of Psychiatry*, 158(1), 103–105.

Melville, C.A. (2003). A critique of the *Diagnostic Criteria for Psychiatric Disorders for Use with Adults with Learning Disabilities/Mental Retardation (DC-LD)* chapter on non-affective psychotic disorders. *Journal of Intellectual Disability Research*, 47(Suppl.1), 16–25.

Moore, T.H.M., Zammit, S., Lingford-Hughes, A., et al. (2007). Cannabis use and risk of psychotic or affective mental health outcomes: a systematic review. *Lancet*, 370(9584), 319–328.

Moorhead, T.W.J., Stanfield, A., Spencer, M., et al. (2009). Progressive temporal lobe grey matter loss in adolescents with schizotypal traits and mild intellectual impairment. *Psychiatry Research: Neuroimaging*, 174(2), 105–109.

Morgan, V.A., Leonard, H., Bourke, J., et al. (2008). Intellectual disability co-occurring with schizophrenia and other psychiatric illness: population-based study. *British Journal of Psychiatry*, 193(5), 364–372.

Moss, S., Patel, P., Prosser, H. (1993). Psychiatric morbidity in older people with moderate and severe learning disability. I: Development and reliability of the patient interview (PAS-ADD). *British Journal of Psychiatry*, 163, 471–480.

Moss, S., Prosser, H., Goldberg, D. (1996). Validity of the schizophrenia diagnosis of the psychiatric assessment schedule for adults with developmental disability (PAS-ADD). *British Journal of Psychiatry*, 168(3), 359–367.

National Institute for Health and Care Excellence. (2014). *Psychosis and Schizophrenia in Adults: Treatment and Management. NICE Guideline [CG178]*. At: http://www.nice.org.uk/guidance/cg178/chapter/recommendations

Newcomer, J.W. (2007). Metabolic considerations in the use of antipsychotic medications: a review of recent evidence. *Journal of Clinical Psychiatry*, 68(1), 20–27.

O'Dwyer, J.M. (1997). Schizophrenia in people with intellectual disability: the role of pregnancy and birth complications. *Journal of Intellectual Disability Research*, 41(3), 238–251.

Oliver, P.C., Piachaud, J., Done, J., et al. (2002). Difficulties in conducting a randomized controlled trial of health service interventions in intellectual disability: implications for evidence-based practice. *Journal of Intellectual Disability Research*, 46(4), 340–345.

Ousley, O.Y., Smearman, E., Fernandez-Carriba, S., et al. (2013). Axis I psychiatric diagnoses in adolescents and young adults with 22q11 deletion syndrome. *European Psychiatry*, 28(7), 417–422.

Owen, M.J., O'Donovan, M.C., Thapar, A., et al. (2011). Neurodevelopmental hypothesis of schizophrenia. *British Journal of Psychiatry*, 198(3), 173–175.

Perälä, J., Suvisaari, J., Saarni, S.I., et al. (2007). Lifetime prevalence of psychotic and bipolar I disorders in a general population. *Archives of General Psychiatry*, 64(1), 19–28.

Pharoah, F., Mari, J.J., Rathbone, J., et al. (2010). Family intervention for schizophrenia. *Cochrane Database of Systematic Reviews*, 12, CD000088.

Pickard, M. and Paschos, D. (2005). Pseudohallucinations in people with intellectual disabilities: two case reports. *Mental Health Aspects of Developmental Disabilities*, 8(3), 91–93.

Raja, M. and Azzoni, A. (2010). Autistic spectrum disorders and schizophrenia in the adult psychiatric setting: diagnosis and comorbidity. *Psychiatria Danubina*, 22(4), 514–521.

Royal College of Psychiatrists (2001). *Diagnostic Criteria for Psychiatric Disorders for Use with Adults with Learning Disabilities/Mental Retardation (DC-LD).* London: Royal College of Psychiatrists.

Sanderson, T.L., Best, J.J.K., Doody, G.A., et al. (1999). Neuroanatomy of comorbid schizophrenia and learning disability: a controlled study. *Lancet,* 354(9193), 1867–1871.

Schneider, M., Debbané, M., Bassett, A.S., et al. (2014). Psychiatric disorders from childhood to adulthood in 22q11.2 deletion syndrome: results from the International Consortium on Brain and Behavior in 22q11.2 Deletion Syndrome. *American Journal of Psychiatry,* 171(6), 627–639.

Shprintzen, R.J. (2008). Velo-cardio-facial syndrome: 30 Years of study. *Developmental Disabilities Research Reviews,* 14(1), 3–10.

Singh, A.N., Matson, J.L., Hill, B.D., et al. (2010). The use of clozapine among individuals with intellectual disability: a review. *Research in Developmental Disabilities,* 31(6), 1135–1141.

Sinnema, M., Boer, H., Collin, P., et al. (2011). Psychiatric illness in a cohort of adults with Prader–Willi syndrome. *Research in Developmental Disabilities,* 32(5), 1729–1735.

Soni, S., Whittington A., Holland, A.J., et al. (2008). The phenomenology and diagnosis of psychiatric illness in people with Prader–Willi syndrome. *Psychological Medicine,* 38(10), 1505–1514.

Spiller, M.J., Costello, H., Bramley, A., et al. (2007). Consumption of mental health services by people with intellectual disabilities. *Journal of Applied Research in Intellectual Disabilities,* 20(5), 430–438.

Starling, J. and Dossetor, D. (2009). Pervasive developmental disorders and psychosis. *Current Psychiatry Reports,* 11(3), 190–196.

Steen, R.G., Mull, C., McClure, R., et al. (2006). Brain volume in first-episode schizophrenia. Systematic review and meta-analysis of magnetic resonance imaging studies. *British Journal of Psychiatry,* 188(6), 510–518.

Stein, L.I. and Test, M.A. (1980). Alternative to mental hospital treatment: I. Conceptual model, treatment program, and clinical evaluation. *Archives of General Psychiatry,* 37(4), 392–397.

Sussmann, J.E., McIntosh, A.M., Lawrie, S.M., et al. (2009). Obstetric complications and mild to moderate intellectual disability. *British Journal of Psychiatry,* 194(3), 224–228.

Teeluckdharry, S., Sharma, S., O'Rourke, E., et al. (2013). Monitoring metabolic side effects of atypical antipsychotics in people with an intellectual disability. *Journal of Intellectual Disabilities,* 17(3), 223–235.

Thalayasingam, S., Alexander, R.T., Singh, I. (2004). The use of clozapine in adults with intellectual disability. *Journal of Intellectual Disability Research,* 48(6), 572–579.

Tsakanikos, E., Bouras, N., Costello, H., et al. (2007). Multiple exposure to life events and clinical psychopathology in adults with intellectual disability. *Social Psychiatry and Psychiatric Epidemiology,* 42(1), 24–28.

Tsakanikos, E., McCarthy, J., Kravariti, E., et al. (2010). The role of ethnicity in clinical psychopathology and care pathways of adults with intellectual disabilities. *Research in Developmental Disabilities,* 31(2), 410–415.

Van Os, J., Rutten, B.P.F., Poulton, R. (2008). Gene–environment interactions in schizophrenia: review of epidemiological findings and future directions. *Schizophrenia Bulletin,* 34(6), 1066–1082.

Waldeck, T., Wyszynski, B., Medalia, A. (2001). The relationship between Usher's syndrome and psychosis with Capgras syndrome. *Psychiatry: Interpersonal and Biological Processes,* 64(3), 248–255.

Warner, R., (2009). Recovery from schizophrenia and the recovery model. *Current Opinion in Psychiatry,* 22(4), 374–380.

Welch, K.A., Lawrie, S.M., Muir, W., et al. (2011). Systematic review of the clinical presentation of schizophrenia in intellectual disability. *Journal of Psychopathology and Behavioral Assessment,* 33(2), 246–253.

White, P., Chant, D., Edwards, N., et al. (2005). Prevalence of intellectual disability and comorbid mental illness in an Australian community sample. *Australian and New Zealand Journal of Psychiatry,* 39(5), 395–400.

Chapter

Mood disorders

Anna M. Palucka, Pushpal Desarkar, and Yona Lunsky

Introduction

Mood disorders in those with intellectual disabilities (ID) can be thought of as "under-recognized yet over-treated." They are under-recognized in that clinicians and caregivers can fail to recognize signs of mood disorders in those with ID. Instead, their behaviors are attributed to their disability, and when they are treated, because of misdiagnosis and the late stage at which they are addressed, the main treatment is medication, with polypharmacy being a risk. This chapter describes the main clinical features of mood disorders in people with ID and the similarities and differences in clinical presentation that occur when compared to the general population. It also reviews what is known about etiology and treatment for mood disorders in the ID population.

Diagnostic features

The *Diagnostic Manual – Intellectual Disability* (DM-ID; Fletcher et al., 2007) makes very limited adaptations to the standard diagnostic criteria, but does provide useful behavioral descriptions of symptoms of each disorder. In contrast, the *Diagnostic Criteria for Psychiatric Disorders for Use with Adults with Learning Disabilities/Mental Retardation* (DC-LD; Royal College of Psychiatrists, 2001) makes significant modifications to include symptoms commonly reported in individuals with ID not featured in the standard diagnostic criteria, such as the onset of or increase in aggression or other problem behaviors.

Depression

Individuals with ID are a highly heterogeneous group in relation to cognitive, communication, and social skills, even when comparing individuals with the same level of ID (Harris, 1998). The existing body of literature suggests that individuals at higher levels of intellectual ability present with psychiatric symptoms typically seen in the general population. The diagnosis in those with more severe levels of disability, however, is more complicated and is also more reliant on caregiver report due to challenges in communication. Consequently, the observational skills of the caregiver greatly affect the accuracy of the diagnosis. For example, Hurley (2008) found that depressed mood was infrequent as the chief complaint for patients with ID who were diagnosed with

Psychiatric and Behavioral Disorders in Intellectual and Developmental Disabilities, ed. Colin Hemmings and Nick Bouras. Published by Cambridge University Press. © Cambridge University Press 2016.

depression. It was instead the behavioral disturbance that prompted referral for psychiatric assessment. This suggests that caregivers may fail to recognize symptoms of depression and not seek psychiatric consultation in the absence of disturbed behavior.

The DM-ID (Charlot et al., 2007a), thus, recommends using a developmental approach to support diagnosis of depression, as has been done for children without ID. Such an approach considers how one's developmental level impacts how depression is manifested, and includes irritable mood, for example, as a diagnostic symptom.

Mild/moderate ID

There is a general consensus that people with mild ID show a full range of mood symptoms and can be assessed with minimal adjustment to diagnostic criteria, providing the clinician has an understanding of the developmental level and adaptive skills of the individual, as even within the mild ID population, individual differences exist in the ability to identify and report internal states and thoughts. Furthermore, although individuals with mild and moderate ID are often grouped together in research studies, individuals with moderate ID may have significantly more difficulty reporting cognitive symptoms such as diminished ability to concentrate or excessive guilt compared to individuals with mild ID.

Severe/profound ID

Identification of depressive symptoms in individuals with severe or profound disability can be very challenging due to the intrinsic cognitive and communication limitations and atypical presentation of this population. Cognitive symptoms such as feelings of guilt, hopelessness, or suicidal ideation are rarely described (Ross and Oliver, 2003), and consequently these individuals are less likely to meet the **full** diagnostic criteria (Cain et al., 2003; Charlot et al., 2007b). Behavioral (or depressive) equivalents have been proposed as atypical symptoms of depression in individuals with severe disabilities. Self-injury, screaming, and aggression were identified as distinct symptoms of depression in Marston et al. (1997), but this finding has not been replicated (Tsiouris et al., 2003; Sturmey et al., 2010a). Furthermore, externalizing behaviors do not appear to be specific to mood disorders and research in this area suggests caution in using symptoms substitution. Instead, improving the reliability at the assessment level is recommended (Charlot et al., 2007b), with focus on core diagnostic features that can be observed (all symptoms excluding cognitive ones). Alterations in mood can manifest as a person crying every day, a decrease in laughing/smiling, and/or vegetative symptoms such as changes in eating (weight), sleeping, and motor activity (Lowry, 1998). Tsiouris et al. (2003) identified eight most frequently reported depressive symptoms in a research study where nearly half the subjects had severe/profound ID. These symptoms included: anxiety, depressed affect, irritability, loss of interest, social isolation, lack of emotion, sleep disturbance, and lack of confidence.

Bipolar disorders

Individuals with ID are more frequently diagnosed with a rapid cycling form of bipolar disorder (four or more episodes per year) than the general population. Abnormal mood states in individuals with ID diagnosed with bipolar disorder appear to be correlated with aggression. Given the recent inclusion of a new disorder of disruptive mood dysregulation (DSM-5) to mitigate overdiagnosis of bipolar disorder in young children, and the importance of considering developmental effects on mood disorders, there is a clear need to further investigate the course and nature of bipolar symptomatology in individuals with ID.

Mild/moderate ID

Similar to the presentation of depressive disorders, it appears that individuals with mild ID and good expressive language skills will show a full range of symptoms, and minimal adjustments to the diagnostic criteria will be required. The content of cognitive symptoms of mania (inflated self-esteem or grandiosity) may be simplified reflecting the developmental stage of the individual, such as a belief that the person can drive or is getting married when they do not have a partner. The mood may also be more irritable than expansive.

Severe/profound ID

The diagnosis of bipolar disorder is more difficult in individuals with severe or profound ID and affective symptoms may be difficult to distinguish from those related to developmental disabilities (Evans et al., 1995). The challenge is to "detect syndrome-specific affective behavior against a background of nonspecific behavioral responses triggered by a multiplicity of physiological, psychological, and social stimuli" (Sovner and Pary, 1993). While further work on symptom identification in this population is needed, a picture of core clinical features is slowly emerging. For example, psychomotor agitation, disturbed sleep patterns, and changes in mood and aggression correlated with the diagnosis of mania in a group of 15 adults with ID diagnosed with a bipolar disorder (Matson et al., 2007). Similarly, Sturmey et al. (2010b) found that a decreased need for sleep, restlessness, agitation, and irritability were associated with mania in adults with ID.

In this group, full diagnostic criteria for bipolar disorder will likely not be met due to limitations in verbal and cognitive abilities. Diagnosis could be made, however, based on observable criteria/behavioral correlates (Lowry, 1998). For instance, pressured speech may appear as increased vocalization or gesturing, and distractibility as moving from one activity to another, or not being able to complete activities of daily living.

Epidemiology

Considerable heterogeneity exists in the reported prevalence estimates of mood disorders among individuals with ID. Studies have reported prevalence rates of mood disorder ranging from 1.7% to 6.6% (Corbett, 1979; Lund, 1985; Cooper and Bailey, 2001; Cooper et al., 2007). A recent large-scale population-based Australian study with improved design found the prevalence rate of unipolar depression to be lower (0.9%; Morgan et al., 2008) than previously reported rates (2.2% –Deb et al., 2001; 4.1% – Cooper et al., 2007). An accurate assessment of psychopathology in ID is challenging for various reasons, and existing epidemiological studies suffer from significant methodological limitations, which impair generalizability of findings. Examples of such limitations include: (i) failure to report differences in the rates among mood disorders and its subtypes; (ii) failure to report if the rates are point prevalence or lifetime prevalence;

(iii) inadequate or unclear case ascertainment; (iv) application of inadequate or variable screening instruments; and (v) variable composition and size of the study population. In a Scottish epidemiological study (Cooper et al., 2007), the prevalence rate increased when an ID-specific diagnostic instrument, the DC-LD (Royal College of Psychiatrists, 2001), was used, rather than relying on clinical diagnosis.

Some studies have suggested that mood disorders are more common in those with ID than those without ID (Richards et al., 2001), and that prevalence increases with age (Lund, 1985). However, other studies have not supported these findings (Deb et al., 2001; Cooper et al., 2007; Morgan et al., 2008)). The prevalence of depression is higher in women than men (Cooper et al., 2007), as has been found for the general population. No association has been reported between level of ID and depression (Cooper et al., 2007).

The reported prevalence of bipolar disorder (1.3%) is within general population estimates (Morgan et al., 2008). The prevalence of cyclothymia is about 0.3% (Cooper et al., 2007). A recent study examining hospitalized bipolar patients reported that compared to bipolar patients without ID, patients with ID tend to be younger and have significantly longer length of stay (Wu et al., 2013).

There is a considerable dearth of studies examining prevalence rates of mood disorders in children. Existing studies report varying prevalence rates of depression ranging from 1.5% to 4.4% (Dekker and Koot, 2003; Emerson, 2003); thus, very similar to the adult prevalence rates. No parallel epidemiological research has been conducted with regard to bipolar disorder in children.

Suicide. Existing studies clearly support the existence of suicidal behavior and completed suicide among individuals with ID (Lunsky, 2004; Lunsky et al., 2012), albeit the rates tend to be lower than in the general population (see Merrick et al., 2006 for review). Common methods include poisoning or cutting/stabbing. Individuals with ID who attempt suicide tend to be younger and are more likely to visit emergency departments than those who only express suicidal thoughts (Lunsky et al., 2012). Risk factors for attempted/threatened suicide in this population include female gender, a higher level of functioning, previous history of self-harm behaviors (Lunsky et al., 2012), unemployment, perceived stress, loneliness, depression, and anxiety (Merrick et al., 2006).

Etiology
Biological
The etiopathogenesis of mood disorders in ID is yet to be understood. Unfortunately, this has been generally a largely neglected topic in the contemporary psychiatric neuroscience research. The previously hypothesized direct association (Hurley et al., 2003) between ID and depression is yet to be confirmed. Important leads have mainly come from genetic research, and a few genetic syndromes have so far been associated with mood disorder in ID such as Fragile X syndrome, 22q11 deletion syndrome, tuberous sclerosis, Rubinstein–Taybi syndrome, Down syndrome, neurofibromatosis, phenylketonuria (Hassiotis et al., 2014), Prader–Willi syndrome, and Smith–Magenis syndrome (Kerner, 2014). Both depression and bipolar disorder have been associated with these genetic syndromes and, at this point, it is unclear if any of these syndromes has a specific association with any mood disorder subtypes. A recent literature review conducted by

Walker et al. (2011) questioned the previous suggestion that depression is more common in people with Down syndrome.

Psychosocial

Psychosocial variables play an important role in the onset of mood disorders. Symptoms of depression have been associated with negative life events, low social support and stressful interpersonal relationships, and poor self-esteem (Esbensen and Benson, 2006). Negative social experiences including stigmatization, peer rejection, infantilization, and restricted access to employment opportunities have also been identified as risk factors for depression in the ID population (Morin et al., 2010). Trauma, more prevalent in those with ID than in those without, may also be a precursor to mood disorders (Wigham et al., 2011)

Assessment

The diagnosis of mood disorder depends on accurate identification of aspects of feeling and thinking, **and** observable behavior. Establishing baseline functioning, gathering information from multiple sources about diagnostically relevant changes in the mental status or behavior, and allowing a longer period of time for assessment, especially for bipolar disorder, are essential for accurate diagnosis of mood disorders in individuals with ID, particularly in those who cannot self-report. Use of assessment tools validated in the ID population is recommended.

Instruments for assessment of symptoms of depression

Several assessment measures have been developed to assess depressive symptoms specifically in individuals with ID. Two recent exhaustive reviews (Perez-Achiaga et al., 2009; Hermans and Evenhuis, 2010) compared psychometric properties of existing measures, including self-reporting, informant-based, and observation schedules. They concluded that most instruments require further research, particularly regarding sensitivity and specificity in the ID population; however, several promising instruments were highlighted.

Self-reporting

- The Glasgow Depression Scale for people with a Learning Disability (GDS; Cuthill et al., 2003)is a 20-item scale for adults with mild to moderate ID. It also has a 16-item Carer Supplement (GDS-CS) that provides additional clinical information.
- The Self-Report Depression Questionnaire (SRDQ; Reynolds and Baker, 1988) is a 32-item self-report questionnaire developed for individuals with mild ID.

Informant-based

Informant-based depression scales tend to be encompassed in instruments assessing broader psychopathology:

- The Reiss Screen for Maladaptive Behaviour (RSMB; Reiss, 1998) is a 38-item questionnaire of psychiatric symptoms in adolescents and adults with mild to severe ID with two 5-item depression subscales, behavioral signs, and physical signs.
- The Assessment of Dual Diagnosis (ADD; Matson and Bamburg, 1998) is a 79-item screen for psychiatric disorders in individuals with mild to moderate ID with an 8-item depression scale.

- The Psychiatric Assessment Schedule for Adults with Developmental Disabilities Checklist (PAS-ADD Checklist; Moss et al., 1998) is a broad screen for mental health problems in individuals with ID with a 25-item affective/neurotic subscale.

Note: Instruments designed for use with the general population have been used with and without modifications with individuals with ID; however, their validation in this population is limited (Hermans and Evenhuis, 2010).

Instruments for assessment of symptoms of mania/affective disorder

There are several informant-based measures including the six-item Mania subscale of the Assessment of Dual Diagnosis (ADD; Matson and Bamburg, 1998); the five-item Manic/Hyperactive Behaviour subscale of the Anxiety, Depression and Mood Scale (ADAMS; Esbensen et al., 2003), suitable for all levels of ability; and the seven-item Mania scale of the Diagnostic Assessment for the Severely Handicapped–Revised (DASH-II; Matson, 1995), for use with individuals with severe/profound ID. Tools such as the Monthly Sleep Chart (Carr et al., 1998) and the Bipolar Mood Chart (Sovner and Desnoyers-Hurley, 1990) can also aid in the diagnostic process by documenting fluctuations in sleep and mood.

In addition, structured or semi-structured interviews based on the ICD or DSM criteria such as the Psychiatric Assessment Schedule for Adults with Developmental Disabilities (PAS-ADD; Moss et al., 1997) and the Mood and Anxiety Semi-Structured interview (MASS; Charlot et al., 2007a) can assist clinicians in evaluating both depressive and bipolar disorders.

Intervention and treatment

Pharmacological

See also Chapter 14.

Robust evidence of efficacy or safety regarding use of individual agents is lacking, as individuals with ID are either under-represented or excluded from clinical trials. Furthermore, it has been suggested that idiosyncratic and paradoxical reactions tend to occur at a higher rate in people with ID (Antochi and Stavrakaki, 2004; Stavrakaki et al., 2004), and recognition of adverse effects can be difficult in those who have limited communication abilities. Due to these factors, pharmacotherapy should be used cautiously and referral to specialist services should be considered for all complex cases.

The UK's National Institute for Health and Care Excellence (NICE) recommends that when treating individuals with mild ID for depression, where possible offer the same evidence-based interventions utilized in the general population. Due to the favorable risk–benefit ratio, selective serotonin reuptake inhibitors (SSRIs) should be used as the first line of treatment for unipolar depression. Among SSRIs, the efficacy and safety of citalopram and fluoxetine are supported by open-label clinical trials in adults with ID (Howland, 1992; Verhoeven et al., 2001). The efficacy of paroxetine in the treatment of depressed adolescents with ID was also supported in one open-label study (Masi et al., 1997). With regard to bipolar disorder, the main treatment options include mood stabilizers and atypical antipsychotics. There is some evidence through case series that clozapine might be well tolerated and efficacious. Among mood stabilizers, valproic acid/divalproex has the most anecdotal support through case series and chart reviews (Buzan et al., 1998; Ruedrich et al., 1999; see also Chapter 13).

Psychological

See also Chapter 16.

With regard to psychosocial interventions for mood disorder in individuals with ID, the area with the strongest empirical support is cognitive-behavioral therapy (CBT) for depression. Studies have been published in the USA, UK, and Australia, including a recent randomized controlled trial (RCT) focused on individual treatment for anxiety or depression (Hassiotis et al., 2013), and group intervention with a no-treatment control group (McCabe et al., 2006), and a related group-intervention study where the same treatment was delivered by direct care staff (McGillivray et al., 2008). CBT can clearly be modified successfully for this population (see the systematic review by Vereenooghe and Langdon, 2013), but there is agreement that it is not appropriate for individuals with more severe disability due to the difficulty accessing and modifying cognitions. That said, some of the behavioral principles in these types of interventions, such as scheduling pleasurable events, should have utility regardless of cognitive ability. With increased disability severity, the role of caregiver and context become even more important and there is some literature on the use of CBT with caregivers (Kushlick et al., 1997), but not specifically caregivers of individuals with ID and mood disorders. Caregivers can assist the individual to adhere with treatment, which should assist with generalizability and maintenance of treatment gains (see also Chapter 15).

Issues associated with depression etiology can also be intervention targets. If loneliness triggers depression, for example, enhancing the individual's social circle might be beneficial. If depression is caused by stress, removing stressors or providing improved coping strategies can be helpful. However, these types of interventions have yet to receive formal evaluation, with the exception of one study evaluating group treatment for grief (Dowling et al., 2006). No studies of psychosocial treatment for bipolar disorder in ID have been published. That being said, it has been suggested that multimodal interventions, which include behavioral elements, interventions with caregivers, and medication management, can help individuals with these types of difficulties. Further research is warranted.

Conclusions

Mood disorders are common in individuals with ID, although not always well recognized. It remains challenging to assess these disorders in individuals with more severe disabilities and continued efforts are required to develop valid assessment instruments (Adams and Oliver, 2011). While the relationship between challenging behavior, particularly aggression, and mood disturbance in individuals with ID needs to be further investigated, it may be useful to consider the diagnosis of affective disorders in the presence of self-injurious or aggressive behaviors (Hemmings et al., 2006). There are both biological and psychosocial contributors to mood disorders, similar to what has been reported in the general population. More research is required on the effectiveness of pharmacotherapy for this population, particularly around bipolar disorder treatment. There is a growing evidence base for CBT and depression, but psychological interventions for bipolar disorder have been less studied.

Key summary points

- Despite significant advances, mood disorders in ID may still be underdiagnosed.
- Core symptoms can be identified even at severe levels of ID.
- Symptom substitution should be avoided. Externalizing behaviors may be a manifestation of underlying distress and are not diagnostically specific. While not diagnostically specific, challenging behavior seems a key atypical feature of mood disorder in ID.
- Assessment should be multidisciplinary and include information from different sources including the individual.

References

Adams, D. and Oliver, C. (2011). The expression and assessment on emotions and internal states in individuals with severe or profound intellectual disabilities. *Clinical Psychology Review*, 31, 293–306.

Antochi, R. and Stavrakaki, C. (2004). Determining pharmacotherapy options for behavioral disturbances in patients with developmental disabilities. *Psychiatric Annals*, 34, 205–212.

Buzan, R.D., Dubovsky, S.L., Firestone, D., et al. (1998). Use of clozapine in 10 mentally retarded adults. *Journal of Neuropsychiatry and Clinical Neurosciences*, 10, 93–95.

Cain, N.N., Davidson, P.W., Burhan, A.M., et al. (2003). Identifying bipolar disorders in individuals with intellectual disability. *Journal of Intellectual Disability Research*, 47, 31–38.

Carr, E.G., Neumann, J.K., Darnell, C.L. (1998). The clinical importance of sleep data collection: a national survey and case reports. *Mental Health Aspects of Developmental Disabilities*, 1, 39–43.

Charlot, L., Deutsch, C.K., Fletcher, K., et al. (2007a). Validation of the Mood and Anxiety Semi-Structured (MASS) interview for patients with intellectual disabilities. *Journal of Intellectual Disability Research*, 51, 821–834.

Charlot, L., Fox, S., Silka, V.R., et al. (2007b). Mood disorders in individuals with intellectual disability. In R. Fletcher, E. Loschen, C. Stavrakaki, et al. (eds.), *Diagnostic Manual – Intellectual Disability:*

A Textbook of Diagnosis of Mental Disorders in Persons with Intellectual Disability. Kingston, NY: NADD Press.

Cooper, S.A. and Bailey, N.M. (2001). Psychiatric disorders amongst adults with learning disabilities-prevalence and relationship to ability level. *Irish Journal of Psychological Medicine*, 18, 45–53.

Cooper, S.A., Smiley, E., Morrison, J., et al. (2007). Mental ill-health in adults with intellectual disabilities: prevalence and associated factors. *British Journal of Psychiatry*, 190, 27–35.

Corbett, J.A. (1979). Psychiatric morbidity and mental retardation. In F.E. James and R.P. Snaith (eds.), *Psychiatric Illness and Mental Handicap*. London: Gaskell Press.

Cuthill, F.M., Espie, C.A., Cooper, S.A. (2003). Development and psychometric properties of the Glasgow Depression Scale for people with a learning disability. Individual and carer supplement versions. *British Journal of Psychiatry*, 182, 347–353.

Deb, S., Thomas, M., Bright, C. (2001). Mental disorder in adults with intellectual disability. I: prevalence of functional psychiatric illness among a community-based population aged between 16 and 64 years. *Journal of Intellectual Disability Research*, 45, 495–505.

Dekker, M.C. and Koot, H.M. (2003). DSM-IV disorders in children with borderline to moderate intellectual disability. I: prevalence and impact. *Journal of the American Academy of Child and Adolescent Psychiatry*, 42, 915–922.

Dowling, S., Hubert, J., White, S., Hollins, S. (2006) Bereaved adults with intellectual disabilities: a combined randomized controlled trial and qualitative study of two community-based interventions. *Journal of Intellectual Disability Research*, 50(4), 277–287.

Emerson, E. (2003). Prevalence of psychiatric disorders in children and adolescents with and without intellectual disability. *Journal of Intellectual Disability Research*, 47, 51–58.

Esbensen, A.J. and Benson, B.A. (2006). A prospective analysis of life events, problem behaviours and depression in adults with intellectual disability. *Journal of Intellectual Disability Research*, 50, 248–258.

Esbensen, A.J., Rojahn, J., Aman, M.G., et al. (2003). Reliability and validity of an assessment instrument for anxiety, depression, and mood among individuals with mental retardation. *Journal of Autism and Developmental Disorders*, 33, 617–629.

Evans, D.L., Byerly, M.J., Greer, R.A. (1995). Secondary mania: diagnosis and treatment. *Journal of Clinical Psychiatry*, 56, 31–37.

Fletcher, R., Loschen, E., Stavrakaki, C., et al. (eds.) (2007). *Diagnostic Manual – Intellectual Disability: A Textbook of Diagnosis of Mental Disorders in Persons with Intellectual Disability*. Kingston, NY: NADD Press.

Harris, J. (1998). *Developmental Neuropsychiatry Volume II: Assessment, Diagnosis, and Treatment of Developmental Disorders*. New York, NY: Oxford University Press.

Hassiotis, A., Serfaty, M., Azam, K., et al. (2013). Manualised individual cognitive behavioural therapy for mood disorders in people with mild to moderate intellectual disability: a feasibility randomized controlled trial. *Journal of Affective Disorders*, 151, 186–195.

Hassiotis, A., Stueber, K., Thomas, B., et al. (2014). Mood and anxiety disorders. In E. Tsakanikos and J. McCarthy (eds.), *Handbook of Psychopathology in Intellectual Disability: Research, Practice, and Policy*. New York, NY: Springer Science.

Hemmings, C.P., Gravestock, S., Pickard, M. et al. (2006). Psychiatric symptoms and problem behaviours in people with intellectual disabilities. *Journal of Intellectual Disability Research*, 50, 269–276.

Hermans, H. and Evenhuis, H.M. (2010). Characteristics of instruments screening for depression in adults with intellectual disabilities: systematic review. *Research in Developmental Disabilities*, 31, 1109–1120.

Howland, R.H. (1992). Fluoxetine treatment of depression in mentally retarded adults. *Journal of Nervous and Mental Disease*, 180, 202–205.

Hurley, A.D. (2008). Depression in adults with intellectual disability: symptoms and challenging behaviour. *Journal of Intellectual Disability Research*, 52, 905–916.

Hurley, A.D., Folstein, M., Lam, N. (2003). Patients with and without intellectual disability seeking outpatient psychiatric services: diagnoses and prescribing pattern. *Journal of Intellectual Disability Research*, 47, 39–50.

Kerner, B. (2014). Genetics of bipolar disorder. *Application of Clinical Genetics*, 12, 33–42.

Kushlick, A., Trower, P., Dagnan, D. (1997). Applying cognitive-behavioural approaches to the carers of people with learning disabilities who display challenging behaviour. In B. Stenfert Kroese, D. Dagnan, K. Loumidis (eds.), *Cognitive-Behaviour Therapy for People with Learning Disabilities*. London: Routledge.

Lowry, M. (1998). Assessment and treatment of mood disorders in persons with developmental disability. *Journal of Developmental and Physical Disability*, 10, 387–406.

Lund, J. (1985). The prevalence of psychiatric morbidity in mentally retarded adults. *Acta Psychiatrica Scandinavica*, 72, 563–570.

Lunsky, Y. (2004). Suicidality in a clinical and community sample of adults with mental retardation. *Research in Developmental Disabilities*, 25, 231–243.

Lunsky, Y., Raina, P., Burge, P. (2012). Suicidality among adults with intellectual disability. *Journal of Affective Disorders*, 140, 292–295.

Marston, G.M., Perry, D., Roy, A. (1997). Manifestations of depression in people with intellectual disabilities. *Journal of Intellectual Disability Research*, 41, 476–480.

Masi, G., Marcheschi, M., Pfanner, P. (1997). Paroxetine in depressed adolescents with intellectual disability: an open label study. *Journal of Intellectual Disability Research*, 41, 268–272.

Matson, J.L. (1995). *Diagnostic Assessement for the Severely Handicapped-II.* Baton Rouge, LA: Disability Consultants.

Matson, J.L. and Bamburg, J.W. (1998). Reliability of the Assessment of Dual Diagnosis (ADD). *Research in Developmental Disabilities*, 19, 89–95.

Matson, J.L., Gonzalez, M.L., Terlonge, C., et al. (2007). What symptoms predict the diagnosis of mania in persons with severe/profound intellectual disability in clinical practice? *Journal of Intellectual Disability Research*, 51, 25–31.

McCabe, M.P., McGillivray, J.A., Newton, D.C. (2006). Effectiveness of treatment programmes for depression among adults with mild/moderate intellectual disability. *Journal of Intellectual Disability Research*, 50, 239–247.

McGillivray, J., McCabe, M., Kershaw, M. (2008) Depression in people with intellectual disability: an evaluation of a staff-administered treatment program. *Research in Developmental Disabilities*, 29, 524–536.

Merrick, J., Merrick, E., Lunsky, Y., et al. (2006). A review of suicidality in persons with intellectual disability. *Israel Journal of Psychiatry and Related Sciences*, 43, 258–264.

Morgan V.A., Leonard H., Bourke J., et al. (2008). Intellectual disability co-occurring with schizophrenia and other psychiatric illness: population-based study. *British Journal of Psychiatry*, 193, 364–372.

Morin, D., Rivard, M., Cobigo, V., et al. (2010). Intellectual disabilities and depression: how to adapt psychological assessment and intervention. *Canadian Psychology*, 51, 185–193.

Moss, S., Ibbotson, B., Prosser, H., et al. (1997). Validity of the PSA-ADD for detecting psychiatric symptoms in adults with learning disability (mental retardation). *Social Psychiatry and Psychiatric Epidemiology*, 32, 344–354.

Moss, S., Prosser, H., Costello, H., et al. (1998). Reliability and validity of the PAS-ADD checklist for detecting psychiatric disorders in adults with intellectual disability. *Journal of Intellectual Disability Research*, 42, 173–183.

Perez-Achiaga, N., Nelson, N., Hassiotis, A. (2009). Instruments for the detection of depressive symptoms in people with intellectual disabilities: a systematic review. *Journal of Intellectual Disabilities*, 13, 55–76.

Reiss, S. (1988). *The Reiss Screen for Maladaptive Behavior: Test Manual.* Worthington, OH: IDS Publishing.

Reynolds, W.M. and Baker, J.A. (1988). Assessment of depression in persons with mental retardation. *American Journal on Mental Retardation*, 93, 93–103.

Richards, M., Maughan, B., Hardy, R., et al. (2001). Long-term affective disorder in people with mild learning disability. *British Journal of Psychiatry*, 179, 523–527.

Ross, E. and Oliver, C. (2003). The assessment of mood in adults who have severe or profound mental retardation. *Clinical Psychology Review*, 23, 225–245.

Royal College of Psychiatrists (2001). *Diagnostic Criteria for Psychiatric Disorders for Use with Adults with Learning Disabilities/Mental Retardation (DC-LD).* London: Royal College of Psychiatrists.

Ruedrich, S., Swales, T.P., Fassaceca, C., et al. (1999). Effect of divalproex sodium on aggression and self-injurious behaviour in adults with intellectual disability: a retrospective review. *Journal of Intellectual Disability Research*, 43, 105–111.

Sovner, R. and Desnoyers-Hurley, A.D. (1990).
Bipolar mood chart. *Habilitative Healthcare
Newsletter*, 9, 96.

Sovner, R. and Pary, R. (1993). Affective
disorders in developmentally disabled
persons. In J.L. Matson and R.P. Barrett
(eds.), *Psychopathology in the Mentally
Retarded*. Needham Heights, MA: Allyn
and Bacon.

Stavrakaki, C., Antochi, R., Emery, C. (2004).
Olanzapine in the treatment of pervasive
developmental disorders: a case series
analysis. *Journal of Psychiatry and
Neuroscience*, 29, 57–60.

Sturmey, P., Laud, R.B., Cooper, C.L., et al.
(2010a). Challenging behaviors should not
be considered depressive equivalents in
individuals with intellectual disabilities.
II. A replication study. *Research in
Developmental Disabilities*, 31, 1002–1007.

Sturmey, P., Laud, R.B., Cooper C.L., et al.
(2010b). Mania and behavioral equivalents:
a preliminary study. *Research in
Developmental Disabilities*, 31, 1008–1014.

Tsiouris, J.A., Mann, R., Patti, P.J., et al.
(2003). Challenging behaviours should not
be considered as depressive equivalents in
individuals with intellectual disability.

Journal of Intellectual Disability Research,
47, 14–21.

Vereenooghe, L. and Langdon, P.E. (2013).
Psychological therapies for people with
intellectual disabilities: a systematic review
and meta-analysis. *Research in
Developmental Disabilities*, 34, 4085–4102.

Verhoeven, W.M., Veendrik-Meekes, M.J.,
Jacobs, G.A., et al. (2001). Citalopram in
mentally retarded patients with depression:
a long-term clinical investigation. *European
Psychiatry: Journal of the Association of
European Psychiatrists*, 16, 104–108.

Walker, J.C., Dosen, A., Buitelaar, J.K., et al.
(2011). Depression in Down syndrome: a
review of the literature. *Research in
Developmental Disabilities*, 32, 1432–1440.

Wigham, S., Hatton, C., Taylor, J.L. (2011).
The effects of traumatizing life events on
people with intellectual disabilities: a
systematic review. *Journal of Mental Health
Research in Intellectual Disabilities*, 4, 19–39.

Wu, C.S., Desarkar, P., Palucka, A., et al.
(2013). Acute inpatient treatment,
hospitalization course and direct costs in
bipolar patients with intellectual disability.
Research in Developmental Disabilities,
34, 4062–4072.

Anxiety disorders

Jane McCarthy and Eddie Chaplin

Introduction

Anxiety disorders as defined in the *Diagnostic and Statistical Manual of Mental Disorders, Fifth Edition* (DSM-5; American Psychiatric Association, 2013) "include disorders that share features of excessive fear and anxiety and related behavioral disturbance. Fear is the emotional response to real or perceived imminent threat, whereas anxiety is the anticipation of future threat." The fear or anxiety is not transient but persistent, usually lasting six months or more. Within DSM-5 the chapter on anxiety disorders includes disorders that occur in childhood, namely separation anxiety disorders and selective mutism, but also specific phobias, social anxiety disorder (social phobia), panic disorder, agoraphobia, and generalized anxiety disorder. The focus of this chapter is to cover conditions that are commonly diagnosed in adult life and so come under sections F40 and F41 within the *International Classification of Diseases and Related Health Problems, Tenth Revision* (ICD-10; World Health Organization, 1992), and include phobic anxiety disorders, panic disorders, and generalized anxiety disorder. Anxiety disorders do occur in people with ID but may be missed (Stavrakaki and Lunsky, 2007; Davis et al., 2008). Due to the limitations of DSM-5 and ICD-10 in diagnosing mental disorders in people with ID the *Diagnostic Manual – Intellectual Disability* (DM-ID; Fletcher et al., 2007) was developed in the USA and the *Diagnostic Criteria for Psychiatric Disorders for Use with Adults with Learning Disabilities/Mental Retardation* (DC-LD) was developed in the UK to complement the ICD-10 (DC-LD; Royal College of Psychiatrists, 2001). The use of an adapted diagnostic system can increase the rates of diagnosing anxiety and other mental disorders in people with ID (Cooper et al., 2007).

Anxiety disorders are estimated to occur in 2–17% of people with ID (Reid et al., 2011), and it is generally accepted that rates of anxiety disorders are comparable to the wider population. The prevalence in the wider population for generalized anxiety disorder over a 12-month period is estimated to be 3.1%, and for agoraphobia 0.8% (Kessler et al., 2005), with a lifetime prevalence of 1.7% for agoraphobia in adolescents and adults (American Psychiatric Association, 2013). This compares to a point prevalence of 4% of anxiety disorders in a recent large-scale population study of people with ID in Glasgow, Scotland (Reid et al., 2011). Generalized anxiety disorder was the most common disorder at a rate of 1.7%, followed by agoraphobia at a prevalence of 0.7%. The participants in this study underwent a structured mental health assessment and the

Psychiatric and Behavioral Disorders in Intellectual and Developmental Disabilities, ed. Colin Hemmings and Nick Bouras. Published by Cambridge University Press. © Cambridge University Press 2016.

diagnosis was made using ICD-10 criteria. Another cross-sectional study of those with mild ID using ICD-10 criteria and in those with severe ID using the Diagnostic Assessment for the Severely Handicapped scale found a prevalence rate of 2.2% for generalized anxiety disorder (Deb et al., 2001).

History-taking and presentation

People with ID may present with anxiety symptoms in an atypical way in terms of complaining of physical symptoms or presenting with a form of challenging behavior. It is important to recognize that developmental level may affect the presentation, and to be a disorder the fear or anxiety must be in excess or persist beyond what is expected for that developmental level. A full physical examination is required to identify any conditions that can be wrongly diagnosed as anxiety, such as thyroid disease or caffeine-induced anxiety disorder. For people with mild to moderate ID, the history should be taken in the same way as for the wider population, which is by direct enquiry of their symptoms. For those with severe ID, then additional observations from informants on behavior, such as sleep pattern, irritability, and aggression, is needed to aid diagnosis. There are no recommended investigations except those needed in the ruling out of medical conditions.

Generalized anxiety disorder presents as excessive anxiety, worry, and apprehension occurring for most days for six months (DM-ID; Fletcher et al., 2007), which the person finds difficult to control. The symptoms present as restlessness or feeling on edge, irritability, mind going blank, being easily fatigued, muscle tension, sleep difficulties, such as problems with getting off to sleep or remaining asleep, or having a restless night. Anxiety disorders also present with somatic or autonomic symptoms such as dry mouth, difficulty swallowing, sweating, shaking, chest pain, headache, fatigue, and urinary frequency. The behavioral response of anxiety is avoidance of situations, for example in those with agoraphobia, to be hypervigilant, to show a startle response, a reduced libido, and problems with concentrating. Anxiety can present as an episode such as panic disorder, be continuous in a generalized anxiety disorder, or in response to a specific stressful event such as moving to a new placement. Generalized anxiety disorder peaks in middle age and declines across the later years of life. There is no evidence to say this pattern is different for people with ID.

Panic disorder presents as a discrete period of intense fear or discomfort. In panic disorder, people have symptoms of palpitations in which the heart feels as if it is racing and pounding. The person can be observed to be sweating and trembling, with difficulty breathing, and may hyperventilate. The person may complain of chest pain, feeling dizzy, or look gray in color as if they are going to collapse. They can sometimes have feelings of unreality such as derealization, or being detached from oneself that is depersonalization, or fear that they are going to lose control. Symptoms of depersonalization and derealization may be difficult to detect in those with moderate to severe ID (Cooray et al., 2007). The person with ID may complain of a fear of dying or numbness sensations with observed chills or hot flushes. Extreme panic may result in aggression and destructive behavior.

Phobic anxiety disorders can present as specific phobias in which the person has persistent fear of specific things, such as blood, having an injection, or animals. The individual may have a phobia for a specific situation, such as going in an elevator, enclosed places, or going on an aeroplane. In agoraphobia, people have anxiety around a place or situation usually outside the home, such as an open market place or traveling in a train, in which escape may be difficult. Agoraphobia can start in childhood but peaks in late adolescence and early adulthood.

Social phobia is fear of failing in social situations or performing in front of other people. Social phobias may happen when people are exposed to unfamiliar people or maybe scrutiny by others. The individual fears being negatively evaluated by others or being rejected or humiliated by others. They may express this fear or anxiety in those with severe ID through tantrums, freezing, or shrinking from social situations with unfamiliar people (Cooray et al., 2007).

Risk factors

Females have higher rates of anxiety disorders than men, and this possibly may be due to women being subjected to more stressful life events. Reports of childhood experiences of sexual and physical abuse are more common in panic disorder than in certain other anxiety disorders. A third of the risk of experiencing generalized anxiety disorder is genetic and overlaps with the risk for negative affectivity (American Psychiatric Association, 2013).

There are a number of reasons why people with ID might be vulnerable to developing anxiety disorders. This could be due to people with ID having high rates of physical health problems, being more socially excluded, and being more at risk of experiencing adversity (Hassiotis et al., 2014). In the Glasgow Study, Reid et al. (2011) found not having daytime employment and a recent history of life events were associated with having an anxiety disorder, but that previously being a long-term hospital resident was not linked with having an anxiety disorder in adults with ID. A life event such as a bereavement has also been reported to increase the risk for both anxiety and depressive symptoms in people with ID (Dodd et al., 2005; see also Chapter 9).

Some genetic conditions associated with ID, such as tuberous sclerosis and Williams syndrome, report anxiety to be common (Paschos et al., 2014). Anxiety is reported to occur frequently in people with autism and ID (Helverschou and Martinsen, 2011). Structural parts of the brain system, such as the amygdala and hippocampus, have been implicated in the development of the anxiety disorders, as have neurotransmitters, such as serotonin and gamma-aminobutyric acid (GABA), which are also implicated in the brains of those with autism spectrum disorders (Romanczyk et al., 2006).

Diagnostic tools

There are a number of tools and instruments for identifying and diagnosing individuals with anxiety disorders in people with ID (Moss and Hurley, 2014).

These can include instruments that are based on interview with an informant to obtain the history, or tools can be used directly with the individual to elicit self-report symptoms.

Informant-based tools

The Psychiatric Assessment Schedule for Adults with Developmental Disabilities (PAS-ADD; Moss et al., 1993) is a semi-structured interview of an informant that produces a psychiatric diagnosis using ICD-10 criteria. There are smaller, related measures, such as the Mini PAS-ADD and the PAS-ADD Checklist. The PAS-ADD Checklist (Moss et al., 1998) serves as a screening tool to identify people with depressive or anxiety symptoms. The Mini PAS-ADD contains a subscale for anxiety and can be used by people who are not mental health specialists (Prosser et al., 1998).

The Diagnostic Assessment for the Severely Handicapped–II (DASH-II) schedule was developed for those with severe and profound ID (Matson, 1995). The DASH-II has demonstrated good inter-rater reliability and validity and contains 13 subscales, which includes anxiety.

The Developmental Behavior Checklist (DBC) was initially developed for use with children and adolescents (Einfeld and Tonge, 2002), but now has an adult version (DBC-A) with 107 items. The DBC-A is designed to assess behavioral and emotional problems of adults with ID. This instrument has been widely used and has six subscales, including anxiety.

Another tool with reported psychometric properties that has been used to assess anxiety is the Psychopathology Inventory for Mentally Retarded Adults (PIMRA; Aman et al., 1986). This is used to support making a diagnosis and, although it is able to recognize symptoms, it may overestimate rates of the disorder (Gustafsson and Sonnander, 2005). An earlier Swedish study of those with ID in contact with mental health services reported a prevalence rate of anxiety of 26.8% using the PIMRA (Gustafsson and Sonnander, 2004).

Self-report tools

The Glasgow Anxiety Scale for people with an ID (GAS-ID; Mindham and Espie, 2003) is one of the only anxiety scales developed specifically for people with ID. It consists of 27 items broken down into three subscales: worries, physiology, and phobias. The GAS-ID has demonstrated good reliability and validity and is easy to administer in clinical practice.

The Fear Survey for Adults with Mental Retardation (FSAMR) is an instrument designed to measure current fears that are specific to people with ID given their experience. The FSAMR is administered verbally to the individual (Ramirez and Lukenbill, 2007) and includes 73 fear items from which fear frequency and intensity scores are calculated.

Other tools include the Beck Depression Inventory (BDI), which is widely used in clinical practice in the wider population and has been modified to be used with people with intellectual disabilities (Lindsay and Skene, 2007). The Hospital Anxiety and Depression Scale (HADS) has been used in assessing adults with ID, but needs adaptation of wording with further evaluation of the psychometric properties (Dagnan et al., 2008).

Management and treatment

The key first task is to undertake a multidisciplinary assessment. It is important not only to assess the presenting symptoms and behaviors but also how the person is functioning at home or in the day-service or at work and to review their current medication, including any evidence of substance misuse. It is important to obtain a history of current social supports, including their living situation, family relationships, and the level of support they are receiving. In addition, any other comorbid conditions that occur, such as depression or dementia, need to be identified, as do any physical health problems. When anxiety is comorbid with depression then the first priority should be to treat the depression. Often people with generalized anxiety disorder have sleep disturbance, and it is important to advise them around regular sleep and wake times, taking physical exercise, and ensuring proper environment for sleep. Substance misuse needs to be assessed as a possible comorbid condition and within DSM-5, substance/medication-induced anxiety disorder is recognized as a specific condition. Anxiety disorders may occur in the context of autism spectrum disorders in adults with ID, but there are challenges in making the diagnosis (Hagopian and Jennett, 2008), and the physiological symptoms of anxiety may be more difficult to recognize in those with autism (Helverschou and Martinsen, 2011).

Medication

See also Chapter 13.

The first choice of antidepressant for anxiety disorders will often be a selective serotonin reuptake inhibitor (SSRI; for example, sertraline), and if the person's anxiety does not respond to one antidepressant then this can be changed to a different SSRI antidepressant. Alternatively, antidepressants from a different class can be used, such as serotonin noradrenaline reuptake inhibitors (SNRI), as advised in guidelines from the UK's National Collaborating Centre for Mental Health (2011). There is little evidence for the prescription of antipsychotics used on their own or in combination with an anti-depressant for anxiety disorders (Pies, 2009). Benzodiazepines or antipsychotic drugs should not be offered for the treatment of anxiety disorders in a primary care setting but only be prescribed with specialist advice. The prescriber needs to show caution with anxiolytics in adults with ID as they may cause paradoxical excitement and disinhibition (King, 2007). Pregabalin can also be offered if the person cannot tolerate an antidepressant. The patient may not respond to a psychological intervention alone, so combining an antidepressant with cognitive-behavioral therapy (CBT) is recommended in national guidance, as described below.

The NICE guidelines from the Department of Health in England covering general anxiety disorder recommend a stepped-care model (National Institute for Health and Clinical Excellence, 2011). The stepped-care model considers anxiety in increasing intensity in each of the steps, outlining the appropriate treatment, treatment location and support needed, and how services are organized to deliver the most effective interventions according to individual clinical presentation. Intervention is designed to "relieve symptoms, restore function and prevent relapse" (National Institute for Health and Clinical Excellence, 2011) by targeting the triggers and factors that maintains the condition. The guidelines state that when assessing people with moderate to severe ID, clinicians need to consult with the relevant specialist.

It is now generally accepted that people with ID can benefit from psychological treatments, although some still cast aspersions as to its effectiveness in this group (Hassiotis et al, 2011). Adaptation of CBT may be required on an individual basis depending on the individual's level of ability with regards to language, communication, memory, and planning. For those with mild ID, the same interventions apply as for the general population but may need to take into account the delivery and duration of the intervention (see also Chapter 15). In the early steps of treatment, NICE guidelines recommend the use of interventions such as individual guided self-help (GSH) or psychoeducational groups. All these treatments are based on the principles of CBT but involve minimal therapist contact. For severe anxiety, the options are individual high-intensity psychological interventions, such as CBT, or applied relaxation and/or drug treatment.

Improving Access to Psychological Therapies (IAPTs) teams have been created in the UK to provide psychological assessment and management of anxiety disorders. The reality is, however, that many IAPTs services still do not take referrals of people with ID (Burke 2014), even though UK policy advocates equal access to mental health services for this group. In some areas, specialist IAPTs teams for individuals with ID have been developed (Improving Access to Psychological Therapies teams, 2009).

There are a number of psychological interventions available to treat anxiety and, according to the severity of individual clinical presentations, psychological interventions are split into high- and low-intensity interventions. Low-intensity interventions are embedded in the stepped-care approach and are used in cases of mild to moderate anxiety. This type of intervention is delivered usually within primary care settings, but can be seen in use in secondary and tertiary settings where anxiety coexists with other mental illness. Low-intensity interventions normally use cognitive-behavioral therapy and rely on helping the person understand their condition and to teach strategies aimed at self-management. This is in the form of non-facilitated help where the person is directed to appropriate self-help materials according to their needs. This differs from GSH, which is facilitated by a healthcare professional who guides, monitors, and supports the person in treatment. The systematic review of non-facilitated help reported a "significant moderate effect" size for anxiety scores and rates of relapse when compared to non-active controls for generalized anxiety disorder (National Institute for Health and Clinical Excellence, 2011). The NICE review on GSH reported on four RCTs with some improvement in the treatment groups, but the evidence was of insufficient quality to draw any inferences (National Institute for Health and Clinical Excellence, 2011). However, there is no evidence reported in these reviews relating to individuals with ID.

High-intensity interventions are used to treat moderate to severe forms of anxiety, including phobias and generalized anxiety disorder, and for those who have not responded to treatment using low-intensity interventions. High-intensity interventions include applied relaxation, where the person manages their anxiety whilst exposed to the situation which triggers anxiety, and a number of psychotherapeutic approaches. Of these, CBT is the most common and, working with a therapist, the individual works on set goals that are informed by a shared formulation relating to the presented problem. The NICE systematic review of 12 RCTs reported significant improvements in response and remission rates (indicated by a 75% response rate using a validated anxiety measure) in treating anxiety for those receiving CBT compared to waiting-list controls. There is not the same strength of evidence for the use of CBT for anxiety disorders in populations of people with ID. The best evidence evaluating psychological interventions in populations of people with ID has come from systematic and general reviews (Hatton, 2002; Hassiotis and Hall, 2008; Brown et al., 2011), but with little evidence on how interventions work and are delivered (Wilner, 2005). Hassiotis et al. (2011) has developed a manual of CBT for individuals with ID that covers the treatment of common mental disorders in an attempt to define and standardize what is a modified approach. This manual is freely available at www.ucl.ac.uk/psychiatry/cbt. There is less evidence on the clinical effectiveness of low-level psychological interventions in people with ID, and what is available is mostly anecdotal.

In recent years there has been an increasing interest in the use of GSH (Chaplin et al., 2012, 2013; Chester et al., 2013). This has included publication of the SAINT, which is the first GSH manual and resources publicly available to have been developed specifically for people with ID (Chaplin et al., 2014). A single-case experimental design (SCED) (A–B–A–B) was used in the SAINT study. Twelve participants completed all four phases with nine (75%) demonstrating decreased symptom scores in both intervention phases for depression and three (25%) for anxiety. Two of the participants and a control replicated the SCED over a longer period with the intention to see if the results could be replicated over a longer period. All three of the participants showed a decrease in anxiety symptoms in both intervention phases and two (66.6%) had decreased depression scores. Overall, those with a history of affective disorders ($N = 8$) showed the most consistent improvement (Chaplin, 2014).

Conclusions

It appears that individuals with ID are not evidently at increased risk of anxiety disorders compared to the general population. However, the limited studies have reported variable prevalence rates depending on diagnostic system used and the population under study. When anxiety symptoms occur in people with ID they are often not recognized by health professionals to be a condition that needs further assessment and treatment (Hassiotis et al., 2014). The NICE guidelines (National Institute for Health and Clinical Excellence, 2011) from the UK provide evidence of the stepped-care approach to the assessment and treatment of anxiety disorders. However, there is limited evidence of the effectiveness of these approaches for individuals with ID who experience barriers when trying to access the psychological treatments available. There are still those that question the ability of people with ID to engage in such treatments, but in the last few years resources for both CBT and GSH specifically developed for people with ID have become available (Hassiotis et al., 2011; Chaplin et al., 2014). There needs to be a focus on supporting people with ID and carers to recognize when they have anxiety, so they can access interventions with emerging evidence of effectiveness (Hassiotis et al., 2011) and have more control over their mental and physical well-being (Burke, 2014; Taggart and Cousins, 2014). Future research is needed on the application of these adapted treatment manuals in different clinical settings, with evaluation of their effectiveness in combination with psychopharmacological treatments in adults with ID.

Key summary points

- Anxiety disorders are estimated to occur in 2–17% of adults with ID, and these rates are comparable to the wider population.
- Life events, such as bereavement, increase the risk of anxiety disorders in adults with ID.
- There are an increasing number of self-report tools and measures that have been developed specifically for the diagnosis of anxiety disorders in adults with ID.
- There are treatments that have been developed in recent years for adults with ID and anxiety disorders, including manualized approaches to CBT and GSH.

References

Aman, M.G., Watson, J.E., Singh, N.N., et al. (1986). Psychometric and demographic characteristics of the psychopathology instrument for mentally retarded adults. *Psychopharmacology Bulletin*, 22, 1072–1076.

American Psychiatric Association. (2013). *Diagnostic and Statistical Manual of Mental Disorders, Fifth Edition*. Washington, DC: American Psychiatric Association.

Brown, M., Duff, H., Karatzias, T., Horsburgh, D. (2011). A review of the literature relating to psychological interventions and people with intellectual disabilities: issues for research, policy, education and clinical practice. *Journal of Intellectual Disabilities*, 15, 31–45.

Burke, C.-K. (2014). *Feeling Down: Improving the Mental Health of People with Learning Disabilities*. London, Foundation for People with Learning Disabilities.

Chaplin, E. (2014). Is guided self help a treatment option for people with intellectual disability? PhD thesis. London: Institute of Psychiatry, King's College London.

Chaplin, E., Craig, T., Bouras, N. (2012). Using service user and expert opinion, to identify and review items for the SAINT: a guided self-help pack for adults with intellectual disability. *Advances in Mental Health and Intellectual Disabilities*, 6(1), 17–25.

Chaplin, E., Chester, R., Tsakanikos, E., et al. (2013). Reliability and validity of the SAINT: a guided self-help tool for people with intellectual disabilities. *Journal of Mental Health Research in Intellectual Disabilities*, 6(3), 245–253.

Chaplin, E., McCarthy, J., Hardy, S., et al. (2014). *Guided Self-help for People with Intellectual Disabilities and Anxiety and Depression*, Brighton, UK: Pavilion.

Chester, R., Chaplin, E., Tsakanikos, E., et al. (2013). Gender differences in self-reported symptoms of depression and anxiety in adults with intellectual disabilities. *Advances in Mental Health and Intellectual Disabilities*, 7(4), 191–200.

Cooper, S.-A., Smiley, E., Morrison, J., Williamson, A., Allan, L. (2007). Mental ill-health in adults with intellectual disability: prevalence and associated factors. *British Journal of Psychiatry*, 190, 27–35.

Cooray, S., Cooper, S.-A., Gabriel, S., Gaus, V. (2007). Anxiety disorders. In R. Fletcher, E. Loschen, C. Stavrakaki (eds.), *Diagnostic Manual – Intellectual Disability (DM-ID): A Textbook of Diagnosis of Mental Disorders in Persons with Intellectual Disability*. Kingston, NY: NADD Press.

Dagnan, D., Jahoda, A., McDowell, K., et al. (2008). The psychometric properties of the hospital anxiety and depressions scales adapted for use with people with intellectual disabilities. *Journal of Intellectual Disability Research*, 52, 942–949.

Davis, E., Saeed, S.A., Antonacci, D.J. (2008). Anxiety disorders in persons with developmental disabilities: empirical informed diagnosis and treatment. *Psychiatr Q*, 79, 249–263.

Deb, S., Thomas, M., Bright, C. (2001). Mental disorder in adults with intellectual disability: prevalence of functional psychiatric illness among a community-based population aged between 16 and 64 years. *Journal of Intellectual Disability Research*, 45, 495–505.

Dodd, P., Dowling, S., Hollins, S. (2005). A review of the emotional, psychiatric and behavioural responses to bereavement in people with intellectual disabilities. *Journal of Intellectual Disability Research*, 49, 537–543.

Einfeld, S.L. and Tonge, B.J. (2002). *Manual for the Developmental Behaviour Checklist*, second edition. Clayton: Monash University Center for Developmental Psychiatry and School of Psychiatry, University of New South Wales.

Fletcher, R., Loschen, E., Stavrakaki, C., et al. (eds.) (2007). *Diagnostic Manual – Intellectual Disability: A Textbook of Diagnosis of Mental Disorders in Persons with Intellectual Disability*. Kingston, NY: NADD Press.

Gustafsson, C. and Sonnander, K. (2004). Occurrence of mental health problems in Swedish sample of adults with intellectual disabilities. *Social Psychiatry and Psychiatric Epidemiology*, 39, 448–456.

Gustafsson, C. and Sonnander, K. (2005). A psychometric evaluation of a Swedish version of the psychopathology inventory for mentally retarded adults (PIMRA). *Research in Developmental Disabilities*, 26, 183–201.

Hagopian, L.P. and Jennett, H.K. (2008). Behavioural assessment and treatment of anxiety in individuals with intellectual disabilities and autism. *Journal of Developmental and Physical Disabilities*, 20, 467–483.

Hassiotis, A. and Hall, I. (2008). Behavioural and cognitive-behavioural interventions for outwardly-directed aggressive behaviour in people with learning disabilities. *Cochrane Database of Systematic Reviews*, 3, CD003406.

Hassiotis, A., Serfaty, M., Azam, K., et al. (2011). Cognitive behaviour therapy (CBT) for anxiety and depression in adults with mild intellectual disability (ID): a pilot randomised controlled trial. *Trials*, 12: 95.

Hassiotis, A., Stueber, T.B., Charlot, L. (2014). Depressive and anxiety disorders in intellectual disability. In E. Tsakanikos and J. McCarthy (eds.), *Handbook of Psychopathology in Intellectual Disability: Research, Policy and Practice*. New York, NY: Springer Science.

Hatton, C. (2002). Psychosocial interventions for adults with intellectual disabilities and mental health problems: a review. *Journal of Mental Health*, 11, 357–374.

Helverschou, S.B. and Martinsen, H. (2011). Anxiety in people diagnosed with autism and intellectual disability: recognition and phenomenology. *Research in Autism Spectrum Disorders*, 5, 377–387.

Improving Access to Psychological Therapies (IPATs) teams (2009) *Improving Access to Psychological Therapies: Learning Disability Positive Practice Guide*. At: http://www.iapt .nhs.uk/silo/files/learning-disabilities-positive-practice-guide-2013.pdf

Kessler, R.C., Chiu, W.T., Demler, O., et al. (2005). Prevalence, severity and comorbidity of 12-month DSM-IV disorders in the National Comorbidity Survey Replication. *Archives of General Psychiatry*, 62, 617–627.

King, B. (2007). Psychopharmacology in intellectual disabilities. In N. Bouras and G. Holt (eds.), *Psychiatric and Behavioural Disorders in Intellectual and Developmental Disabilities*, second edition. Cambridge: Cambridge University Press.

Lindsay, W.R. and Skene, D.D. (2007). The Beck Depression Inventory II and the Beck Anxiety Inventory in people with intellectual disabilities: factor analyses and group data. *Journal of Applied Research in Intellectual Disabilities*, 28, 401–408.

Matson, J.L. (1995). *Diagnostic Assessment for the Severely Handicapped Scale (DASH-II)*. Baton Rouge, LA: Disability Consultants.

Mindham, J. and Espie, C.A. (2003). Glasgow Anxiety Scale for people with an Intellectual Disability (GAS-ID): development and psychometric properties of a new measure for use with people with mild intellectual disability. *Journal of Intellectual Disability Research*, 47, 22–30.

Moss, S. and Hurley, A.D. (2014). Integrating assessment instruments within the diagnostic process. In E. Tsakanikos and J. McCarthy (eds.), *Handbook of Psychopathology in Intellectual Disability: Research, Policy and Practice*. New York, NY: Springer Science.

Moss S., Patel P., Prosser H., et al. (1993). Psychiatric morbidity in older people with moderate and severe learning disability (mental retardation). Part I: development and reliability of the patient interview (the PAS-ADD). *British Journal of Psychiatry*, 163, 471–480.

Moss, S., Prosser, H., Costello, H., et al. (1998). Reliability and validity of the PAS-ADD checklist for detecting psychiatric disorders in adults with intellectual disability. *Journal of Intellectual Disability Research*, 42, 173–183.

National Collaborating Centre for Mental Health. (2011). *Guidelines Number 123 – Common*

Mental Health Disorders: the NICE Guidelines on Identification and Pathways in Care. London: British Psychological Society and Royal College of Psychiatrists.

National Institute for Health and Clinical Excellence. (2011). *Generalised Anxiety Disorder (With or Without Agoraphobia) in Adults. NICE Guideline [CG113].* London: National Institute for Health and Clinical Excellence.

Paschos, D., Bass, N., Strydom, A. (2014). Behavioural phenotypes and genetic syndromes. In E. Tsakanikos and J. McCarthy (eds.), *Handbook of Psychopathology in Intellectual Disability: Research, Policy and Practice.* New York, NY: Springer Science.

Pies, R. (2009). Should psychiatrists use atypical antipsychotics to treat nonpsychotic anxiety? *Psychiatry*, 6, 29–37.

Prosser, H., Moss, S.C., Costello, H., et al. (1998). Reliability and validity of the Mini PAS-AOD for assessing psychiatric disorders in adults with intellectual disability. *Journal of Intellectual Disability Research*, 42, 264–272.

Ramirez, S.Z. and Lukenbill, J.F. (2007). Development of the fear survey for adults with mental retardation. *Research in Developmental Disabilities*, 28, 225–237.

Reid, K.A., Smiley, E., Cooper, S.A. (2011). Prevalence and associations of anxiety disorders in adults with intellectual disability. *Journal of Intellectual Disability Research*, 55, 172–181.

Romanczyk, R.G., Gillis, J.M., Barron, M.G., et al. (2006). *Autism and the Physiology of Stress and Anxiety. Stress and Coping in Autism.* New York, NY: Oxford University Press.

Royal College of Psychiatrists (2001). *Diagnostic Criteria for Psychiatric Disorders for Use with Adults with Learning Disabilities/Mental Retardation (DC-LD).* London: Royal College of Psychiatrists.

Stavrakaki, C. and Lunsky, Y. (2007). Depression, anxiety and adjustment disorder in people with intellectual disability. In N. Bouras and G. Holt (eds.), *Psychiatric and Behavioural Disorders in Intellectual and Developmental Disabilities,* second edition. Cambridge: Cambridge University Press.

Taggart, L. and Cousins, W. (2014). *Health Promotion for People with Intellectual Disabilities.* Maidenhead, UK: McGraw Hill/Open University Press.

Willner, P. (2005). The effectiveness of psychotherapeutic interventions for people with learning disability: a critical overview. *Journal of Intellectual Disability Research*, 49, 73–85.

World Health Organization (1992). *International Classification of Diseases (ICD-10).* Geneva: World Health Organization.

Stress, traumatic, and bereavement reactions

Philip Dodd and Fionnuala Kelly

Introduction

In the time since Reiss et al. (1982) discussed the impact of diagnostic overshadowing on the under-recognition of psychiatric illness in people with intellectual disabilities (ID), significant work has been done to look at the impact of the developmental level of the individual with ID on the expression of the common psychiatric illnesses. Pathological reactions to stress, trauma, and bereavement in people with ID is an area of study that has attracted relatively sparse research activity. This chapter will look at the pathological reactions that people with ID can experience following an adverse life event. Particular emphasis will be made on recent trauma- and bereavement-related research.

Stress

Stress is a state of mental or emotional strain or tension resulting from adverse or demanding circumstances (*Pocket Oxford English Dictionary*, 2013). Alternatively put, stress usually occurs "when we feel we have too much to do and too much on our minds, or other people are making unreasonable demands on us, or we are dealing with situations that we do not have control over" (Mind, 2014).

Anxiety and stress are part of the definition of the universal human experience, often in response to life events. Stress and anxiety are distressing emotions, consisting of both psychological and somatic manifestations and hyper-arousal, frequently accompanied by behavioral reactions. At optimal levels, psychological stress and anxiety are normal, motivational, and protective, helpful in coping with adversity (the Yerkes–Dodson law; Yerkes and Dodson, 1906).

Of course, people with ID are not immune from the experience and consequences of stress. People with ID frequently contend with a lifetime of adversity, inadequate social supports, and poor coping skills (Bradley et al., 2012). These factors contribute to increased vulnerability to stressful life events, which may trigger mental illness (Esbensen and Benson, 2006).

Life events

While the experience of adverse life events does not always result in long-term difficulties (Bonanno, 2004) within the general population, the impact of adverse or traumatic life events on mental health has been well described (Tennant, 2002). Historically, it was erroneously believed that people with ID were in some way immune to the effects of adverse or traumatic life events, based on their perceived intellectual limitations, which "protected" the individual from the realization that the life event was traumatic (Bradley et al., 2012). However, it is now generally accepted that people with ID experience more adverse life events than the general population (Hollins and Sinason, 2000), with significant mental health and behavioral sequelae (Bradley et al., 2012), and with some adverse life events, such as sexual abuse, occurring more frequently than with the general population (Turk and Browne, 1993).

It is important to distinguish a trauma reaction (that might lead to post-traumatic stress disorder (PTSD); see below) from other reactions to adverse life events, for example, acute stress reaction. In general, the study of the impact of life events on people with ID has suffered from a lack of objective measures of life events and trauma that have been specifically designed for this population (Wigham et al., 2011a), and much of the research has been based on informant accounts of the effects of adverse life events (Wigham et al., 2011a).

There have been few large-group studies into the experience of life events and its effect on mental health and well-being. Hatton and Emerson (2004), by analyzing survey data, found that children with ID experience more frequent and a wider range of negative life events than children without a disability, and that the experiences are associated with the development of emotional, psychiatric, and conduct disorders. There is evidence that the effects of some life events appear to be cumulative. Correlation data on life events and psychiatric symptoms with a large sample of adults with ID ($N = 1155$) were carried out by Hastings et al. (2004). Affective disorder was predicted by chronological age, type of residence, and exposure to one or more life events in the previous 12 months. Younger adults and people living in residential institutions were at increased risk. Common life events included moving residence (16%), serious illness of a close relative or friend (9%), and serious problems with a close friend, neighbor, or relative (9%).

This research was extended by Owen et al. (2004) who reported on a population of adults in a long stay residential institution. The participants had frequently been exposed to three or four life events in the previous 12 months. Life-event exposure was associated with aggressive/destructive behavior and an increased risk of affective/neurotic disorder. Males were exposed to more frequent life events than females, as were participants with relatively high levels of adaptive behaviors. Common events experienced included change of staff in the residence (88%), minor physical illness (37%), and the inclusion of a new resident (36%).

Specifically looking at the correlation of behavioral problems with the experience of life events, a large survey-based study ($N = 624$) by Hamilton et al., (2005) demonstrated predictive variables including severe ID, mild ID with Down syndrome, cerebral palsy, and moderate ID, as well as the experience of multiple life events.

Finally, a recent longitudinal study of 68 subjects with ID identified associations between life events and affective, neurotic, and psychotic problems, and with anger and aggression (Hulbert-Williams et al., 2014).

Acute stress disorder and acute stress reaction

Acute stress disorder was introduced into *Diagnostic and Statistical Manual of Mental Disorders, Fourth Edition, Text Revision* (DSM-IV-TR; American Psychiatric Association,

2000) to describe acute stress reactions that occur in the initial month after the exposure to a traumatic event and before the possibility of diagnosing PTSD, and to identify trauma survivors in the acute phase who are at high risk for PTSD (Bryant, 2011). A review of 22 studies in the general population concluded that, overall, the acute stress disorder diagnosis is sensitive in predicting PTSD, in that the majority of individuals with a diagnosis of acute stress disorder do subsequently develop PTSD (Bryant et al., 2011). In contrast, the acute stress disorder diagnosis has low specificity, whereby most people who eventually experience PTSD do not initially display acute stress disorder.

In people with ID, dissociative symptoms may be difficult to apply, particularly in people in the severe to profound range of ID: the person may be observed to be "in a daze." Avoidance may be observed, but may be attributed by carers as oppositional behavior (Fletcher et al., 2007). Cognitive phenomena, such as depersonalization and derealization, are difficult for people with ID to describe and are, therefore, excluded. It is also noted that avoidance may also not be as prominent in people with ID, who may have limited opportunities to make and display such choices.

There is very limited evidence of research specifically looking at the diagnosis of acute stress disorder in people with ID. An interesting study carried out looking at 746 adults with ID who had experienced a crisis, found that individuals experiencing life events in the past year were more likely to visit the emergency department in response to crisis than those who had not experienced any life events (Lunsky and Elserafi, 2011). Six specific life events were associated with use of emergency departments – (i) move of house or residence; (ii) serious problems with family, friend, or caregiver; (iii) problems with police or other authority; (iv) unemployed for more than a month; (v) recent trauma or abuse; or (vi) a drug or alcohol problem (Lunsky and Elserafi, 2011).

Adjustment disorders

Several of the diagnostic criteria for adjustment disorders present challenges for the clinician treating people with ID. The first is that the stressor must be identifiable. It is imperative to understand the expected sources of stress in the lives of people with ID, and of the significance to a person with ID of "stressors" (for example, the change of a staff member) that would be considered innocuous in the lives of persons without ID (Levitas and Gilson, 2001). In general, a stressor can be anything in the life of a person with ID that is "beyond the person's power to resolve alone" (Levitas and Gilson, 2001).

There may be a difficulty in taking a reliable account regarding the stressor, as the stressor itself may not be noted or known about by carers. It is important for the clinician to be aware of the baseline mood and functioning of the individual and to recognize the significance of the change in mood, anxiety, and function. The criteria are applicable, assuming that the clinician has sufficient understanding of the manner in which people with ID of different levels can present with anxiety and depressive symptoms (Fletcher et al., 2007). The research literature on adjustment disorders in people with ID is extremely limited. A retrospective outpatient psychiatric chart review of information in the first psychiatric diagnostic evaluation for the most recent 100 adult patients with mild ID, 100 patients with moderate, severe, or profound ID, and 100 matching non-ID patients found rates of adjustment disorder at 1% (mild ID), 2% (moderate to profound ID), and 2% non-ID (Hurley et al., 2003). However, some authors have concluded that adjustment disorder is probably underdiagnosed in the ID population (Raitasuo et al., 1999). In a study to validate the use of the Psychiatric Assessment Schedule for Adults with Developmental Disabilities (PAS-ADD) Checklist (Moss et al., 1998), 8% of psychiatric clinic attenders were diagnosed with adjustment disorder. The sample comprised of 226 individuals who were referred over a three-year period to a specialist mental health service for people with ID (Sturmey et al., 2005).

Post-traumatic stress disorder

There are no definitive boundaries between the stress associated with adverse life events and trauma; however, the experience of trauma is subjective, based upon the person's perception (Weathers and Keane, 2007). One of the principal outcomes of psychological trauma is PTSD. This is a trauma-related chronic anxiety disorder, it is often cyclic, and can have profound impact on the general functioning of the individual. Awareness of the condition, and clinical efficacy with the general population, has improved in more recent times (Bisson and Andrew, 2007). Reflective of this, research of the condition with people with ID is growing.

Presentation and diagnosis

The prevalence of PTSD in ID is most reliably reported as 16% (Ryan, 1994). The diagnosis of PTSD in people with ID is complicated by the level of disability and it's influence on the clinical manifestation of the trauma, as well as the issue of what constitutes an extreme traumatic stressor in the context of the ID (McCarthy, 2001; Fletcher et al., 2007).

For caregivers of people with ID, who are not in a position to independently self-report, traumatic events may not be known, reported, or recognized. In addition, it is important to be able to distinguish a trauma reaction from other possible reactions to adverse life events, such as depression, given the centrality of the trauma to the treatment of the condition. Recently, a self-report and informant-based screening tool has been developed (Wigham et al., 2011b). The Lancaster and Northgate Trauma Scales (LANTS; Wigham et al., 2011b, 2014) are made up of a 29-item self-report scale and a 43-item informant scale. The *Diagnostic Manual – Intellectual Disability* (DM-ID) devotes a complete chapter to PTSD (Fletcher et al., 2007), giving adaptation details of possible presentation differences and points out that evaluation of some areas may be difficult in people with verbal limitations, such as avoidance of talking about an incident, and describing feelings such as depersonalization and derealization. Looking at the re-experiencing cluster, frightening dreams without recognizable content are more likely in individuals with a lower developmental age, or with severe or profound ID (McCarthy, 2001). Avoidance can present with problems with recall; this may also appear solely as a function of the individual's developmental age and require careful assessment. Avoidance behaviors and diminished participation may be reported as "non-compliance." Caregivers may report that the individual isolates him or herself, or avoids physical contact (Sequeira and Hollins, 2003; Tomasulo and Razza, 2007).

The hyper-arousal cluster of symptoms in people with ID can present as agitated or acting-out behavior, including self-injurious behavior as referenced in DM-ID (Toma-sulo and Razza, 2007), and are emphasized as a possible presentations for people with more severe ID and PTSD (McCarthy, 2001; Mitchell and Clegg, 2005). Behavioral acting out of traumatic experiences is more common for individuals with lower developmental age. These episodes require judicious assessment in that they can appear to be symptoms of psychosis in adults. Some cases of self-injurious behavior may be symptomatic of traumatic exposure and hyper-arousal. Finally, reduction in daily living skills as a symptom of PTSD is emphasized in DM-ID (Tomasulo and Razza, 2007) as described in research (Murphy et al., 2007).

Bereavement

Complicated grief involves the experience of certain grief-related symptoms and emotions at a time, and severity, beyond which could be considered adaptive. These symptoms include separation distress-type symptoms, such as longing and searching for the deceased; loneliness, preoccupation with thoughts of the deceased, in addition to symptoms of traumatic distress, such as feelings of disbelief, mistrust, anger, shock, detachment from others, and experiencing somatic symptoms of the deceased (Prigerson et al., 1999). In addition, the death of a close attachment figure can be directly associated with the onset of more non-specific mental health difficulties, such as depression, anxiety, and self-blame, among others (Parkes, 2006).

In the general population, prolonged grief disorder is the main complicated grief presentation described in the literature. Prolonged grief disorder is made up of symptoms of "separation distress" and "traumatic distress," coupled with evidence of poor social and occupational performance (Prigerson et al., 2009). It is generally agreed that symptoms of separation distress are at the core of prolonged grief disorder, relating to the idea that prolonged grief is a form of an attachment difficulty resulting from separation, as originally described by Bowlby (1980). Traumatic distress symptoms represent bereavement-specific manifestations of being traumatized by the death. The proposed traumatic distress symptoms included efforts to avoid reminders of the deceased, feelings of purposelessness about the future, a sense of numbness, feeling shocked and stunned, difficulty acknowledging the death, feeling life is empty without the deceased, an altered sense of trust and security, in addition to anger over the death.

Complicated grief with intellectual disabilities
Ability to grieve

It was long considered impossible for people with ID to experience grief. A possible result of this is the fact that little empirical research work has been done to specifically look at the normal or complicated grief response in people with ID. Much of the work describing people with ID and their reaction to bereavement has been based on descriptive case reports (Lannen et al., 2008).

Research has previously been carried out looking at the individual's understanding of the concept of death, to assess whether an individual has a cognitive understanding of grief and bereavement. Concept of death is made up of finality (death is final), non-functionality (functioning ends at the time of death), causality (death occurs for many reasons), and universality (death is a certainty) (Speece and Brent, 1984). Research suggests that people with ID have limited concept of death, and that this is related to the level of cognitive functioning (McEvoy et al., 2002; MacHale et al., 2009).

The impact of bereavement on emotion, behavior, and mental health in people with ID

Psychiatric illness

To date, a comprehensive prospective grief study has not been carried out in people with ID. Hence, our understanding of the impact of bereavement is largely based on case studies, or small-scale case-control studies (Dodd et al., 2005; Brickell and Munir, 2008; Dodd and Guerin, 2009).

Hollins and Esterhuyzen (1997) carried out a systematic study of the reaction of people with ID to bereavement. They recruited adult subjects ($N = 50$) from day centers, who had lost a parent in the preceding two years, and compared them to a non-bereaved matched control group. The authors point out that although increased symptoms of psychopathology were found, this does not automatically indicate pathological grief, since many of these symptoms form part of what we understand to be "normal grief."

Behavior and emotion

Harper and Wadsworth (1993) carried out 43 structured direct interviews with adults with moderate to severe ID, using the Iowa Loss Instrument, designed by the authors. They found 25 of the individuals questioned reported that at least one death was very disruptive to their lives, complaining of symptoms of anger, anxiety, confusion, and discomfort thinking about the death. Eighteen of the individuals for whom the loss had occurred at least a year previous to the interview reported continuing problems in their lives, including feelings of loneliness, anxiety, sadness, and behavior problems.

In the study by Hollins and Esterhuyzen (1997), a significant increase in irritability, lethargy, inappropriate speech, and hyperactivity was demonstrated in the bereaved group compared to the control group. At follow-up, general behavior was found to have deteriorated between the initial assessment and the follow-up approximately five years after the reference bereavement, suggesting continued difficulties, possibly related to the bereavement.

Complicated grief

As previously reported, prolonged grief disorder is now the most widely used term within the general population when describing complicated grief (Prigerson et al., 2009). However, it has not been used to date in any research with people with ID. The terms pathological or complicated grief are more common in this body of literature. In general, little emphasis is made in the reporting of research with people with ID emphasizing the distinction between typical and pathological grief, in contrast to the research with the general population. There are many challenges that exist in trying to examine complicated grief in this population, including the fact that many of the screening questionnaires looking at prolonged grief disorder in the general population assess psychological responses that are often difficult to establish in people with ID (Brickell and Munir, 2008). However, it is generally agreed that people with ID are at a greater risk of developing pathological grief responses due to communication difficulties, secondary losses, such as loss of the family home/move to live with paid carers, cognitive difficulties in achieving an understanding of the meaning of the loss, an important coping strategy used by many individuals in the general population. This can be made more difficult when people with ID are not provided with appropriate grief and bereavement psychoeducation, sometimes compounded then by being excluded from grief and bereavement rituals (Brickell and Munir, 2008).

Given the need to identify people with ID who are experiencing difficulties following a bereavement, some research has been carried out looking at complicated grief symptoms in people with ID (Dodd et al., 2008). The research found that bereaved individuals experience complicated grief symptoms following the death of a parent, with one-third of the bereaved group experiencing 10 or more clinically apparent symptoms. Separation distress symptoms (for example, yearning, distrust of others) occurred more frequently than traumatic grief-type symptoms (for example, disbelief or bitterness over the loss). This, of course, is in keeping with the view that attachment difficulties are at the center of the experience of loss for people with ID. The authors also found evidence of a correlation between increased bereavement ritual involvement and the development of symptoms. The authors speculate that the individuals in the study may have taken part in bereavement rituals without appropriate preparation or previous experience of such rituals (for example, with bereaved friends or more distant family). Therefore, this lack of ritual context may contribute to the development of symptoms.

A self-report measure of complicated grief symptoms has recently been developed (O'Keeffe et al., 2012). Preliminary data analysis has identified differences in the frequency of symptoms as reported in self- and proxy reports, with some evidence that paid carers report internal symptoms, such as experience of auditory and visual hallucinations, less frequently. In addition, people with ID may be more likely to experience criteria associated with separation distress rather than traumatic grief (Guerin et al., 2014).

Conclusions

A key challenge for clinicians working with people with ID with mental health or behavioral problems is constant alertness to possible psychiatric diagnoses, in the context of the developmental level of the individual. This is a particular challenge when looking at possible stress, trauma, or bereavement reactions of people with ID. The adverse life event may not be recognized by the clinician as significant, and the clinical presentation of the reaction may not resonate with what would be expected in general population clinical presentations.

In recent times, evidence-based adaptations are being made to general population diagnostic criteria that will serve to enhance the accuracy of clinical assessments, with the potential of developing and providing more specific treatment approaches.

Key summary points

- Stress, trauma, and bereavement reactions are frequently experienced by people with ID. Adverse and traumatic life events are also experienced more often than the general population. There is a lack of measures of life events and trauma specifically adapted for the ID population.
- Acute stress reactions in people with ID is an under-researched area. Diagnostic criteria have, however, been developed that reflect some differences in the presentation in people with ID.

- The rate of adjustment disorders in people with ID is probably underestimated, and needs more research in epidemiological studies. Clinical experience in psychiatric assessment of people with ID, therefore, is important in making this diagnosis.
- For PTSD in people with ID, traumatic events may not be known, reported, or recognized. The development of validated assessment tools, such as the LANTS, will serve to develop the empirical evidence in support of the diagnostic criteria.
- People with ID can present with significant complicated grief reactions. The concept of death may be limited. Preparation for the death of loved ones is important.

References

American Psychiatric Association. (2000). *Diagnostic and Statistical Manual of Mental Disorders – Text Revision, Fourth Edition.* Washington, DC: American Psychiatric Association.

Bisson, J. and Andrew, M. (2007). Psychological treatment of post-traumatic stress disorder (PTSD). *Cochrane Database of Systematic Reviews,* 18, CD003388.

Bonanno, G. (2004). Loss, trauma, and human resilience: have we underestimated the human capacity to thrive after extremely aversive events? *American Psychologist,* 59, 20–28.

Bowlby, J. (1980). *Attachment and Loss, Vol. 3. Loss – Sadness and Depression.* London: The Hogarth Press.

Bradley, E., Sinclair, L., Greenbaum, R. (2012). Trauma and adolescents with intellectual disabilities: interprofessional clinical and service perspectives. *Journal of Child and Adolescent Trauma,* 5, 33–46.

Brickell, C. and Munir, K. (2008). Grief and its complications in individuals with intellectual disability. *Harvard Review of Psychiatry,* 16(1), 1–12.

Bryant, R.A. (2011). Acute stress disorder as a predictor of posttraumatic stress disorder: a systematic review. *Journal of Clinical Psychiatry,* 72, 233–239.

Bryant, R.A., Friedman, M.J., Spiegel, D., Ursano, R., Strain, J. (2011). A review of acute stress disorder in DSM-5. *Depression and Anxiety,* 28(9), 802–817.

Dodd, P. and Guerin, S. (2009) Grief and bereavement in people with intellectual disabilities. *Current Opinion in Psychiatry,* 22(5), 442–446.

Dodd, P., Dowling, S., Hollins, S. (2005). A review of the emotional, psychiatric and behavioural responses to bereavement in people with intellectual disabilities. *Journal of Intellectual Disability Research,* 49, 537–543.

Dodd, P., Guerin, S., McEvoy, J., et al. (2008). A study of complicated grief symptoms in people with intellectual disabilities. *Journal of Intellectual Disabilities,* 52, 415–425.

Esbensen, A.J. and Benson, B.A. (2006). A prospective analysis of life events, problem behaviours and depression in adults with intellectual disability. *Journal of Intellectual Disability Research,* 47, 51–58.

Fletcher, R., Loschen, E., Stavrakaki, C. (eds.) (2007). *Diagnostic Manual – Intellectual Disability (DM-ID): A Textbook of Diagnosis of Mental Disorders in Persons with Intellectual Disability.* Kingston, NY: NADD Press.

Guerin, S., Lockhart, K., McEvoy, J., Dodd, P. (2014). Fit for purpose? Examining the occurance of persistent complex bereavement related disorder in persons with intellectual disability. *Journal of Applied Research in Intellectual Disabilities,* 27(4), 327.

Hamilton, D., Sutherland, G., Iacono, T. (2005). Further examination of relationships between life events and psychiatric symptoms in adults with intellectual disabilities. *Journal of Intellectual Disability Research,* 49, 839–844.

Harper, D.C. and Wadsworth, J.S. (1993). Grief in adults with mental retardation: preliminary findings. *Research in Developmental Disabilities,* 14, 313–330.

Hastings, R., Hatton, C., Taylor, J., Maddison, C. (2004). Life events and psychiatric symptoms in adults with intellectual disabilities. *Journal of Intellectual Disability Research*, 48, 42–46.

Hatton, C. and Emerson, E. (2004). The relationship between life events and psychopathology amongst children with intellectual disabilities. *Journal of Applied Research in Intellectual Disabilities*, 17, 109–117.

Hollins, S. and Esterhuyzen, A. (1997). Bereavement and grief in adults with learning disabilities. *British Journal of Psychiatry*, 170, 497–502.

Hollins, S. and Sinason, V. (2000). Psychotherapy, learning disabilities and trauma: new perspectives. *British Journal of Psychiatry*, 176, 32–36.

Hulbert-Williams, L., Hastings, R., Owen, D.M., et al. (2014). Exposure to life events as a risk factor for psychological problems in adults with intellectual disabilities: a longitudinal design. *Journal of Intellectual Disability Research*, 58, 48–60.

Hurley, A.D., Folstein, M.F., Lam, N. (2003). Patients with and without intellectual disabilities seeking outpatient psychiatric services: diagnoses and prescribing pattern. *Journal of Intellectual Disability Research*, 47, 39–50.

Lannen, P., Wolfe, J., Prigerson, H.G., Onelov, E. (2008). Unresolved grief in a national sample of bereaved parents: impaired medical and physical health 4–9 years later. *Journal of Clinical Oncology*, 26, 5870–5876.

Levitas, A. and Gilson, S.F. (2001). Predictable crises in the lives of persons with mental retardation. *Mental Health Aspects of Developmental Disabilities*, 4, 89–100.

Lunsky, Y. and Elserafi, J. (2011). Life events and emergency department visits in response to crisis in individuals with intellectual disabilities. *Journal of Intellectual Disability Research*, 55(7), 714–718.

MacHale, R., McEvoy, J., Tierney, E. (2009). Caregiver perceptions of the understanding of death and need for bereavement support in adults with intellectual disabilities.

Journal of Applied Research in Intellectual Disabilities, 22, 6, 574–581.

McCarthy, J. (2001). Post-traumatic stress disorder in people with learning disability. *Advances in Psychiatric Treatment*, 7, 163–169.

McEvoy, J., Reid, Y., Guerin, S. (2002). Emotion recognition and concept of death in people with learning disabilities. *British Journal of Learning Disabilities*, 48, 83–89.

Mind. (2014). *How to Manage Stress*. At: http://www.mind.org.uk/information-support/tips-for-everyday-living/stress-guide

Mitchell, A. and Clegg, J. (2005). Is post-traumatic stress disorder a helpful concept for adults with intellectual disability? *Journal of Intellectual Disability Research*, 49, 552–559.

Moss, S., Prosser, H., Costello, H., et al. (1998). Reliability and validity of the PAS–ADD Checklist for detecting psychiatric disorders in adults with intellectual disability. *Journal of Intellectual Disability Research*, 42, 173–183.

Murphy, G.H., O'Callaghan, A.C., Clare, I.C.H. (2007). The impact of alleged abuse on behaviour in adults with severe intellectual disabilities. *Journal of Intellectual Disability Research*, 51, 741–749.

O'Keeffe, L., Dodd, P., Guerin, S., Lockhart, K., McEvoy, J. (2012). Developing a self-report measure of complicated grief in people with intellectual disability. *Journal of Applied Research in Intellectual Disability*, 56, 663.

Owen, D.M., Hastings, R.P., Noone, S.J., et al. (2004). Life events as correlates of problem behaviour and mental health in a residential population of adults with developmental disabilities. *Research in Developmental Disabilities*, 25, 309–320.

Parkes, C.M. (2006). *Love and Loss: The Roots of Grief and its Complications*. London: Routledge.

Pocket Oxford English Dictionary, 11th edition. (2013). Oxford: Oxford University Press.

Prigerson, H., Shear, K., Jacobs, S., Reynolds, C., Maciejewski, P. (1999). Consensus criteria for traumatic grief: a preliminary empirical test. *British Journal of Psychiatry*, 174, 67–73.

Prigerson, H., Horowitz, M.J., Jacobs, S.C., et al. (2009). Prolonged grief disorder: psychometric validation of criteria proposed for DSM-V and ICD-11. *PLoS Medicine*, 6, e1000121.

Raitasuo, S., Taiminen, T., Salokangas, R.K. (1999). Characteristics of people with intellectual disability admitted for psychiatric inpatient treatment. *Journal of Intellectual Disability Research*, 43(2), 112–118.

Reiss, S., Levitan, G.W., Szyszko, J. (1982). Emotional disturbance and mental retardation: diagnostic overshadowing. *American Journal of Mental Deficiency*, 86, 567–574.

Ryan, R. (1994). Post-traumatic stress disorder in persons with developmental disability. *Community Mental Health Journal*, 30(1), 45–54.

Sequeira, H. and Hollins, S. (2003). Clinical effects of sexual abuse on people with learning disability. *British Journal of Psychiatry*, 182, 13–19.

Speece, M.W. and Brent, S.B. (1984). Children's understanding of death: a review of three components of the death concept. *Child Development*, 55, 1671–1686.

Sturmey, P., Newton, J.T., Cowley, A., et al. (2005). The PAS-ADD Checklist: independent replication of its psychometric properties in a community sample. *British Journal of Psychiatry*, 186, 319–323.

Tennant, C. (2002). Life events, stress, and depression: a review of the findings. *Australian and New Zealand Journal of Psychiatry*, 36, 173–182.

Tomasulo, D.J. and Razza, N.J. (2007). Posttraumatic stress disorder. In R. Fletcher, E. Loschen, C. Stavrakaki (eds.), *Diagnostic Manual – Intellectual Disability (DM-ID): A Textbook of Diagnosis of Mental Disorders in Persons with Intellectual Disability*. Kingston, NY: NADD Press.

Turk, V. and Browne, H. (1993). The sexual abuse of adults with learning disabilities: results of a two year incidence study. *Mental Handicap Research*, 6(3), 193–216.

Weathers, F.W. and Keane, T.M. (2007). The Criterion A problem revisited: controversies and challenges in defining and measuring psychological trauma. *Journal of Traumatic Stress*, 20, 107–121.

Wigham, S., Hatton, C., Taylor, J.L. (2011a). The effects of traumatizing life events on people with intellectual disabilities: a systematic review. *Journal of Mental Health in Intellectual Disabilities*, 4, 19–39.

Wigham, S., Hatton, C., Taylor, J.L. (2011b). The Lancaster and Northgate Trauma Scales (LANTS): the development and psychometric properties of a measure of trauma for people with mild to moderate intellectual disabilities. *Research in Developmental Disabilities*, 32, 2651–2659.

Wigham, S., Taylor, J.L., Hatton, C. (2014). A prospective study of the relationship between adverse life events and trauma in adults with mild to moderate intellectual disabilities. *Journal of Intellectual Disability Research*, 58(12), 1131–1140.

Yerkes, R.M. and Dodson, J.D. (1906). The relation of strength of stimulus to rapidity of habit formation. *Journal of Comparative Neurology and Psychology*, 18, 459–482.

Chapter 10

Personality disorders

William R. Lindsay and Regi Alexander

Introduction

Early studies on personality disorder (PD) and people with intellectual disabilities (ID) noted that, similar to studies in the general population, there was likely to be comorbidity with other mental disorders and illnesses (Earl, 1961; Blackburn, 2000). One of the first systematic investigations into PD and ID was conducted by Corbett (1979). He identified a prevalence rate of 25.4%, of which almost half was immature and unstable PD. The extent to which one can separate the effects of developmental delay as a result of ID from immature and unstable personality illustrates some of the difficulties inherent in the diagnosis of PD. Eaton and Menolascino (1982) reported a prevalence rate of 27% for PD in a community-based sample of people with ID. Ballinger and Reid (1987) used the Standardized Assessment of Personality (SAP; Mann et al., 1981) and reported a prevalence rate of severe PD in 22% of a sample of individuals with mild or moderate ID. These authors, along with Gostasson (1987), also commented on the difficulty in applying diagnostic criteria for PD to individuals with severe and profound ID. Early studies established that PD could be assessed and was prevalent to some extent in this population. They identified some of the difficulties concerning comorbidity and diagnosis in more severe levels of ID and pointed out some confusion with immaturity and dependence.

Khan et al. (1997) also used the SAP and reported that 50% of their sample had personality abnormalities and 31% had a degree of impairment sufficient to warrant a diagnosis of PD. Of those diagnosed, the specific disorders were as follows: schizoid 10%; impulsive 7%; paranoid 5%; dependent 3%; dissocial 3%; histrionic 1%; anxious 1%; and ankastic 1%. Goldberg et al. (1995) reported very high levels of PD in people with ID. They found abnormal personality traits in 57% of individuals in an institutional sample and 91% of individuals in a community sample.

Flynn et al. (2002) studied a hospital inpatient sample and reported that 92% were diagnosed with PD using ICD-10 criteria. In contrast, working with the same ICD-10 criteria, Naik et al. (2002) found PD in 7% of a community sample, while Alexander et al. (2002) found PD in 58% of a sample of patients referred to a forensic hospital.

A turning point in research on PD and ID came with Alexander and Cooray's (2003) review of studies. They noted that there was a lack of reliable diagnostic instruments, the use of different diagnostic systems, a confusion of definition and personality theory, and

Psychiatric and Behavioral Disorders in Intellectual and Developmental Disabilities, ed. Colin Hemmings and Nick Bouras. Published by Cambridge University Press. © Cambridge University Press 2016.

difficulty in distinguishing PD from other problems integral to ID, such as communication problems, sensory disorders, and developmental delay. They concluded that "the variation in the co-occurrence of PD in ID with prevalence ranging from less than 1% to 91% in a community sample and 22% to 92% in hospital settings, is very great and too large to be explained by real differences." They recommended tighter diagnostic criteria and greater use of behavioral observation and informant information. Reid et al. (2004) made similar recommendations and made initial attempts to integrate mainstream work on personality with the small amount of work available investigating PD and ID. These authors used the NEO-PI-R, the standard questionnaire measure of the Five Factor Model (FFM) of personality structure (Costa and McCrae, 1985). This is one of the most widely accepted assessments for personality, with considerable empirical support. It has also been one of the bases for the alternative model to assess PD in DSM-5. In a series of case illustrations, Reid et al. (2004) found that those individuals who scored high on psychopathy (Psychopathy Checklist–Revised; Hare 1991) had low scores on the agreeableness and conscientiousness scale of the NEO-PI-R. This finding is similar to that reported in mainstream personality research (Blackburn 2000).

Lindsay et al. (2005) employed the recommendations made by Alexander and Cooray (2003) in a study of 164 males with ID in three forensic settings – high-secure, medium/low-secure, and community forensic services. They employed four independently rated measures of PD: a DSM-IV criteria checklist completed, firstly, from file review; secondly, by a clinician; thirdly, from nurse observations; and, finally, the SAP completed by care staff. A consensus rating was derived from the four assessments and a total prevalence of PD in this forensic sample was 39.5%. They reported that the ratings had high levels of reliability. As would be expected in a forensic population, antisocial PD was the largest category at 22% of cases, and rates of PD across the other categories were between 1% and 3%. It should be noted that care was taken in these guidelines to avoid the confusion first mentioned by Corbett (1979), that of confusing developmental delay with immature or dependent PD. There were no cases with dependent PD in the entire sample. It is also interesting that a previous, more general, file review of mental disorder in this sample (Hogue et al. 2006) had found PD recorded at 22.6% in the case files. By far the highest level of underrecording was in the community forensic sample, which was 1.4% in the case files and 33% in the carefully organized assessment study (Hogue et al. 2006). These authors noted that even the highest figures found in this forensic ID sample were lower than the figures of over 90% in studies on community samples reviewed by Alexander and Cooray (2003).

Lindsay et al. (2007) reported a factor analysis of the PD categories. In mainstream PD research, Blackburn et al. (2005) had previously investigated higher-order dimensions with 168 male forensic psychiatric patients and found two higher-order factors that appeared to underlie personality structure. They labeled these two factors as "acting-out" and "anxious-inhibited," which was similar to higher-order structures identified by Morey (1988). In a similar confirmatory factor analysis on offenders with ID, Lindsay et al. (2007) produced a two-factor solution similar to that found previously with an "avoidant/inhibition" factor with high loadings from schizotypal PD, avoidant PD, obsessive-compulsive PD, and a lower loading from schizoid PD; and an "acting-out" factor with high loadings from borderline, narcissistic, and paranoid PD, with a smaller loading from antisocial PD. Therefore, the higher-order dimensions of PD in this study (Lindsay et al., 2007) in forensic participants with ID were similar to those found in populations with mental disorder found in other studies (Blackburn et al., 2005).

Alexander et al., (2006) reported on the outcome of 65 patients with ID treated in medium-secure forensic hospital settings. They found that the main associations with reconviction were a previous offense of theft or burglary, age of less than 27 years, and the presence of a PD. This relationship between PD and crime has been shown repeatedly with mainstream offending populations (Monahan et al., 2001; Fazel and Danesh, 2002). Indeed, one of the main reasons promoting the study of PD has been, on the one hand, the predictive relationship between antisocial PD and crime, while, on the other, the predictive relationship between borderline PD and psychiatric patient status (Widiger and Frances, 1989). Using the same population as Lindsay et al. (2006), Morrissey et al. (2007) found that the Psychopathy Checklist–Revised (PCL-R) was significantly associated with negative treatment progress in terms of a move to more restricted treatment conditions. The PCL-R is strongly associated with antisocial PD. These authors have consistently made the caution that the construct of PD is a highly devaluing label and should be used very carefully with the population of people with ID who are already highly devalued.

Most of the more recent work on PD and ID has been done on forensic populations. Alexander et al. (2010) compared the progress of 138 patients with ID in a secure setting over a six-year period, 77 with a dissocial or emotionally unstable PD (ICD-10) and 61 without. They found that previous histories of aggression and violence were no different in the two groups, but convictions for violent offenses and compulsory detentions were significantly more common in the group with PD. However, there were no clinically significant differences in terms of outcome for the groups, and the authors concluded that patients with PD and ID could be successfully treated in a general service for people with ID and a range of mental disorders. In a further comparison, Alexander et al. (2012) compared the progress of three groups following treatment in a secure hospital system, one with ID, a second with ID and PD, and a third with PD only. The two groups with ID appeared to follow similar treatment and management trajectories, while the group with PD followed a very different trajectory. Both ID groups had lower rates of post-release conviction and lower rates of violent reoffenses at two-year follow-up.

Three small treatment studies have used an adapted version of dialectical behavior therapy (DBT) in small groups of people with ID. Sakdalan et al. (2010) used a 13-week program with six participants and, although the sample size was very small, they found significant improvements on dynamic risk assessment. Morrissey and Ingamells (2011) developed a longer 60-session DBT program and reported anecdotal improvements in four out of six participants, 12 months following treatment. Mason (2007) reported a single case where assessment of personality and PD guided successful treatment.

The assessment of personality and people with ID

The authors of DSM-5 have considered carefully the relationship between PD and normal personality, concentrating exclusively on the FFM of personality (McCrae and Costa, 1991). Beginning with Cattell (1946), factor models were developed and refined, with five robust factors emerging most consistently (Norman, 1963; Goldberg., 1981; McCrae and Costa, 1987). These factors are extraversion/introversion, agreeableness, conscientiousness, neuroticism, and openness to experience, and the FFM is a comprehensive statistical summary of personality traits.

The FFM of personality assumes a trait theory perspective, in that individual differences characterize a person, and these, in turn, will influence thoughts, feelings, and behaviors (McCrae and Costa, 1991). The five factors are thought to be fully comprehensive and generally agreed to be the basic dimensions of a "normal" personality (Emmons, 1995). Neuroticism (N) is the most consistent domain and runs on a continuum from neurotic to stable. A tendency to feel negative affect, for example, fear, guilt, or anger, is at the core of N. Extraversion (E) runs on a continuum from extraversion to introversion. E is sometimes known as the "sociable" domain; however, it also includes factors such as sensation-seeking and assertiveness, which do not necessarily have a sociable component. Openness (O) refers to the individual's openness to experience and covers a wide range of attributes including intellect, imagination, and values. The Agreeableness (A) domain focuses most strongly on interpersonal abilities and needs, and runs on a continuum from agreeable to disagreeable. Conscientiousness (C) reflects determination, strong will, and a sense of duty, and is also related to some aspects of N such as impulse control and self-regulation factors (Piedmont and Weinstein, 1993; Costa and McCrae, 1995).

The NEO-PI-R is the most widely accepted and evaluated questionnaire measuring the FFM (Berry et al., 2001), which is the model employed for the alternative diagnostic system in DSM-5. The 241 questions of the NEO-PI-R thoroughly identify the five factors/domains and also the 30 facets which are the defining traits of the domains. The six facets of each domain are grounded in psychological theory and ensure that the domain is widely covered, and that they highlight key individual differences. N's facets are anxiety, anger, hostility, depression, self-consciousness, impulsiveness, and vulnerability. The facets identified with E are warmth, gregariousness, assertiveness, activity, excitement seeking, and positive emotions. O's facets were recognized as being fantasy, aesthetics, feelings, actions, ideas, and values. Trust, straightforwardness, altruism, compliance, modesty, and tender-mindedness are facets of A. Finally, C's facets have been identified as competence, order, dutifulness, achievement, striving, self-discipline, and deliberation. It has been suggested by Roepke et al. (2001) that personality profiles are fairly stable over time, and there is little difference in the profiles of adults aged 50–84 and 85–100. After some criticism regarding the lack of validity scales within the NEO-PI-R (for example, Schinka et al., 1997), Costa and McCrae (1995) included an observer rating (form R) to be taken in addition to the self-rating (form S), which they believe reveals the validity of the responses. This also provides strength for work on people with ID in that there is a check on the self-ratings and also allows comparisons of both sets of results.

Lindsay et al. (2007) adapted and simplified the language of the NEO-PI-R to be suitable for people with ID. They first tested that the adapted assessment produced results very similar to the full questionnaire. They then used the self- and observer versions to assess its applicability for the client group with 40 participants with ID and carers who knew the person well. They found that there were consistent differences between self- and observer ratings, with people with ID rating themselves as significantly more agreeable, extraverted, and conscientious than observers. The difference was less marked in extraversion/introversion where the self-ratings were 5 percentiles above the mean and the observer ratings were 5 percentiles below the mean. However, with the A and C factors, observers rated the participant significantly lower in agreeableness and conscientiousness than the people with ID did themselves.

Given the extent of work on these various models of personality in mainstream literature, it is of surprise that research in the field of personality and ID has developed from an entirely different standpoint. The standpoint of all previous work has been, on the one hand, developmental, reviewing the way in which developmental experiences form personality characteristics in individuals with ID, and, on the other hand, the personality factors behind the way in which people with ID are motivated to interact with their environment. Therefore, in a series of studies with children, Switzky (2001) reviewed the importance of intrinsic motivation in children who worked harder, required less praise for staying on task, and maintained their performance longer when compared with externally motivated children, when working under self-monitored conditions. By contrast, externally motivated children worked better when under closer supervision by teachers. They concluded that self-regulation was an extremely important trait in people with ID when considering relatively independent living in less regulated settings. They felt that motivational orientation (intrinsic vs. extrinsic) was a central concept in personality development in individuals with ID. In a series of studies, (for example, Switzky and Haywood, 1991, 1992) it was found that these differences were most prevalent when there was less external support and guidance. Intrinsically motivated individuals worked as well in situations of higher supervision as they did in lower supervision situations.

In another model, Reiss and Havercamp (1997) outlined 16 basic values that provide motivation for all individuals, including people with ID. They developed an assessment to use these values, and Reiss and Havercamp (1997, 1998), in factor analytic studies, found a 16-factor solution that conformed to the basic values in their theoretical construction. They also found that people with and without ID showed the same motivational profiles in relation to achieving these basic values. In other words, people with and without ID pursue happiness through motivation for the same needs, which they specified as social contact, curiosity, honor, family, independence, power, order, idealism, status, vengeance, romance, exercise, acceptance, tranquillity, eating, and saving. Aberrant environments that did not satisfy ordinary desires and psychological needs are likely to produce personality difficulties, while aberrant motivation (for example, desire for excessive amounts of positive reinforcement) is similarly likely to result in distortions of personality.

A further personality approach based on a developmental perspective is that of Zigler and colleagues (Zigler 2001; Zigler et al. 2002), who have derived an alternative personality structure based on informant reports. Incorporating earlier developmental work, Zigler et al. (2002) described five traits as follows: positive reaction tendency ("heightened motivation ... to both interact with and be dependent upon a supportive adult"); negative reaction tendency ("initial wariness shown when interacting with strange adults"); expectancy of success ("the degree to which one expects to succeed or fail when presented a new task"); outer directedness ("tendency ... to look to others for the cues to solutions of difficult or ambiguous tasks"); and efficacy motivation ("the pleasure derived from tackling and solving difficult problems"). When compared with their typically developing peers, people with ID tend to have lower expectancy of success and efficacy motivation, and higher positive and negative reaction tendencies and outer directedness.

These conceptualizations of development and motivation are interesting and wide-ranging in their view of personality, but clearly quite distinct from the way in which personality theory has developed in mainstream populations.

We have reviewed these systems of personality assessment because normal personality has been a focus for the DSM-5 alternative system of classification. As mentioned, DSM-5 has emphasized the primary assessment system – the FFM. While there is little research on this system in people with ID, it is the case that there is a wealth of disparate research on personality and very little research substantiating the use of the FFM with this population.

Psychiatric disorders, PD, and personality

Over the last two decades there has been a steady clinical and research interest in the relationship between the assessment of psychiatric disorders in clinical settings, the assessment of PDs, and their relationship to normal personality dimensions (Reynolds and Clark 2001; Quirk et al., 2003; Caperton et al., 2004; Edens, 2009). High levels of neuroticism and low levels of extroversion feature strongly in a variety of psychiatric populations (Zuckerman 1999). As an example, Quirk et al. (2003) examined the relationship between assessed psychiatric problems, personality features, and PD in 1342 inpatients. Neuroticism scores were strongly related to anxiety disorders and borderline PD, while introversion was related to post-traumatic stress disorder and borderline PD. The strongest relationships to emerge in this field are between coercive personality characteristics and acting-out PDs (antisocial, narcissistic, aggressive) (Edens, 2009); neurotic personality characteristics and several psychiatric disorders such as depression, paranoia, social introversion, anger, obsessiveness, and schizophrenia (Reynolds and Clark 2001; Caperton et al., 2004); externalizing psychopathology and antisocial and paranoid traits; and, finally, internalizing psychopathology and borderline PD traits (Edens, 2009).

Lindsay et al. (2010) studied these relationships using a forensic sample of 212 male participants with ID. They previously established the validity of assessments of normal personality and used these to study the relationship between personality, PD, and risk, using validated risk assessments. The findings suggested an orderly convergence of emotional problems, personality, and risk. Externalizing emotional problems had a significant relationship with antisocial PD and narcissistic PD, while internalizing emotional problems correlated significantly with avoidant PD. There were similar strong relationships between externalizing emotional problems and dominant personality characteristics, and significant negative correlations between externalizing emotional problems and nurturant personality dimensions. There was a strong relationship between narcissistic PD and dominant personality characteristics, and further negative statistical relationships between avoidant PD and dominant personality characteristics, and negative correlations between antisocial PD and nurturant personality characteristics.

Conclusions

There has been a significant increase in the range and amount of substantive research on people with ID. In a previous chapter (Lindsay 2006, in Bouras and Holt, 2007) much of the available knowledge consisted of recommendations for diagnosis and extrapolation from mainstream research. All of the research in this chapter has been conducted on people with moderate and mild ID. It does show an emerging literature on the reliability and validity of a PD diagnosis with this client group, and also demonstrates an orderly relationship between PD, underlying personality constructs, and emotional difficulties.

There continues, however, to be significant limitations in the extent and breadth of research in the field, and it is an obvious drawback that most of the recent studies have come from two principal research groups (Alexander and colleagues and Lindsay and colleagues).

Key summary points

- There has been a significant increase recently in research on PD in people with ID.
- Most of the more recent work on PD and ID has been done on forensic populations.
- Treatment studies have increased in number, including those on the use of DBT.

References

Alexander, R.T. and Cooray, S. (2003). Diagnosis of personality disorders in learning disability. *British Journal of Psychiatry*, 182(44), S28–S31.

Alexander, R.T., Piachaud, J., Odebiyi, L., Gangadharan, S.K. (2002). Referrals to a forensic service in the psychiatry of learning disability. *British Journal of Forensic Practice*, 4, 29–33.

Alexander, R.T., Crouch, K., Halstead, S., Pichaud, J. (2006). Long-term outcome from a medium secure service for people with intellectual disability. *Journal of Intellectual Disability Research*, 50, 305–315.

Alexander, R.T., Green, F.N., O'Mahony, B., et al. (2010). Personality disorders in offenders with intellectual disability: a comparison of clinical, forensic and outcome variables and implications for service provision. *Journal of Intellectual Disability Research*, 54(7), 650–658.

Alexander, R.T., Chester, V., Gray, N.S., Snowden, R.J. (2012). Patients with personality disorders and intellectual disability – closer to personality disorders or intellectual disability? A three-way comparison. *Journal of Forensic Psychiatry and Psychology*, 23(4), 435–451.

Ballinger, B.R. and Reid, A.H. (1987). A standardised assessment of personality in mental handicap. *British Journal of Psychiatry*, 150, 108–109.

Berry, D.T.R., Bagby, M.R., Smerz, J., et al. (2001). Effectiveness of the NEO-PI-R research validity scales for discriminating analog malingering and genuine psychopathology. *Journal of Personality Assessment*, 76(3), 496–517.

Blackburn, R. (2000). Classification and assessment of personality disorders in mentally disordered offenders: a psychological perspective. *Criminal Behaviour and Mental Health*, 10(Special Suppl.), S8–S32.

Blackburn, R., Logan, C., Renwick, S.J.D., Donnelly, J.P. (2005). Higher order dimensions of personality disorder: hierarchical and relationships with the Five Factor Model, the interpersonal circle and psychopathy. *Journal of Personality Disorders*, 19, 597–623.

Bouras, N. and Holt, G. (eds.) (2007). *Psychiatric and Behavioural Disorders in Intellectual and Developmental Disabilities*, second edition. Cambridge: Cambridge University Press.

Caperton, J.D., Edens, J.F., Johnson, J.K. (2004). Predicting sex offender institutional adjustment and treatment compliance using the Personality Assessment Inventory. *Psychological Assessment*, 16, 187–191.

Cattell, R.B. (1946). Confirmation and clarification of primary personality factors. *Psychometrika*, 12, 197–220.

Corbett, J.A. (1979). *Psychiatric Illness in Mental Handicap*. London: Gaskell Press.

Costa, P.T., Jr. and McCrae, R.R. (1985). *The NEO Personality Inventory*. Odessa, FL: Psychological Assessment Resources.

Costa, P.T., Jr. and McCrae, R.R. (1995). Domains and facets: hierarchical personality assessment using the revised NEO Personality Inventory. *Journal of Personality Assessment*, 64(1), 21–50.

Earl, C.J.C. (1961). *Subnormal Personalities: Their Clinical Investigation and Assessment.* London: Bailliere, Tindall and Cox.

Eaton, I.F. and Menolascino, F.J. (1982). Psychiatric disorders in the mentally retarded: types, problems and challenges. *American Journal of Psychiatry*, 139, 1297–1303.

Edens, J.F. (2009). Interpersonal characteristics of male criminal offenders: personality, psychopathological and behavioural correlates. *Psychological Assessment*, 21, 89–98.

Emmons, R.A. (1995). Levels and domains in personality: an introduction. *Journal of Personality*, 63(3), 342–364.

Fazel, S. and Danesh, J. (2002). Serious mental disorder among 23,000 prisoners: systematic review of 62 surveys. *Lancet*, 16, 545–550.

Flynn, A., Mathews, H., Hollins, S. (2002). Validity of the diagnosis of personality disorder in adults with learning disability and severe behaviour problems. *British Journal of Psychiatry*, 180, 543–546.

Goldberg, B., Gitta, M.Z., Puddephatt, A. (1995). Personality and trait disturbance in an adult mental retardation population: significance for psychiatric management. *Journal of Intellectual Disability Research*, 39, 284–294.

Goldberg, L.R. (1981). Language and individual differences: the search for universals in personality lexicons. In L. Wheeler (ed.), *Review of Personality and Social Psychology*, Vol. 2. Beverley Hills, CA: Sage.

Gostasson, R. (1987). Psychiatric illness among the mildly mentally retarded. *Journal of Medical Science*, 44(Suppl.), 115–124.

Hare, R.D. (1991). *The Hare Psychopathy Checklist – Revised.* Toronto, ON: Multi Health Systems.

Hogue, T.E., Steptoe, L., Taylor, J.L., et al. (2006). A comparison of offenders with intellectual disability across three levels of security. *Criminal Behaviour and Mental Health*, 16, 13–28.

Khan, A., Cowan, C., Roy, A. (1997). Personality disorders in people with learning disabilities: a community survey. *Journal of Intellectual Disability Research*, 41, 324–330.

Lindsay, W.R., Gabriel, S., Dana, L., Dosen, A., Young, S. (2005). Personality disorders. In R. Fletcher, E. Loschen, C. Stavrakaki (eds.), *Diagnostic Manual – Intellectual Disability (DM-ID): A Textbook of Diagnosis of Mental Disorders in Persons with Intellectual Disability.* Kingston, NY: NADD Press.

Lindsay, W.R., Hogue, T., Taylor, J.T., et al. (2006). Two studies on the prevalence and validity of personality disorder in three forensic learning disability samples. *Journal of Forensic Psychiatry and Psychology*, 17, 485–506.

Lindsay, W.R., Rzepecka, H., Law J. (2007). An exploratory study into the use of the Five Factor Model of Personality with People with Intellectual Disabilities. *Clinical Psychology and Psychotherapy*, 14, 428–437.

Lindsay, W.R., Taylor, J., Hogue, T., et al. (2010). The relationship between assessed emotion, personality, personality disorder and risk. *Psychiatry, Psychology and Law*, 17, 385–397.

Mann, A.H., Jenkins, R., Cutting, J.C., Cowan, P.J. (1981). The development and use of an assessment of abnormal personality. *Psychological Medicine*, 11, 839–847.

Mason, J. (2007). Personality assessment in offenders with mild and moderate intellectual disabilities. *British Journal of Forensic Practice*, 9(1) 31–39.

McCrae, R.R. and Costa, P.T., Jr. (1987). Validation of the Five Factor Model of Personality across instruments and observers. *Journal of Personality and Social Psychology*, 52, 81–90.

McCrae, R.R. and Costa, P.T., Jr. (1991). The NEO Personality Inventory: using the Five Factor Model in counselling. *Journal of Counselling and Development*, 69(4), 367–373.

Monahan, J., Steadman, H., Silver, E., et al. (2001). *Re-thinking Risk Assessment: The MacArthur Study of Mental Disorder and Violence.* New York, NY: Oxford University Press.

Morey, L.C. (1988). The categorical representation of personality disorder: a cluster analysis of DSM III-R personality features. *Journal of Abnormal Psychology*, 97, 314–321.

Morrissey, C. and Ingamells, B. (2011). Adapted dialectical behaviour therapy for male offenders with intellectual disability in a high secure environment: six years on. *Journal of Learning Disabilities and Offending Behaviour*, 2, 11–17.

Morrissey, C., Mooney, P., Hogue, T., Lindsay, W.R., Taylor, J.L. (2007). Predictive validity of psychopathy in offenders with intellectual disabilities in a high security hospital: treatment progress. *Journal of Intellectual and Developmental Disabilities*, 32, 125–133.

Naik, B.I., Gangadharan, S.K., Alexander, R.T. (2002). Personality disorders in learning disability – the clinical experience. *British Journal of Developmental Disabilities*, 48, 95–100.

Norman, W.T. (1963). Towards an adequate taxonomy of, personality attributes: replicated factor structure in peer nomination personality ratings. *Journal of Abnormal and Social Psychology*, 66, 574–583.

Piedmont, R.L. and Weinstein, H.P. (1993). A psychometric evaluation of the new NEO-PI-R facet scales for agreeableness and conscientiousness. *Journal of Personality Assessment*, 60(2), 302–318.

Quirk, S.W., Christiansen, N.D., Wagner, S.H., McNulty, J.L. (2003). On the usefulness of normal measures of personality for clinical assessment: evidence of the incremental validity of the revised NEO personality inventory. *Psychological Assessment*, 15, 311–325.

Reid, A.H., Lindsay, W.R., Law, J., Sturmey, P. (2004). The relationship of offending behaviour and personality disorder in people with developmental disabilities. In W.R. Lindsay, J.L. Taylor, P. Sturmey (eds.), *Offenders with Developmental Disabilities*. Chichester, UK: Wiley and Sons.

Reiss, S. and Havercamp, S.H. (1997). The sensitivity theory of motivation: why functional analysis is not enough. *American Journal on Mental Retardation*, 101, 553–566.

Reiss, S. and Havercamp, S.H. (1998). Towards a comprehensive assessment of functional motivation: factor structure of the Reiss profiles. *Psychological Assessment*, 10, 97–106.

Reynolds, S.K., and Clark, L.A. (2001). Predicting dimensions of personality from domains and facets of the Five Factor Model. *Journal of Personality*, 69, 199–222.

Roepke, S., McAdams, L.A., Lindamer, L.A., et al. (2001). Personality profiles among normal aged individuals as measured by the NEO-PI-R. *Aging and Mental Health*, 5(2), 159–165.

Sakdalan, J.A., Shaw, J., Collier, V. (2010). Staying in the here-and-now: a pilot study on the use of dialectical behaviour therapy group skills training for forensic clients with intellectual disability. *Journal of Intellectual Disability Research*, 54(6), 568–572.

Schinka, J.A., Kinder, B.N., Kremer, T. (1997). Research validity scales for the NEO-PI-R: development and validation. *Journal of Personality Assessment*, 68(1), 127–138.

Switzky H.N. (2001). *Personality and Motivational Differences in Persons with Mental Retardation*. Mahwah, NJ: Lawrence Erlbaum Associates.

Switzky, H.N. and Haywood, H.C. (1991). Self-reinforcement schedules in persons with mild mental retardation. Effects of motivational orientation and instructional demands. *Journal of Mental Deficiency Research*, 35, 221–230.

Switzky, H.N. and Haywood, H.C. (1992). Self-reinforcement schedules in young children: effects of motivational orientation and instructional demands. *Learning and Individual Differences*, 4, 59–71.

Widiger, T.A. and Frances, A.J. (1989). Epidemiology, diagnosis and comorbidity of borderline personality disorder. In A. Tasman, R.F. Hales, A.J. Frances (eds.), *Review of Psychiatry*, Vol. 8. Washington, DC: American Psychiatric Press.

Zigler, E. (2001). Looking back 40 years and still seeing the person with mental retardation as a whole person. In H.N. Switzky (ed.), *Personality and Motivational Differences in Persons with Mental Retardation*. Mahwah, NJ: Lawrence Erlbaum Associates.

Zigler, E., Bennett-Gates, D., Hodapp, R., Henrich, C.C. (2002). Assessing personality traits of individuals with mental retardation. *American Journal on Mental Retardation*, 107, 181–193.

Zuckerman, M. (1999). *The Vulnerability to Psychopathology: A Biosocial Model*. Washington, DC: American Psychological Association.

Mental illness with intellectual disabilities and autism spectrum disorders

Trine L. Bakken, Sissel B. Helvershou, Siv Helene Høidal, and Harald Martinsen

Introduction

People with autism spectrum disorders (ASD) are assumed to be especially vulnerable to developing psychiatric disorders. As in the general population, the distribution of prevalences indicates depression and anxiety as the most frequent disorders reported, while obsessive-compulsive disorder (OCD) and psychoses are less frequently reported (Bakken et al., 2010; Skokauskas and Gallagher, 2010; Helverschou et al., 2011; Steensel et al., 2011; Simonoff et al., 2012; Bakken, 2014). However, the estimates of mental illness vary considerably; some studies report estimates up to 84% (Howlin and Moss, 2012). The variation may be explained by methodological issues, such as biased samples, small sample sizes, differences in the disorders targeted and the populations' characteristics (clinical samples vs. representative samples), differences in assessment methods used and the clinical experience of interviewers, and whether the measures have been validated for participants with autism. Futhermore, the majority of studies encompass children and adolescents, and individuals with IQ within the normal range (Matson and Cervantes, 2014).

In this chapter, we use the shorter term "autism" for ASD; likewise we use "ID only" instead of "intellectual disabilities" without additional ASD.

Autism as a risk for developing mental illness

Autism persistently disturbs the individual's ability to understand life events and to communicate and interact with others. Communication impairments might include echolalia, repetitions of words or phrases, detailed language when explaining, idiosyncratic use of words or expressions, and literal interpretation. Autistic idiosyncrasies may cause communicational misunderstandings. For example, a woman with autism and mild ID had an idiosyncratic way of rating significant others by the size of their kidneys (Bakken et al., 2009). Autism also impacts the ability to regulate emotions in a suitable way, which may elicit negative responses from others. Emotion dysregulation is found to be significantly higher compared to typical controls (Samson et al., 2014).

The features that characterize people with autism and the problems those with autism often experience are associated with a number of problems that are considered as general risk factors when they occur in the general population (Reese et al., 2005). Thus, autism

Psychiatric and Behavioral Disorders in Intellectual and Developmental Disabilities, ed. Colin Hemmings and Nick Bouras. Published by Cambridge University Press. © Cambridge University Press 2016.

seems to imply a significant vulnerability for developing adjustment problems and mental illness (Simonoff et al., 2013).

The environment is often unpredictable and confusing for people with autism due to their autistic comprehension problems. They may experience daily activities as meaningless, have problems with interpreting the activities of others, and not know what is going to happen during the day. Each day they are confronted with challenges they are unable to cope with, and often experience catastrophic reactions and conflicts caused by comprehension difficulties, cognitive inflexibility, and difficulties in distinguishing between importance and non-importance. Three particular problems occur especially often among people with autism. They experience severe stress, are hypersensitive to sensory stimulation, and have large fluctuations in daily functioning. These problems are not part of the syndrome and not exclusively related to autism, but may nevertheless be named *central autism problems*. The magnitude of stress problems has, for example, raised the question: "Is autism a stress disorder?" (Morgan, 2006). These problems contribute to the daily burden experienced by those with autism and may give rise to cognitive overload (Helverschou, 2010). Cognitive overload may arise over time in people with autism when they experience stressful situations related to task solving, sensory difficulties, or demanding social settings (Hill and Frith, 2003; Colvin and Sheehan, 2014). Negative reactions to sensory stimuli, such as noise, light, and smell may exacerbate the stress of everyday life. Sensory disintegration (difficulty with processing sensory information) includes both over- and under-sensitivity (Lane et al., 2010) and occurs especially often in those with autism; prevalences up to 95% are found in children with autism (Schaaf et al., 2014). Anxiety reactions may be attributed to sensory over-responsivity (Green et al., 2012).

Confounding between autism and mental illness

The large variation in prevalences of mental illness in people with autism is probably explained mainly by the problems of delineation between autism and mental illness (Helverschou, 2010). The considerable overlap between autism and psychiatric constructs result in symptom overlap and problems in distinguishing between autism and psychiatric disorders (Helverschou et al., 2008). The clearest symptom overlap is found for autism and schizophrenia, and for autism and OCD. Lack of social interaction is both a feature of autism and a symptom of schizophrenia (Bakken and Høidal, 2013). Odd and unusual features in people with autism and idiosyncratic preoccupations can be mistaken for delusions or other positive signs of schizophrenia, and language problems, like literal comprehension, in people with autism may be confused with thought disorder (Bakken and Høidal, 2013). The ritualistic and repetitive behaviors that are among the core characteristics of autism may also be symptoms of OCD, but the compulsion-driven quality that characterizes OCD goes beyond the core features of autism (Scahill et al., 2006; Helverschou et al., 2013). Nervousness and anxiety symptoms were included in the first descriptions of autism, and despite the fact that anxiety symptoms are not included in the features that define autism, anxiety has been suggested as an integral component of the disorder (Helverschou and Martinsen, 2011). Symptoms of depression may be overlooked in people with autism due to the difficulties of observing mood changes, which are among the main symptoms of depression. Symptoms of depression may also be overshadowed by and wrongly attributed to autism, since social withdrawal, limited facial expression, and flattened affect may be indicators of both disorders. Similarly, sleeping and eating problems may be interpreted as related to autism or as symptoms of depression (Skokaukas and Gallagher, 2010; Helverschou et al., 2011).

The considerable overlap in symptoms may explain both why a complex autistic condition may be diagnosed as mental illness, and why mental illness frequently is attributed to the autism diagnosis (Helverschou et al., 2011). The large variation in prevalences, thus, indicates that mental illness is both under- and overdiagnosed in people with autism.

There are two main pitfalls. The first is to interpret features of autism as mental illness. By using measurements not adjusted for people with autism, such as instruments for the general population or for people with ID only, autism features are likely to be misinterpreted as psychiatric symptoms. This may be the case for the studies reporting the highest prevalence rates (e.g., Simonoff, et al., 2008). The second pitfall is to overlook mental illness in people with autism, which may explain the lower rates of depression and anxiety reported (e.g., Tsakanikos et al., 2006; Melville et al., 2008). Likewise, when some studies report that people with ID-only more often suffer from psychiatric disorders compared to those with both autism and ID, these reports may be explained by psychiatric symptoms in those with autism being overshadowed by autism features.

Identifying mental illness in people with autism and ID

Differentiating between autism and mental illness may entail more valid psychiatric diagnoses. A previous study demonstrated that clinicians were able to identify symptoms of four groups of mental illness that do not overlap with the core characteristics of autism (Helverschou et al., 2008). The items scored were included in a carer-completed screening checklist, the Psychopathology in Autism Checklist (PAC). The first validation study of the PAC demonstrated that it is possible to differentiate between people with autism and ID diagnosed with and without mental illness (Helverschou et al., 2009). The results suggest that co-occurring mental illness can be identified by changes or deterioration in the patterns of behavior typical of autism (Ghaziuddin, 2005; Hutton et al., 2008).

Reduced capacity for introspection and problems in communicating personal state add to the complex process of identifying mental health problems in individuals with autism and ID.

In people with both autism and ID, the diagnostic process is further complicated by the combination of the comprehension and communication difficulties related to autism and the problems in self-reporting related to ID.

At present, there is no consensus about use of criteria diagnosing mental illness in people with autism. There are few instruments (Underwood et al., 2011). The diagnostical complexity indicates that standard diagnostic manuals may not be used unmodified. Thus, identification of mental illness in people with autism and ID requires comprehensive expertise in both autism and mental illness, and requires information comparing the person's changes in behavior and mood over time (Helverschou, 2010; Helverschou et al., 2011).

Anxiety: overlooked and undertreated?

A high prevalence of anxiety symptoms and disorders has been reported in the last decade (Helverschou, 2010; Helverschou et al., 2011). This may have contributed to increased awareness about interventions (Matson and Nebel-Schwalm, 2007; Helverschou et al., 2013; White et al., 2013). Individuals with autism seem to be especially vulnerable to developing anxiety related to problems associated with autism (Gillott and Stranden, 2007). Cognitive comprehension difficulties may lead to confusion and stress-coping difficulties. Features that characterize autism, like rituals and repetitive behavior, have been considered as related to anxiety or as strategies for coping with anxiety (Helverschou, 2010). Thus, anxiety in individuals with autism has been interpreted as an effect of having autism as well as a cause of some of the characteristics of autism.

Comparisons across autism subtypes have yielded conflicting results, but the majority of studies suggest an interaction effect between higher levels of anxiety and higher levels of cognitive capacity (MacNeil et al., 2009; White et al., 2013). However, this assumption may be due to the difficulties related to anxiety recognition in people with autism and ID (MacNeil et al., 2009). For example, in a comparison between checklist assessment and individual clinical assessment, it was found that physiological arousal may be difficult to observe in people with autism and ID (Helverschou and Martinsen, 2011). Anxiety reactions, both usual and idiosyncratic reactions, seem more easily recognized. Thus, anxiety disorders may be identified in individuals with autism and ID with the same or similar symptoms as in non-autistic individuals. To be able to identify the anxiety symptoms, further psychiatric examinations are recommended, using both checklists and systematic observations, as well as signs of general adjustment problems (Helverschou, 2010).

Prevalence of mental illness in people with ID and autism

A representative study of mental illness among adolescents and adults in Norway screened prevalence of mental illness in people with ID and autism – the "autism group," compared to people with "ID only" (Bakken et al., 2010). Sixty-two autism and 132 ID-only participants were screened for mental illness with the PAC (Helverschou et al., 2009). The PAC encompasses 42 items: 30 items representing four diagnostic groups (psychosis, depression, anxiety, and OCD) and 12 items representing general adjustment problems – GAP (passivity, unrest, sleeping and eating problems, social avoidance, aggression, and self-harm).

The screening procedure required severe GAP scores concomitantly with above cutoff scores for one of the four mental illness categories to screen for a psychiatric disorder. General adjustment problems also occur concomitantly with symptoms of mental illness in the general population. In people with autism and ID who suffer from mental illness, such symptoms are found to be prominently present (Helverschou et al., 2009).

Severe GAP prevalence was found to be high both in the autism group – 56.5%, and ID-only group – 22.7%. The prevalence of severe adjustment problems was very high in the autism group and markedly lower in the ID-only group. Most of the individuals with severe GAP were also found to have a psychiatric disorder. The screened prevalence of the four diagnostic groups varied markedly in both the autism and the ID-only group. The relative frequency of depression was highest in the ID-only group – 87% of the participants with severe GAP scores, compared to 70% in the autism group (not statistically significant). The lowest prevalence found in both groups was for OCD; about 24% of those with autism and 17% of those without. More than a quarter of the participants with autism screened for psychosis, compared to about 9% in the ID-only group. About 64% in the autism group screened for anxiety.

Generally, those screened with one of the psychiatric diagnoses also had high scores corresponding to the other disorders. Thus, it seems that signs of *all* the psychiatric disorders were widespread among those who scored for at least one disorder. In the total group screened with mental illness, the differences between the psychosis and the depression scores on one hand, and the anxiety and the OCD scores on the other hand, were statistically significant.

The results from the study suggested an interaction effect between autism/ID and mental illness. Especially the prevalence of anxiety seemed to be relatively higher in the autism than in the ID-only group, though all four diagnostic groups had a substantially higher screened prevalence in the autism than in the ID-only group. The result suggested that having anxiety problems is an important characteristic of the adult autism population, and anxiety problems are probably involved in the development of psychiatric disorders in this population (Helverschou et al., 2011). It is suggested that the occurrence of psychiatric disorders in autism constitutes an intrinsic feature of an autistic liability, due to the poor association between psychiatric disorders and language skills or level of IQ (Hutton et al., 2008).

Implications for clinical practice

Mental illness in people with autism and ID is linked to the risk factors of adjustment problems, anxiety, and breaks of continuity. Adjustment problems are directly and indirectly caused by main characteristics of autism. Most basic is an inadequate understanding of the social context; for example, deficient social understanding and social skills, failure to know how to perform some ordinary tasks, and an inability to meet the expectations of others. There is an indirect link with *structure dependency*. ID and mental illness strengthen and add to the adjustment problems, which may increase their autistic traits in number and severity.

Diagnostic assessment

Research indicates that, even in countries where research addresses mental illness in people with autism, there is probably extensive underdiagnosis of mental illness in this group (Bakken et al., 2010; Bradley et. al., 2011). However, recent studies showing an increased prevalence indicate that more people with autism are being acknowledged as suffering from mental illness (Joshi et al., 2010; Helverschou et al., 2011).

Understanding the patients' symptoms, colored by idiosyncratic speech and behavior, is a prerequisite for valid diagnoses. For example, to distinguish between idiosyncratic ways of expressing feelings and psychotic delusions, information about characteristics and symptoms must be collected from preschool childhood onwards (Bakken and Høidal, 2013). Information including psychometrics, interviews with formal and informal caregivers, observations, and physiological measures is crucial (MacNeil et al., 2009; Bakken and Høidal, 2013).

Confounding between autism and mental illness may cause diagnostic shadowing both ways; mental illness may be overlooked when symptoms are attributed to impairments caused by autism, and autism may be overlooked by mental illness symptoms overshadowing characteristics of autism (Geurts and Jansen, 2011; Cholemkery et al., 2014).

Services and treatment

Evidence is sparse for best clinical practice for adults and adolescents with autism and ID and additional mental illness (Helverschou et al., 2011). Services, especially psychosocial interventions, are understudied (Helverschou et al., 2011). An important period regarding mental health for persons with autism is transition from childhood to adulthood, as most services are still provided for children (McConachie et al., 2011). As the average onset age for major psychiatric disorders like psychosis and affective disorder is in adolescence and early adulthood, this is a critical phase (McConachie et al., 2011).

As psychiatric treatment in this area is a neglected area of research, approaches so far have for the most part been adapted methods from general psychiatry or from patients with ID only (Bakken et al., 2008b; Bakken, 2014; White et al., 2013). Cognitive impairments are aggravated when individuals with autism are affected by mental illness, and, therefore, treatment should be provided in a timely and systematic manner and individually tailored (Simonoff et al., 2008). Communication deficits and impaired ability for introspection disqualify insight-oriented psychotherapy aimed at uncovering inner conflicts, especially in the presence of psychotic ideas or behavior (Ghaziuddin, 2005). Therapy, therefore, is often psychoeducative and supportive.

For psychotic or affective disorders, a combination therapy of medication and psychosocial intervention is recommended beside a plan for crisis intervention (Helverschou et al., 2011); the clients may also profit from inpatient admission (Bakken and Martinsen, 2013). In the acute phase, individuals with autism and psychosis or affective disorder may show severe global functional deterioration and disorganized behavior, and, hence, not be able to uphold basic self-care tasks such as eating, going to the bathroom or dressing, and upholding social relationships (Bakken, 2014). They may appear agitated and active. This restlessness may "mask" their energy loss, irritability, and aggression in depression. Such misinterpretations regularly lead to demands for task solving, which are impossible for clients to perform, and which at the same time they are incapable of communicating verbally (Bakken et al., 2008a). However, according to clinical experience, individuals with autism and ID will again master previously learned skills when the most acute phase has passed (Bakken et al., 2008b). Hence, therapeutic variables include the elimination of demands and tasks that the client is not capable of performing. Effective staff communication, including *responding meaningfully*, achieving *joint attention, task sustainment, and emotional support*, is a prerequisite for therapeutic interaction with the client, especially if he or she is psychotic (Bakken et al., 2008a). Unless staff know the patient's idiosyncratic use of words and phrases, and also idiosyncratic behavior, they cannot provide adequate staff response to the patient's utterances.

The emotional climate in treatment settings has important effects on patient outcome. Professional caregivers ought to be sensitive to the clients' symptoms (Bakken, 2014).

Due to cognitive impairments, the client may feel uneasy and stressed when a caregiver is talking and he or she does not understand. Instructions might be perceived as criticism (stressful) by the patient, even when caregivers try to help the patient to master the task. Caregiver communication should be characterized by low expressed emotion without criticism, hostility, and over-involvement (Bakken, 2014).

Anxiety symptoms displayed by clients with other psychiatric disorders like depression and psychoses may benefit from interventions specifically directed to clients with anxiety disorders (Helverschou, 2010; Mohiuddin et al., 2011; Steensel et al., 2011; Wood et al., 2015). Studies including people with autism and anxiety disorders and control groups indicate that cognitive-behavioral therapy (CBT) approaches, adapted to the individual's level of functioning, are most frequently recommended for this group (White et al., 2013). There is consensus in this field that CBT has to be adjusted to the communication and comprehension difficulties and specific needs that characterize individuals with ASD. Additionally, the clients should not be exposed to unplanned events or unfamiliar people. A rehabilitation plan should include well-known activities in order to avoid stress. In order to prevent and reduce anxiety, staff–client intereraction should uphold structure and predictability, strategies similar to those typically recommended for people with autism (Helverschou, 2006). Clinical experience underpins that anxiety reactions are especially frequent in the acute phases of psychoses and mood disorders.

Interventions towards people with autism and post-traumatic stress disorder have barely been studied. In a recently published case study, psychosocial interventions towards people with more severe ID were studied (Bakken et al., 2014). The study suggested that interventions require a therapist as well. Exposure therapy may be contraindicated in patients with more severe ID in addition to autism. Hence, protection from anxiety triggers may be more feasible (Bakken et al., 2014).

Among adults with autism, psychotropic medication is common, although there is no evidence that psychotropic medication is effective related to core features of autism (Stachnik and Nunn-Thompson, 2007). However, case reports imply that relevant medication is essential also in autism populations with regard to anxiety disorders, OCD, psychosis, mania, and depression (Ghaziuddin, 2005). It is recommended that pharmacotherapy should be provided only for specific target symptoms (Volkmar, 2014). People with ID and autism tend to report side effects inadequately (Tveter et al., 2014).

Conclusions

It is vital that professionals involved in diagnostics and treatment have broad expertise in both autism and mental illness. When autism appears in combination with ID, which particularly represent special challenges related to diagnostics and treatment, specialized experience with this issue is additionally required.

Key summary points

- Mental illness may easily be missed in people with ID due to diagnostic overshadowing, especially with regard to the symptoms of schizophrenia and OCD, which resemble the characteristics of ASD.
- At present there is no consensus on diagnostic practice and criteria for the purpose of diagnosing mental illness in people with ASD.
- Diagnostic criteria needs to be modified to successfully diagnose mental illness in people with ASD and ID.
- General adjustment problems, such as passivity, unrest, sleeping and eating problems, social avoidance, aggression, and self-harm, may be caused by mental illness. When people with ASD and ID show adjustment problems, mental illness should be ruled out.

- Few interventions especially developed for this group of clients exist. At this point, adapted interventions used for the general population or for individuals with ID should be provided.
- Interventions must be adapted individually regarding the client's cognitive capacity, personal communication style and behavior, and additional impairments such as dysfunctional sensory integration.

References

Bakken, T.L. (2014). Psychosis and disorganized behavior in adults with autism and intellectual disability: case identification and staff–patient interaction. In V.B. Patel, V.R. Preedy, C.R. Martin (eds.), *Comprehensive Guide to Autism.* New York, NY: Springer Science.

Bakken, T.L. and Høidal, S.H. (2013). Asperger syndrome or schizophrenia, or both? Case identification of 12 adults in a specialised psychiatric inpatient unit. *International Journal of Developmental Disabilities*, 60(4), 215–225.

Bakken, T.L. and Martinsen, H. (2013). Adults with intellectual disabilities and mental illness in psychiatric inpatient units. Empirical studies of patient characteristics and psychiatric diagnoses from 1996–2011. *International Journal of Developmental Disabilities*, 59(3), 179–190.

Bakken, T.L., Eilertsen, D.E., Smeby, N.A., Martinsen, H. (2008a). Effective communication related to psychotic disorganised behaviour in adults with intellectual disability and autism. *Nordic Journal of Nursing Research and Clinical Studies*, 28(88), 9–13.

Bakken, T.L., Foss, N.E., Helverschou, S.B., et al. (2008b). *Mental Illness in Adults with Autism and ID – Experiences from 19 Case Management Projects.* Oslo: The National Autism Unit, Oslo University Hospital.

Bakken, T.L., Eilertsen, D.E., Smeby, N.A., Martinsen, H. (2009). The validity of disorganised behaviour as an indicator of psychosis in adults with autism and intellectual disability: a single case study. *Mental Health Aspects of Developmental Disabilities*, 12(1), 17–22.

Bakken, T.L., Helverschou, S.B., Eilertsen, D.E., et al. (2010). Psychiatric disorders in adolescents and adults with autism and intellectual disability: a representative study in one county in Norway. *Research in Developmental Disabilities*, 31, 1669–1677.

Bakken, T.L., Kildahl, A.N., Gjersoe, V., et al. (2014). PTSD in adults with intellectual disabilities: stabilisation during inpatient stay. *Advances in Mental Health and Intellectual Disabilities*, 8(4), 237–247.

Bradley, E., Lunsky, Y., Palucka, A., Homitidis, S. (2011). Recognition of intellectual disabilities and autism in psychiatric inpatients diagnosed with schizophrenia and other psychotic disorders. *Advances in Mental Health and Intellectual Disabilities*, 5(6), 4–18.

Cholemkery, H., Mojica, L., Rohrmann, S., et al. (2014). Can autism spectrum disorder and social anxiety disorders be differentiated by the social responsiveness scale in children and adolescents? *Journal of Autism and Developmental Disorders*, 44, 1168–1182.

Colvin, G. and Sheehan, M.R. (2014). *Managing the Cycle of Meltdown for Students with Autism.* New York, NY: Skyhorse Publishing.

Geurts, H.M. and Jansen, M.D. (2011). A retrospective chart study: the pathway to a diagnosis for adults referred for ASD assessment. *Autism*, 16(3), 299–305.

Ghaziuddin, M. (2005). *Mental Health Aspects of Autism and Asperger Syndrome.* London: Jessica Kingsley.

Gillott, A. and Stranden, P.J. (2007). Levels of anxiety and sources of stress in adults with autism. *Journal of Intellectual Disabilities*, 11, 359–370.

Green, S.A., Ben-Sasson, A., Soto, T.W., Carter, A.S. (2012). Anxiety and sensory over-responsivity in toddlers with autism spectrum disorders: bidirectional effects across time. *Journal of Autism and Developmental Disorders*, 42(6), 1112–1119.

Helverschou, S.B. (2006). Structure, predictability and manual sign teaching as strategies in regulation of emotions and anxiety. In S. von Tetzchner, E. Grindheim, J. Johannessen, et al. (eds.), *Biological Presuppositions to Culturalization*. Oslo: The Autism Society and University of Oslo.

Helverschou, S.B. (2010). Identification of anxiety and other psychiatric disorders in individuals with autism and intellectual disability. PhD thesis. Oslo: Department of Psychology, University of Oslo.

Helverschou, S.B. and Martinsen, H. (2011). Anxiety in people diagnosed with autism and intellectual disability: recognition and phenomenology. *Research in Autism Spectrum Disorders*, 5, 377–387.

Helverschou, S.B., Bakken, T.L. Martinsen, H. (2008). Identifying symptoms of psychiatric disorders in people with autism and intellectual disability: an empirical conceptual analysis. *Mental Health Aspects of Developmental Disabilities*, 11(4), 105–115.

Helverschou, S.B., Bakken, T.L., Martinsen, H. (2009). The Psychopathology in Autism Checklist (PAC): a pilot study. *Research in Autism Spectrum Disorders*, 3, 179–195.

Helverschou, S.B., Bakken, T.L., Martinsen, H. (2011). Psychiatric disorders in people with autism spectrum disorders: phenomenology and recognition. In J.L. Matson and P. Sturmey (eds.), *International Handbook of Autism and Pervasive Developmental Disorders*. New York, NY: Springer.

Helverschou, S.B., Utgaard, K., Wandaas, P.C. (2013). The challenges of applying and assessing cognitive behavioural therapy for individuals on the autism spectrum in a clinical setting: a case study series. *Good Autism Practice*, 14(1), 17–27.

Hill, E. and Frith, U. (2003). Understanding autism: insights from mind and brain. *Philosophical Transactions of the Royal Society of London. Series B, Biological Sciences*, 358, 281–289.

Howlin, P. and Moss, P. (2012). Adults with autism spectrum disorders. *Canadian Journal of Psychiatry*, 57, 275–283.

Hutton, J., Goode, S., Murphy, M., et al. (2008). New-onset psychiatric disorders in individuals with autism. *Autism*, 12, 373–390.

Joshi, G., Petty, C., Wozniak, J., et al. (2010). The heavy burden of psychiatric comorbidity in youth with autism spectrum disorders: a large comparative study of a psychiatrically referred population. *Journal of Autism and Developmental Disorders*, 40, 1361–1370.

Lane, A.E., Young, R.L., Baker, A.E.Z., Angley, M.T. (2010). Sensory processing subtypes in autism: association with adaptive behaviour. *Journal of Autism and Developmental Disorders*, 40, 112–122.

MacNeil, B.M., Lopes, V.A., Minnes, P.M. (2009). Anxiety in children and adolescents with autism spectrum disorders. *Research in Autism Spectrum Disorders*, 3, 1–21.

McConachie, H., Hoole, S., Le Couteur, A.S. (2011). Improving mental health transitions for young people with autism spectrum disorder. *Child: Care, Health and Development*, 37(6), 764–766.

Matson, J. and Cervantes, P.E. (2014). Commonly studied comorbid psychopathologies among persons with autism spectrum disorders. *Research in Developmental Disabilities*, 35, 952–962.

Matson, J.L. and Nebel-Schwalm, M.S. (2007). Comorbid psychopathology with autism spectrum disorder in children: an overview. *Research in Developmental Disabilities*, 28(4), 341–352.

Melville, C.A., Cooper, S.A., Morrison, J., et al. (2008). The prevalence and incidence of mental ill-health in adults with autism and intellectual disability. *Journal of Autism and Developmental Disorders*, 38, 1676–1688.

Mohiuddin, S., Bobak, A., Gih, D., Ghaziuddin, M. (2011). Autism spectrum disorders: comorbid psychopathology and treatment. In J.L. Matson and P. Sturmey (eds.), *International Handbook of Autism and Pervasive Developmental Disorders*. New York, NY: Springer.

Morgan, K. (2006). Is autism a stress disorder? What studies of nonautistic populations can tell us. In M.G. Baron, J. Groden, G. Groden, L.P. Lipsitt (eds.), *Stress and Coping in Autism*. Oxford: Oxford University Press.

Reese, R.M., Richman, D.M., Belmont, J.M., Morse, P. (2005). Functional characteristics of disruptive behaviour in developmental disabled children with and without autism. *Journal of Autism and Developmental Disorders*, 35, 419–428.

Samson, A.C., Phillips, J.M., Parker, K.J. (2014). Emotion dysregulation and the core features of autism spectrum disorder *Journal of Autism and Developmental Disorders*, 44, 1766-1772.

Scahill, L., McDougle, C.J., Williams, S., et al. (2006). Children's Yale–Brown Obsessive Compulsive Scale modified for pervasive developmental disorders. *Journal of American Academy of Child and Adolescent Psychiatry*, 45, 1114–1123.

Schaaf, R.C., Benevides, T., Mailloux, Z., et al. (2014). An inventory for sensory difficulties in children with autism: a randomized trial. *Journal of Autism and Developmental Disorders*, 44, 1493–1506.

Simonoff, E., Pickles, A., Charman, T., et al. (2008). Psychiatric disorders in children with autism spectrum disorders: prevalence, comorbidity, and associated factors in a population-derived sample. *Journal of the American Academy of Child and Adolescent Psychiatry*, 47(8), 921–929.

Simonoff, E., Jones, C.R.G., Pickles, A., et al. (2012). Severe mood problems in adolescents with autism spectrum disorder. *Journal of Child Psychology and Psychiatry*, 53(11), 1157–1166.

Simonoff, E., Jones, C.R.G., Baird, G., et al. (2013). The persistence and stability of psychiatric problems in adolescents with autism spectrum disorders. *Journal of Child Psychology and Psychiatry*, 54(2), 186–194.

Skokauskas, N. and Gallagher, L. (2010). Psychosis, affective disorders and anxiety in autistic spectrum disorder: prevalence and nosological considerations. *Psychopathology*, 43, 8–16.

Stachnik, J. and Nunn-Thompson, C. (2007). Use of atypical antipsychotics in the treatment of autistic disorder. *Annals of Pharmacotherapy*, 41, 626–634.

Steensel, F.J.A., Bögels, S.M., Perrin, S. (2011). Anxiety disorders in children and adolescents with autistic spectrum disorders: a meta-analysis. *Clinical Child and Family Review*, 14, 302–317.

Tsakanikos, E., Costello, H., Holt, G., et al. (2006). Psychopathology in adults with autism and intellectual disability. *Journal of Autism and Developmental Disorders*, 36, 1123–1129.

Tveter, A.L., Bakken, T.L., Bramness, J.G., Røssberg, J.I. (2014). Adjustment of the UKU Side Effect Rating Scale for adults with intellectual disabilities. A pilot study. *Advances in Mental Health and Intellectual Disabilities*, 8(4), 260–267.

Underwood, L., McCarthy, J., Tsakanikos, E. (2011). Assessment of comorbid psychopathology. In J.L. Matson and P. Sturmey (eds.), *International Handbook of Autism and Pervasive Developmental Disorders*. New York, NY: Springer.

Volkmar, F. (2014). Practice parameter for the assessment and treatment of children and adolescents with autism spectrum disorder. *Journal of the American Academy of Child and Adolescent Psychiatry*, 53(2), 237–257.

White, S., Ollendick, T., Albanmo, A.M. (2013). Randomized controlled trial: multimodal anxiety and social skill intervention for adolescents with autism spectrum disorder. *Journal of Autism and Developmental Disorders*, 43, 382–394.

Wood, J.J. Ehrenreich-May, J., Alessandri, M., et al. (2015). Cognitive behavioral therapy for early adolescents with autism spectrum disorders and clinical anxiety: a randomized, controlled trial, behavior therapy. *Behavior Therapy*, 46(1), 7–19.

12 Attention-deficit/hyperactivity disorder (ADHD)

Elizabeth Evans and Julian Trollor

Introduction

Mounting evidence suggests that attention-deficit/hyperactivity disorder (ADHD) is more common in people with ID than in the general population (Fox and Wade, 1998; O'Brien, 2000; Baker et al., 2010; Neece et al., 2013a). However, diagnostic assessment and management in this population can present significant challenges, and clinicians report feeling less confident in diagnosing ADHD in people with ID compared with those with ADHD alone (Buckley et al., 2006). Within people with ID, ADHD is an additional source of disability which compounds the ID: those with ADHD comorbid to ID show significantly greater impairments in adaptive behavior than those with ID alone (Carmeli et al., 2007), and ADHD diagnoses and symptoms in this population are associated with as high a psychosocial impact as for those without ID (Simonoff et al., 2007), as well as high rates of other psychiatric comorbidities (Neece et al., 2013a).

What is ADHD?

ADHD is a neurodevelopmental disorder with onset in childhood, which is characterized by a persistent pattern of inattention and/or hyperactivity and impulsivity (American Psychiatric Association, 2013). The *Diagnostic and Statistical Manual of Mental Disorders, Fifth Edition* (DSM-5) criteria emphasize the requirements of: symptom onset before the age of 12 years; at least six months duration of symptoms; evidence for symptoms across several settings; significant functional impact; and lack of explanation of symptoms by the presence of another mental disorder (American Psychiatric Association, 2013). Of significance is the requirement for symptoms to be considered with reference to the developmental level of the individual. A lower threshold of inattentive or hyperactive/impulsive symptoms is required for older adolescents and adults (five of nine symptoms in either or both domains) compared to children (six of nine symptoms in either or both domains). However, thresholding of these criteria have not been undertaken for people with an ID. Subtypes are labeled as "combined" or as "predominantly inattentive," or "predominantly hyperactive/impulsive" presentations of the disorder (American Psychiatric Association, 2013). The *International Classification of Diseases and Related Health Problems, Tenth Revision* (ICD-10) uses the term "Hyperkinetic disorder" to refer to a similar disorder, but specifies symptoms must have been apparent no later than seven years of age (World Health Organization, 1992).

Psychiatric and Behavioral Disorders in Intellectual and Developmental Disabilities, ed. Colin Hemmings and Nick Bouras. Published by Cambridge University Press. © Cambridge University Press 2016.

Specific adaptations of ADHD criteria have been published for people with ID. The *Diagnostic Criteria for Psychiatric Disorders for Use with Adults with Learning Disabilities/Mental Retardation* (DC-LD; Royal College of Psychiatrists, 2001) is applicable only to adults, whereas the *Diagnostic Manual – Intellectual Disability* (DM-ID; Fletcher et al., 2007) applies to children, adolescents, and adults with ID. These systems simplify the criteria for ADHD; however, neither the DM-ID nor the DC-LD specify adapted thresholds for symptoms of ADHD in each domain for those with ID, nor do they contextualize the evaluation of such symptoms in the context of ID, beyond stating the need to consider whether symptoms are accounted for by level of ID. External validation and field testing of these criteria for different levels of ID is required.

Epidemiology

Although ADHD appears to be more common in people with ID than in the general population, findings from studies are inconsistent. Prevalence figures in people with ID range from 8.7% to over 40% for children and adolescents (e.g., Strømme and Diseth, 2000; Neece et al., 2013a), and from less than 2% to 55% for adults (e.g., Cooper et al., 2007). Potential reasons for discrepant findings include different sampling strategies resulting in differing age ranges and levels of ID represented in each study, differing assessment methods (e.g., clinician diagnosis vs. criteria-based structured interview schedules, and different approaches to measuring impairment) along with the different diagnostic criteria employed and whether inattentive subtypes are included. Taken together, in keeping with a range of other mental disorders, ADHD is probably over-represented around threefold in people with an ID compared to the general population (Baker et al., 2010; Neece et al., 2011, 2013a).

The relationship between the prevalence of ADHD and ADHD symptoms and level of ID is unclear. For example, O'Brien's (2000) epidemiological study of young adults with ID found increasing rates of ADHD in those with more severe ID, while other studies (e.g., Pearson and Aman, 1994) do not support this observation. These discrepant findings highlight a potential difficulty in identifying ADHD in those with more severe ID (Fox and Wade 1998; Antshel et al., 2006b).

Vulnerability to ADHD is conferred by a number of means, including many biological, environmental, and social risk factors, which give rise to both ADHD and ID. Further, a number of syndromes associated with ID are also associated with an ADHD phenotype. These include tuberous sclerosis complex (De Vries et al., 2007), Williams syndrome (Leyfer et al., 2006), Fragile X syndrome (Hagerman, 2002), Angelman syndrome (Barry et al., 2005), and velocardiofacial syndrome (Antshel et al., 2006a). The added value of diagnosis of ADHD in the setting of a syndrome with a characteristic behavioral phenotype is debatable, but may assist in the prioritization of intervention if clinically meaningful symptoms of ADHD are present.

The impact of ADHD

The functional, social, psychological, and economic impact of ADHD in the general population is well documented (Jensen et al., 2001,). Studies of people with ID have suggested that those with comorbid ADHD experience a "double deficit," which manifests as further impairment of functional skills (Carmeli et al., 2007) and cognitive functions (Di Nuovo and Buono, 2007; Rose et al., 2009). As with the general population, the combination of ADHD and ID in adolescence has significant impact in the educational setting, with ADHD symptoms being predictive of later suspension from school (Handen et al., 1997). In adulthood, the combination of ADHD and ID is associated with increased aggressive and self-injurious behaviors (Cooper et al., 2009a, 2009b), which in turn is likely to be associated with poorer outcomes.

ADHD in the general population is associated with high rates of psychiatric comorbidity, including disorders such as oppositional defiant disorder (ODD), conduct disorder, specific learning disorders, tic disorders, anxiety disorders, affective disorders, and substance-use disorders (e.g., Mayes et al., 2000; Jensen et al., 2001; Biederman et al., 2010). Less is known regarding psychiatric comorbidities in children with ID and ADHD, but emerging evidence suggests very high rates of other mental health problems in this group, particularly ODD (Neece et al., 2013a,). Patterns of additional psychiatric comorbidity in people with both ADHD and ID also appear high in the clinical context, and underscore the complex neuro-behavioral and psychological vulnerabilities of people with both ADHD and ID.

Diagnostic validity in the context of ID

Historically, the question of whether an ADHD diagnosis is valid in the presence of ID has been debated (Burack et al., 2001), and indeed, there is some evidence of a discontinuity between ADHD in people with and without ID, such as differing gender distributions (e.g., Hastings et al., 2005; Neece et al., 2013b). However, validity for the diagnosis is bolstered by several lines of evidence. First, studies which support higher prevalence of ADHD in people with ID (e.g., O'Brien, 2000; Strømme and Diseth, 2000) are consistent with the well-documented, significant negative association between IQ and ADHD symptoms in the general population (Frazier et al., 2004; Antshel et al. 2006b). Second, rates of ADHD symptoms are elevated in people with ID, even after controlling for mental age (e.g., Pearson and Aman, 1994; Hastings et al., 2005), suggesting that lowered IQ alone cannot explain ADHD symptoms. Third, there are consistencies in findings in people with ADHD with and without ID, with respect to the nature of symptoms, their developmental course, the risk factor profiles, and comorbidity profiles (e.g., Antshel et al., 2006b; Neece et al., 2013a, 2013b).

Assessment of ADHD

A multimodal approach is required that follows best practice guidelines for the general population (National Institute for Health and Clinical Excellence, 2008; Royal Australian College of Physicians, 2009), with modifications for the person with ID. Detailed evaluation of current symptoms, an evaluation of their impact across a variety of settings, and the collection of information from multiple different sources is required. The issue of whether to evaluate the individual's symptoms relative to expectations based on chronological age, developmental age, or level of ID has previously been debated (Pearson and Aman, 1994; Seager and O'Brien, 2003). From a clinical perspective, comparing to peers of a similar age *and* level of ID is the most sensible approach (Fletcher et al., 2007). Observational data may assist in determining the severity, frequency, and impact of symptoms, relative to expectation based on level of ID. Detailed evaluation for possible causes or contributors to symptoms, including screening for relevant medical factors (e.g., seizures, sleep disorders, and thyroid disorders) and psychiatric factors is essential.

A thorough developmental assessment and psychiatric history will allow the context-ualization of the symptoms with regard to the person's level of ID, the identification of other relevant psychiatric comorbidities, and if necessary, a review of the etiology of the ID itself. An evaluation of intellectual and adaptive functions may be required if this has not been performed or previous results are unavailable or very old. In the context of mild ID, a psychoeducational assessment may be required if the history suggests the presence of an additional learning disorder. Allied health assessments can assist in determining comorbid speech and language, motor coordination, and sensory problems. Assessing the environmental context to identify possible drivers and moderators of symptoms is important and should take into account the physical environment, adequacy of supports, and dynamics and mental health within the family or cohabitation setting.

Detailed neuropsychological assessment is not routinely recommended but may be of value where there is diagnostic uncertainty in individuals with mild ID, and where more detailed understanding of cognitive strengths and weaknesses is required in planning educational goals. Neurophysiological tests such as the measurement of event-related potentials (ERP) or quantitative analysis of electroencephalogram (EEG) are not recom-mended in people with ID. Structural brain imaging such as magnetic resonance imaging (MRI) of the brain is only recommended if ADHD symptoms are considered to be secondary to a condition associated with underlying structural brain changes. Functional brain imaging such as functional MRI (fMRI) is not recommended in the diagnostic assessment.

For adults with ID who have come for assessment of ADHD symptoms for the first time, a detailed retrospective evaluation for ADHD symptoms in childhood must be performed. Whilst retrospective self-reports of symptoms may be of value, independent verification, preferably from a parent, is important. Other sources of childhood infor-mation, such as previous psychometric assessments, school reports, and information from residential and respite placements, may also be of use.

Symptom rating scales are commonplace in the assessment of ADHD in people without ID. With few exceptions, the validity of these scales in people with ID is either uncertain or questionable: Miller et al. (2004a, 2004b) examined the psychometric properties of popular rating scales assessing symptoms of ADHD in a small sample of children with ID and found very low correlations between parent rating scales. Further, the applicability of such scales in more severe levels of disability appears limited (e.g., Deb et al., 2008). Behavioral rating scales validated for use with people with ID may be more useful (Miller et al., 2004a). The Developmental Behavior Checklist Hyperactiv-ity Index (Einfeld and Tonge, 2002) has been found to have construct validity and discriminant function when used with young people with ID (Einfeld and Tonge, 2002), and to discriminate between children and adolescents with autism spectrum disorders alone and ADHD plus autism spectrum disorders (Gargaro et al., 2014). However, replication with larger samples is required.

Management of ADHD

Current clinical guidelines (National Institute for Health and Clinical Excellence, 2008; Royal Australian College of Physicians, 2009; Canadian ADHD Resource Alliance, 2011) provide comprehensive management recommendations that should be used as a frame-work for the approach to ADHD management in people with ID. These guidelines outline an integrated approach to care that encompasses a broad range of social, personal, educational, and occupational needs. Key principles in the management of ADHD in people with ID include: the adoption of a person-centered approach; promotion of independence whilst acknowledging the age and capacity of the individual; undertaking multidisciplinary assessment and management that engages family and carers; the setting of clear goals for management and monitoring the effectiveness of intervention; and ensuring clinical practice is based on the best available evidence. Significant adaptation of the clinical approach is often required for the assessment and management of ADHD in people with ID. Adaptations may include: preparation and adjustments of consultation processes and length; adaptation of communication; engaging the person and where appropriate the guardian/s in decision-making; and allowing for extended models of working with families and carers.

As with ADHD in the general population, an individual management plan that takes into account specific needs and individual and carer preferences should be developed. However, for individuals with ID and ADHD, consideration of a more complex array of factors is necessary, including: (i) where multiple psychiatric or developmental comorbidities exist, prioritizing interventions, and seeking to minimize impact of ADHD treatments on co-occurring conditions; (ii) careful evaluation of the potential adverse consequences of ADHD pharmacotherapy in the context of individuals with complex medical comorbidities and reduced ability to spontaneously communicate side effects; (iii) determining priorities for intervention in a person-centered manner, including consultation with guardians and family carers as appropriate; (iv) where multiple psychosocial disadvantage exists, carefully prioritizing intervention strategies that are most likely to benefit the mental health and well-being of the individual, thus, avoiding overwhelming the individual or their support networks; and (v) the coordination of clinical care across a potentially more complicated array of settings including educational, vocational, respite, and place of residence.

Education about ADHD for the affected individual, their family, and carers is a core aspect of sound management. For young children with moderately severe ADHD without ID, first-line treatment is parent training/education programs, either as a group or on an individual basis (National Institute for Health and Clinical Excellence, 2008). Although specific evidence for the effectiveness of parent training in children with ID and ADHD is lacking (Reilly and Holland, 2011), parent training can be effective for reducing behavioral difficulties in children with developmental disabilities (Hudson et al., 2003; Tellegen and Sanders, 2013), suggesting it may also be of value in children with ID and ADHD. Cognitive-behavioral therapies, social skills training, and family therapy should be employed where indicated, though direct evidence for their effectiveness in people with ID and ADHD is lacking.

As with the general population, pharmacotherapy in people with ID and ADHD should be limited to those individuals with severe ADHD symptoms and impairments, or where those with moderate symptoms and impairments either refuse non-pharmacological treatments or their symptoms fail to respond to such interventions (Royal Australian College of Physicians, 2009). Stimulants such as methylphenidate and amphetamine salts are the mainstay of drug treatment, but non-stimulant treatments such as atomoxetine or other treatments may also be appropriate (Rowles and Findling, 2010). A small number of short-term randomized controlled trials suggest the effectiveness of methylphenidate at low doses (Aman et al., 2003), higher doses (Pearson et al., 2003), and optimal dosing (Simonoff et al., 2013) in children and adolescents with ADHD. Other types of studies have also added some support for the effectiveness of both methylphenidate (e.g., Handen et al., 1999) and amphetamines (Jou et al., 2004) in ADHD with ID. However, it remains unclear whether stimulants are as effective in people with ID compared to people without ID (e.g., Aman et al., 2003), and whether they are effective in reducing symptoms across all settings (e.g., Pearson et al., 2003). Significant side effects, including sleep disturbance, appetite changes, and weight loss, have been noted in some stimulant studies (Pearson et al., 2003; Simonoff et al., 2013), but not in others (Aman et al., 2003).

In children with ADHD without ID, risperidone treatment is recommended only in the presence of significant conduct disorder with associated aggression (Royal Australian College of Physicians, 2009). No randomized controlled trials on the effectiveness of risperidone have been conducted in people with ADHD and ID. A direct comparison between methylphenidate and risperidone found a more pronounced effect in the latter for reducing ADHD symptoms in children and adolescents with moderate ID (Correia Filho et al., 2005). However, risperidone was associated with significant side effects, including weight gain and somnolence. Risperidone is not, therefore, generally recommended in people with ADHD and ID unless significant comorbidity with severe aggressive behaviors exists.

Areas for future research

Further research is required to establish baseline rates of symptoms of inattentiveness and hyperactivity in people with different levels of ID and in situations where ID is occurring with other developmental disorders, such as autism spectrum disorders. Work in this area will promote greater clarity of the distinction between ADHD "symptoms" versus "disorder." With respect to ADHD diagnosis, neither criteria for the general population nor specific adaptations of criteria that have been developed for people with ID have been validated. Further, it remains unclear whether age adjustment is required for late adolescence and adulthood when considering whether an individual with ID meets threshold for an ADHD diagnosis. The utility of ID-specific and non-specific diagnostic or symptom scales in people with ID of varying levels awaits determination, and attempts should be made to determine their utility in tracking treatment response. Substantial gaps are apparent in the knowledge base regarding the comorbidity of ADHD and ID, and how this varies with level of ID. A more comprehensive evidence base is required on which to base clinical recommendations on both drug and non-drug therapies for ADHD in people with ID. Current research on drug treatments of ADHD largely excludes those with ID in order to control for comorbidities (Correia Filho et al., 2005). The few randomized controlled trials in people with ID have involved small samples (Aman et al., 2003; Pearson et al., 2003), restricted age ranges (Aman et al., 2003; Simonoff et al., 2013) and IQ ranges (Pearson et al., 2003), and brief durations (Pearson et al., 2003). Establishing the effectiveness of non-pharmacological approaches, including parent-training programs and applied behavioral therapy, is critical for this population (Deutsch et al., 2008; Reilly and Holland, 2011; Neece et al., 2013a). Finally, studies which identify risk factors for ADHD in people with ID are also needed (Neece et al., 2013b) in order to design preventative strategies.

Conclusions

Attention-deficit/hyperactivity disorder appears to be much more common in children, adolescents, and adults with ID compared with those without ID. A multimodal approach to diagnosis encompassing information from different sources is essential for people with ID, as is a detailed evaluation for potential medical and psychiatric factors. Symptoms should be assessed relative to both the person's chronological age and their level of ID, and observational data may assist with this. The management of ADHD in those with ID requires an integrated, multidisciplinary approach nestled within the context of the person's overall care. As for those without ID, non-pharmacological interventions should be considered as first-line treatments and pharmacotherapy reserved for those for whom symptoms and their impact are severe, or where non-pharmacological approaches have failed. Where drug therapies are considered, methylphenidate is the mainstay of treatment. However, further research on both pharmacological and non-pharmacological interventions for ADHD in people with ID is needed. Other key gaps in the current literature concern the thresholding of symptoms for diagnosis, the utility of diagnostic and symptom rating scales in this population, and the establishment of baseline rates of symptoms of inattentiveness and hyperactivity associated with different levels of ID.

Key summary points

- ADHD appears to be more common in people with ID compared with those without ID.
- Emerging evidence supports the validity of this diagnosis in some individuals with ID.
- Assessment of ADHD in people with ID requires information from multiple sources. Attention to potential alterative explanations for symptoms, such as medical and psychiatric disorders, is crucial.
- A multimodal approach to treatment is required, with pharmacological treatment being reserved for moderate or severe symptoms, or when non-pharmacological strategies have failed.

References

Aman, M.G., Buican, B., Arnold, L.E. (2003). Methylphenidate treatment in children with borderline IQ and mental retardation: analysis of three aggregated studies. *Journal of Child and Adolescent Psychopharmacology*, 13, 29–40.

American Psychiatric Association. (2013). *Diagnostic and Statistical Manual of Mental Disorders, Fifth Edition*. Washington, DC: American Psychiatric Association.

Antshel, K.M., Fremont, W., Roizen, N.J., et al. (2006a). ADHD, major depressive disorder, and simple phobias are prevalent psychiatric conditions in youth with velocardiofacial syndrome. *Journal of the American Academy of Child and Adolescent Psychiatry*, 45, 596–603.

Antshel, K.M., Phillips, M.H., Gordon, M., et al. (2006b). Is ADHD a valid disorder in children with intellectual delays? *Clinical Psychology Review*, 26, 555–572.

Baker, B.L., Neece, C.L., Fenning, R.M., Crnic, K.A., Blacher, J. (2010). Mental disorders in five-year-old children with or without developmental delay: focus on ADHD. *Journal of Clinical Child and Adolescent Psychology*, 39, 492–505.

Barry, R.J., Leitner, R.P., Clarke, A.R., Einfeld, S.L. (2005). Behavioral aspects of Angelman syndrome: a case control study. *American Journal of Medical Genetics Part A*, 132, 8–12.

Biederman, J., Petty, C.R., Evans, M., Small, J., Faraone, S.V. (2010). How persistent is ADHD? A controlled 10-year follow-up study of boys with ADHD. *Psychiatry Research*, 177, 299–304.

Buckley, S., Dodd, P., Burke, A., et al. (2006). Diagnosis and management of attention-deficit hyperactivity disorder in children and adults with and without learning disability. *Psychiatric Bulletin*, 30, 251–253.

Burack, J.A., Evans, D.W., Klaiman, C., Iarocci, G. (2001). The mysterious myth of attention deficits and other defect stories: contemporary issues in the developmental approach to mental retardation. *International Review of Research in Mental Retardation*, 24, 299–320.

Canadian ADHD Resource Alliance. (2011). *Canadian ADHD Practice Guidelines*, third edition. Toronto, ON: Canadian ADHD Resource Alliance.

Carmeli, E., Klein, N., Sohn, M. (2007). The implications of having attention-deficit/ hyperactivity disorder in male adolescents with intellectual disability. *International Journal of Adolescent Medicine and Health*, 19, 209–214.

Cooper, S.A., Smiley, E., Morrison, J., Williamson, A., Allan, L. (2007). Mental ill-health in adults with intellectual disabilities: prevalence and associated factors. *British Journal of Psychiatry*, 190, 27–35.

Cooper, S.A., Smiley, E., Allan, L.M., et al. (2009a). Adults with intellectual disabilities: prevalence, incidence and remission of self-injurious behaviour, and related factors. *Journal of Intellectual Disability Research*, 53, 200–216.

Cooper, S.A., Smiley, E., Jackson, A., et al. (2009b). Adults with intellectual disabilities: prevalence, incidence and remission of aggressive behaviour and related factors. *Journal of Intellectual Disability Research*, 53, 217–232.

Correia Filho, A.G., Bodanese, R., Silva, T.L., et al. (2005). Comparison of risperidone and methylphenidate for reducing ADHD symptoms in children and adolescents with moderate mental retardation. *Journal of the American Academy of Child and Adolescent Psychiatry*, 44, 748–755.

De Vries, P.J., Hunt, A., Bolton, P.F. (2007). The psychopathologies of children and adolescents with tuberous sclerosis complex (TSC). *European Child and Adolescent Psychiatry*, 16, 16–24.

Deb, S., Dhaliwal, A.J., Roy, M. (2008). The usefulness of Conners' Rating Scales – Revised in screening for attention deficit hyperactivity disorder in children with intellectual disabilities and borderline intelligence. *Journal of Intellectual Disability Research*, 52, 950–965.

Deutsch, C.K., Dube, W.V., McIlvane, W.J. (2008). Attention deficits, attention-deficit hyperactivity disorder, and intellectual disabilities. *Developmental Disabilities Research Reviews*, 14, 285–292.

Di Nuovo, S.F. and Buono, S. (2007). Psychiatric syndromes comorbid with mental retardation: differences in cognitive and adaptive skills. *Journal of Psychiatric Research*, 41, 795–800.

Einfeld, S.L. and Tonge, B.J. (2002). *Manual for the Developmental Behaviour Checklist, second edition – primary carer version (DBC-P) and teacher version (DBC-T)*. Sydney and Melbourne: The University of New South Wales and Monash University.

Fletcher, R., Loschen, E., Stavrakaki, C., et al. (eds.) (2007). *Diagnostic Manual – Intellectual Disability: A Textbook of Diagnosis of Mental Disorders in Persons with Intellectual Disability*. Kingston, NY: NADD Press.

Fox, R.A. and Wade, E.J. (1998). Attention deficit hyperactivity disorder among adults with severe and profound mental retardation. *Research in Developmental Disabilities*, 19, 275–280.

Frazier, T.W., Demaree, H.A., Youngstrom, E.A. (2004). Meta-analysis of intellectual and neuropsychological test performance in attention-deficit/hyperactivity disorder. *Neuropsychology*, 18, 543.

Gargaro, B., May, T., Tonge, B., et al. (2014). Using the DBC-P Hyperactivity Index to screen for ADHD in young people with autism and ADHD: a pilot study. *Research in Autism Spectrum Disorders*, 8, 1008–1015.

Hagerman, R.J. (2002). The physical and behavioral phenotype. In R.J. Hagerman and A. Cronister (eds.), *Fragile X Syndrome: Diagnosis, Treatment, and Research.* Baltimore, MD: The Johns Hopkins University Press.

Handen, B.L., Janosky, J., McAuliffe, S. (1997). Long-term follow-up of children with mental retardation/borderline intellectual functioning and ADHD. *Journal of Abnormal Child Psychology*, 25, 287–295.

Handen, B.L., Feldman, H.M., Lurier, A., Murray, P.J.H. (1999). Efficacy of methylphenidate among preschool children with developmental disabilities and ADHD. *Journal of the American Academy of Child and Adolescent Psychiatry*, 38, 805–812.

Hastings, R.P., Beck, A., Daley, D., Hill, C. (2005). Symptoms of ADHD and their correlates in children with intellectual disabilities. *Research in Developmental Disabilities*, 26, 456–468.

Hudson, A.M., Matthews, J.M., Gavidia-Payne, S.T., et al. (2003). Evaluation of an intervention system for parents of children with intellectual disability and challenging behaviour. *Journal of Intellectual Disability Research*, 47, 238–249.

Jensen, P.S., Hinshaw, S.P., Kraemer, H.C., et al. (2001). ADHD comorbidity findings from the MTA study: comparing comorbid subgroups. *Journal of the American Academy of Child and Adolescent Psychiatry*, 40, 147–158.

Jou, R., Handen, B., Hardan, A. (2004). Psychostimulant treatment of adults with mental retardation and attention-deficit hyperactivity disorder. *Australasian Psychiatry*, 12, 376–379.

Leyfer, O.T., Woodruff-Borden, J., Klein-Tasman, B.P., Fricke, J.S., Mervis, C.B. (2006). Prevalence of psychiatric disorders in 4 to 16-year-olds with Williams syndrome. *American Journal of Medical Genetics Part B: Neuropsychiatric Genetics*, 141, 615–622.

Mayes, S.D., Calhoun, S.L., Crowell, E.W. (2000). Learning disabilities and ADHD overlapping spectrum disorders. *Journal of Learning Disabilities*, 33, 417–424.

Miller, M.L., Fee, V.E., Jones, C.J. (2004a). Psychometric properties of ADHD rating scales among children with mental retardation II: validity. *Research in Developmental Disabilities*, 25, 477–492.

Miller, M.L., Fee, V.E., Netterville, A.K. (2004b). Psychometric properties of ADHD rating scales among children with mental retardation I: reliability. *Research in Developmental Disabilities*, 25, 459–476.

National Institute for Health and Clinical Excellence. (2008). *Attention Deficit Hyperactivity Disorder: Diagnosis and Management of ADHD in Children, Young People and Adults. NICE Guideline [CG 72].* At http://www.nice.org.uk/CG72

Neece, C.L., Baker, B.L., Blacher, J., Crnic, K.A. (2011). Attention-deficit/hyperactivity disorder among children with and without intellectual disability: an examination across time. *Journal of Intellectual Disability Research*, 55, 623–635.

Neece, C.L., Baker, B.L., Crnic, K., Blacher, J. (2013a). Examining the validity of ADHD as a diagnosis for adolescents with intellectual disabilities: clinical presentation. *Journal of Abnormal Child Psychology*, 41, 597–612.

Neece, C.L., Baker, B.L., Lee, S.S. (2013b). ADHD among adolescents with intellectual disabilities: pre-pathway influences. *Research in Developmental Disabilities*, 34, 2268–2279.

O'Brien, G. (2000). Learning disability. In C. Gillberg and G. O'Brien (eds.), *Developmental Disability and Behaviour.* London: MacKeith Press.

Pearson, D.A. and Aman, M.G. (1994). Ratings of hyperactivity and developmental indices: should clinicians correct for developmental level? *Journal of Autism and Developmental Disorders*, 24, 395–411.

Pearson, D.A., Santos, C.W., Roache, J.D., et al. (2003). Treatment effects of methylphenidate on behavioral adjustment in children with mental retardation and ADHD. *Journal of the American Academy of Child and Adolescent Psychiatry*, 42, 209–216.

Reilly, C. and Holland, N. (2011). Symptoms of attention deficit hyperactivity disorder in children and adults with intellectual disability: a review. *Journal of Applied Research in Intellectual Disabilities*, 24, 291–309.

Rose, E., Bramham, J., Young, S., Paliokostas, E., Xenitidis, K. (2009). Neuropsychological characteristics of adults with comorbid ADHD and borderline/mild intellectual disability. *Research in Developmental Disabilities*, 30, 496–502.

Rowles, B.M. and Findling, R.L. (2010). Review of pharmacotherapy options for the treatment of attention-deficit/hyperactivity disorder (ADHD) and ADHD-like symptoms in children and adolescents with developmental disorders. *Developmental Disabilities Research Reviews*, 16, 273–282.

Royal Australian College of Physicians. (2009). *Guidelines on Attention Deficit Hyperactivity Disorder (Draft)*. Sydney: Royal Australian College Of Physicians.

Royal College of Psychiatrists (2001). *Diagnostic Criteria for Psychiatric Disorders for Use with Adults with Learning Disabilities/Mental Retardation (DC-LD)*. London: Royal College of Psychiatrists.

Seager, M.C. and O'Brien, G. (2003). Attention deficit hyperactivity disorder: review of

ADHD in learning disability: *the Diagnostic Criteria for Psychiatric Disorders for Use with Adults with Learning Disabilities/ Mental Retardation[DC-LD]* criteria for diagnosis. *Journal of Intellectual Disability Research*, 47(Suppl. 1), 26–31.

Simonoff, E., Pickles, A., Wood, N., Gringras, P., Chadwick, O. (2007). ADHD symptoms in children with mild intellectual disability. *Journal of the American Academy of Child and Adolescent Psychiatry*, 46, 591–600.

Simonoff, E., Taylor, E., Baird, G., et al. (2013). Randomized controlled double-blind trial of optimal dose methylphenidate in children and adolescents with severe attention deficit hyperactivity disorder and intellectual disability. *Journal of Child Psychology and Psychiatry and Allied Disciplines*, 54, 527–535.

Strømme, P. and Diseth, T.H. (2000). Prevalence of psychiatric diagnoses in children with mental retardation: data from a population-based study. *Developmental Medicine and Child Neurology*, 42, 266–270.

Tellegen, C.L. and Sanders, M.R. (2013). Stepping Stones Triple P – positive parenting program for children with disability: a systematic review and meta-analysis. *Research in Developmental Disabilities*, 34, 1556–1571.

World Health Organization. (1992).*The ICD-10 Classification of Mental and Behavioural Disorders: Clinical Descriptions and Diagnostic Guidelines*. Geneva: World Health Organization.

Chapter 13

Psychopharmacology

Stephen Ruedrich

Introduction

Since the beginning of psychopharmacology, individuals with intellectual disabilities (ID) have been treated with medications (King, 2007). Psychopharmacological practice in persons with ID has been complicated by three different but overlapping approaches:

1. Use of psychotropic medication to address challenging behaviors.
2. Use of psychotropic medication to treat co-occurring psychiatric disorders.
3. Use of medications, some with psychotropic properties, to address ID syndromes themselves, with hope of directly or indirectly addressing associated psychiatric and/ or behavioral disorders.

Surrounding this complexity, many individuals with ID and their families, as well as clinicians and researchers, believe that psychotropics, and particularly antipsychotic medications, have been over-prescribed to persons with ID, often with little clinical justification, and without appropriate monitoring for toxicity (Deb and Unwin, 2007; Tsiouris, 2010).

Today, the use of psychotropic treatment of persons with ID should start with an accurate psychiatric diagnosis (Levitas, 2003). Once a diagnosis is made, psychotropic treatment can usually proceed as it would for a person without ID. Unfortunately, little psychopharmacological literature describes the treatment of specific psychiatric illnesses in persons with ID, surrounding the challenge of valid and reliable psychiatric diagnosis. Current psychotropic practice in persons with ID and psychiatric/behavioral disorders is often symptomatic treatment alone, in the absence of a validly identified psychiatric illness (Fletcher et al., 2007).

Psychopharmacological studies can be separated into three broad types, based on whether they focus primarily on the drug or drug class utilized, on psychiatric diagnosis, or the specific etiology of ID. Early studies presented the use of a particular medication (or class) across a range of diagnoses, and/or across a variety of ID etiologies. Later studies have focused on treatment of a single psychiatric disorder or diagnosis (e.g., depression), across a variety of ID etiologies. Increasingly, researchers are convinced of the importance of ID etiology in diagnosis, and the characterization of behavioral phenotypes (see Chapter 18). Future psychopharmacological studies, to improve validity, would focus on a particular medication or class for the treatment of a specific psychiatric

Psychiatric and Behavioral Disorders in Intellectual and Developmental Disabilities, ed. Colin Hemmings and Nick Bouras. Published by Cambridge University Press. © Cambridge University Press 2016.

disorder, in persons with ID, resulting from a single confirmed etiology (e.g., use of stimulants for attention-deficit/hyperactivity disorder (ADHD) in Fragile X syndrome).

Additionally, very few psychotropic medications have been developed for, or tested in, persons with ID. In new drug development, researchers and regulatory agencies have typically excluded individuals with ID, for a combination of reasons, such as protection of vulnerable research subjects, complex consent issues, metabolic differences, and difficulty of assessing accuracy of treatment response.

There are limited psychotropic studies meeting the contemporary scientific standard of the randomized controlled trial (RCT): double-blind, placebo-controlled methodologies, random assignment of subjects, and standardized measures of efficacy in persons with ID (Courtemanche et al., 2011).

The past

History of the treatment of persons with ID with psychotropic medications

Initial reports focused primarily on the medication utilized, often with little attention paid to psychiatric diagnoses or etiology of ID. As new agents became available, they were given to persons with ID, often in non-specific attempts to ameliorate aggression and self-injurious behavior (SIB); in spite of the suspected fallacy of this practice (Levitas, 2003). Initial agents included the barbiturate anticonvulsants, followed by the first-generation antipsychotics (FGAs), and benzodiazepines; all three have subsequently fallen out of favor (Schroeder et al., 1998). Barbiturates may have significant behavioral side effects (Kalachnik and Hanzel, 2001); similarly, up to 25% of persons with ID treated with benzodiazepines have behavioral disinhibition (Kalachnik et al., 2002). Between the first FGA chlorpromazine (1952) and the first "second-generation" antipsychotic (SGA) clozapine (1989), most FGAs were utilized, although recent use has decreased over concerns regarding efficacy, and propensity for causing serious adverse events (Wilson et al., 1998).

Second-generation antipsychotics have also been widely used, and two (risperidone and aripiprazole) have received approval in the USA for addressing irritability in persons with autism spectrum disorders (ASD) (Ghanizadeh et al., 2014). The hope that other SGAs will be of similar benefit has not yet been supported by systematic research (De Leon et al., 2009). Unwin and Deb (2011) found only six RCTs demonstrating effectiveness of risperidone for problem behaviors in children with ID (with and without ASD); other literature in adults has mostly involved case series (Deb et al., 2007).

Mood stabilizers (particularly anticonvulsants) also have long been used in persons with ID, surrounding frequent co-occurrence of seizure disorders (Harris, 2006). Two recent reviews concluded that both lithium (Deb et al., 2008) and carbamazepine/oxcarbazepine (Jones et al., 2011) appear to have efficacy for aggression/behavioral problems in adults, with methodological limits on interpretation.

Based on efficacy for anxiety, depression, and obsessive-compulsive disorder (OCD) in people with typical IQ, antidepressants have been used in both children and adults with ID, particularly those with comorbid ASD. In ASD, targets have included both core features and repetitive behaviors. In the largest RCT, the selective serotonin reuptake inhibitor (SSRI) citalopram was not better than placebo in addressing repetitive behavior in children with ASD, and produced more adverse events (King et al, 2009); but two smaller studies of SSRIs in adults were more positive for addressing aggression and anxiety (Williams et al., 2010). A recent attempted meta-analysis of tricyclic antidepressants for children with ASD also noted limited and conflicting evidence for efficacy, and significant adverse events (Hurwitz et al., 2012).

Beta-adrenergic blocking medications have been utilized to treat aggression and impulse dyscontrol in persons with ID (Ruedrich and Erhardt, 1999); however, a recent review noted the lack of RCTs supporting this practice (Ward et al., 2013).

Finally, opiate antagonists (naltrexone) have been utilized for high-intensity SIB frequently seen in persons with ID, and several small RCTs have demonstrated efficacy for irritability and hyperactivity in children with ASD (Roy et al., 2015).

The present
Psychotropic treatment of specific psychiatric disorders

Newer studies have focused on the treatment of specific psychiatric disorders, an approach obviously dependent on the validity of the diagnostic process (Fletcher, et al., 2007). Some approaches have utilized objective measures of diagnosis or illness severity, such as cutoff scores on subscales of standardized assessments of psychopathology (e.g., the Behavior Problems Inventory [BPI]; Rojahn et al., 2004), for study inclusion and/or efficacy assessments.

Attention-deficit/hyperactivity disorder

In attention-deficit/hyperactivity disorder (ADHD), stimulants appear effective for motor overactivity, although the response is less robust compared to persons without ID (Aman et al., 2008; Rowles and Findling, 2010). A recent large RCT with methylphenidate was also positive (Simonoff et al., 2013) and atomoxetine use is also supported (Aman et al., 2014). Two small RCTs also supported the alpha-agonists clonidine and guanfacine in children with ADHD and ID (Agarwal et al., 2001; Handen et al., 2008); both drugs caused significant early sedation.

Anxiety disorders

There are no RCTs directly addressing anxiety disorders in persons with ID (King, 2007). Multiple agents have been utilized, including antidepressants, anticonvulsants, benzodiazepines, beta-blockers, buspirone, and antipsychotics; none have an evidence base supporting their use (Davis et al., 2008). The presence of anxiety or OCD did seem to predict benefit from SSRIs used for behavioral disorders (Sohanpal et al., 2007).

Psychotic disorders

Almost no RCTs have attempted to address the treatment of psychotic disorders in persons with ID (De Leon et al., 2009). One early study compared two FGAs for schizophrenia in persons with ID; but methodological problems make interpretation difficult (Menolascino et al., 1985).

Mood disorders

Few studies exist which have focused on drug treatment of mood disorders, particularly in persons with severe ID (Antonacci and Attiah 2008). Although all classes of antidepressants have been utilized for major depression, and mood stabilizers for bipolar disorder in persons with ID, there are no RCTs over the last two decades (Ruedrich et al., 2001).

Self-injurious behavior

There are only a few small RCTs (four with naltrexone, and one with clomipramine) specifically addressing SIB (Gormez et al., 2014), with only weak evidence supporting any of the active drugs over placebo.

Behavior disorders

Oliver-Africano et al. (2009) have described the lack of clinical uniformity of definitions for "challenging behavior" in persons with ID, which may include physical aggression to others, SIB, motor overactivity, property destruction, verbal outbursts, and agitation. Reviews have noted the lack of RCT evidence supporting the use of antidepressants, mood stabilizers, anxiolytics, or opiate antagonists for treating behavioral disorders (Deb and Unwin, 2007) but some support from RCTs for risperidone, particularly in children (Wilner, 2015). However, in a recent multisite RCT comparing haloperidol, risperidone, and placebo for aggression in 80 non-psychotic patients with ID, there were no important differences in efficacy or adverse effects for either antipsychotic medication compared to placebo (Tyrer et al., 2008); nor was active drug cost effective compared to placebo (Tyrer et al., 2009). Still, respondents to a survey of psychiatrists in the UK favored SGAs for aggression and SIB in adults (Unwin and Deb, 2008); although non-medication interventions were favored over any medication.

The future
Drug treatments in ID-related disorders with known etiology
Down syndrome

Surrounding the observation that adults with Down syndrome (DS) develop early-onset Alzheimer-type dementia (Schupf and Sergievsky, 2002); there has been hope that typical treatments for Alzheimer's dementia would be useful in DS, either in delaying or treating dementia, or possibly enhancing cognitive ability in younger persons with DS. Results to date have been disappointing (Costa and Scott-McKean, 2013). One RCT found that donepezil, a cholinomimetic medication approved for Alzheimer's, improved cognition in 21 women with DS (Kondoh et al., 2011); but did not in two larger studies of adolescents and young adults with DS without dementia (Kishnani et al., 2009, 2010); and antioxidant therapy was also ineffective (Lott et al., 2011). Memantine, the other medication currently available for Alzheimer's dementia, did not provide significant cognitive benefit in two other RCTs (Boada et al., 2012; Hanney et al., 2012).

Fragile X syndrome

Attention-deficit/hyperactivity disorder in people with fragile X syndrome (FXS) appears to respond to stimulant medications (Rueda et al., 2009); L-acetylcarnitine (Torrioli et al., 2008) and perhaps divalproex sodium (Torrioli et al., 2010), but not folic acid (Rueda et al. 2009). SSRIs have also been utilized to address anxiety and social aversion in people with FXS (Hagerman et al., 2014). Recent studies have focused on addressing the underlying genetic mechanism of FXS (silencing of the *FMR1* gene, resulting in non-expression of the FX protein), which appears to enhance glutaminergic signaling. Both glutaminergic antagonists and gamma-aminobutyric acid (GABA) agonists have been studied; neither approach has been sufficiently effective to date in controlled trials. Minocycline (a tetracyline antibiotic) has been shown to improve mood and anxiety in people with FXS, presumably by promoting neuronal dendritic spine maturation (Hagerman et al., 2014).

Fetal alcohol spectrum disorder

Although no RCTs are available, ADHD in fetal alcohol spectrum disorder (FASD) may respond to stimulants, with hyperactivity/impulsivity more responsive than inattention (Doig et al., 2008); in an uncontrolled trial, neuroleptics provided some benefit in promoting peer relations (Frankel et al., 2006).

Velocardiofacial syndrome

Methylphenidate was effective (and safe) for ADHD in a RCT trial of 34 children/adolescents with velocardiofacial syndrome (VCFS) (Green et al., 2011), and treating mood and anxiety disorders may delay the onset of psychosis (Gothelf et al., 2013).

Williams syndrome

Although no RCTs are available, treatment of ADHD with methylphendiate was successful in 72% of 38 children/adolescents (Green et al., 2012) and 36% of a large sample of persons with Williams syndrome were receiving antidepressants for anxiety, the majority appearing to benefit (Martens et al., 2012).

Prader–Willi syndrome

Stimulants have not been effective in managing weight (Harris, 2006); and topiramate was ineffective in weight management, but helped compulsive skin picking in a small open-label trial (Shapira et al., 2004). SSRIs may have some efficacy in decreasing skin picking (Dykens and Shah, 2003), and a recent RCT with intranasal oxytocin resulted in increased trust and decreased sadness (Tauber et al., 2011).

Autism spectrum disorders

Medications have been utilized in autism spectrum disorders (ASD) to address both the core features of the disorder, accompanying (non-core) symptoms, and/or comorbid psychiatric disorders. Two (risperidone and aripiprazole) have been found in RCTs to be efficacious for treating irritability in children and adolescents with ASD (Ghanizadeh et al., 2014). Psychostimulants help impulsivity and hyperactivity (Posey et al., 2007) and melatonin has been shown to benefit sleep duration and sleep latency, but not awakenings (Rossignol and Frye, 2013). Other RCTs have provided lack of support for secretin (Williams et al., 2012) and for omega-3 fatty acids (James et al., 2011). Tricyclic antidepressants produced contradictory results and many side effects (Hurwitz et al., 2012). Finally, SSRI antidepressants have also been disappointing, showing some possible efficacy for ASD adults with anxiety and OCD (Williams et al., 2010); but are not effective for repetitive behaviors in children, and poorly tolerated (King et al., 2009).

Newest areas of research are focused on glutamate antagonists, GABA agonists, and oxytocin (Canitano, 2014).

Side effects

Psychotropic medications have physiological effects in addition to their intended effects, some expected, but with others, unexpected and sometimes dangerous (Wilson et al., 1998). Because psychotropic medications and the neurotransmitter systems they affect are not limited to the central nervous system, they have physiological effects on a number of other organ systems (King, 2007). First-generation antispychotics have a long-recognized risk of producing extra-pyramidal adverse effects, including acute dystonias, motor restlessness, Parkinsonism, and, with long-term use, tardive dyskinesia (Harris, 2006). These risks are somewhat less with the SGAs, but the latter can produce an arguably more debilitating set of metabolic changes – weight gain, insulin resistance with type 2 diabetes, and hyperlipidemia (Frighi et al., 2011; De Kuijper et al., 2013). Most antipsychotics, as well as SSRIs and tricyclic antidepressants (TCAs), also carry a risk of QTc prolongation on the electrocardiogram (Beach et al., 2013). Many psychotropics lower the seizure threshold, particularly dangerous in the 25% of persons with ID with comorbid epilepsy (McGrother et al., 2006). The anticonvulsant mood stabilizers carry risks of electrolyte imbalance, ataxia, sedation, and liver toxicity, and with carbamaze-pine and lamotrigine, sometimes dangerous rash (Sipes et al., 2011). Many psychotropics have anticholinergic side effects, resulting in dry mouth, constipation, urinary retention, and oculo-visual symptoms (Wilson et al., 1998). All of the above are complicated by commonplace polypharmacy in persons with ID (Edelsohn et al., 2014).

Individuals with ID present a major additional challenge: the difficulty they have in identifying and communicating any adverse effects to their caregivers or clinicians (Wilson et al., 1998). Persons with ID experiencing adverse events from psychotropic medications, particularly those without communicative language, may demonstrate behavioral problems as a result of orthostatic hypotension, motor restlessness, consti-pation, or a myriad of other distressing adverse events, and are often given additional psychotropic medications, exacerbating the underlying problem (Valdovinos et al., 2005). A number of methodologies involving objective rating scales have been developed to assess for and quantify psychotropic side effects, particularly for the antipsychotic medications, including the Matson Evaluation of Drug Side Effects (MEDS; Matson and Mahan, 2010). Others have offered publications written and illustrated at the develop-mental level of individuals with ID, in order to educate about the risks/benefits of psychotropic medications (Aman et al., 2007).

Conclusions

Decision-making involving psychotropic medications for persons with ID is difficult, with little evidence base guiding therapeutics in particular for psychiatric disorders, and even less for non-syndrome-related behavioral disorders. Several groups have provided clinical consensus to guide treatment teams, notably the *Psychotropic Medications and Developmental Disabilities: The International Consensus Handbook* (Reiss and Aman, 1998), and the Expert Consensus Guideline Series (Rush and Frances, 2000). Deb and colleagues have provided comprehensive reviews of several classes of psychotropics, regarding the strength of evidence supporting use in treating behavioral disorders

(Deb, et al., 2007, 2008; Sohanpal et al., 2007). Finally, the World Psychiatric Association (WPA) Section of the Psychiatry of ID has recently published a series of guidelines outlining best practices with psychotropic medications (Deb et al., 2010). Although specifically aimed at the treatment of behavioral disorders, they offer an excellent framework for all psychotropic practice in ID, highlighting:

1. Completing a comprehensive assessment.
2. Leading to a diagnostic hypothesis.
3. Combining medication with non-medication treatments.
4. Communicating benefits and risks, with full informed consent, to the individual and family.
5. Objectively assessing both efficacy and adverse events with standardized methods.
6. "Starting low and going slow"; with a single agent.
7. Evaluating the risk–benefit profile of medication regularly.
8. Regularly assessing the continued need for medication; and attempting safe withdrawal.
9. Avoiding polypharmacy, particularly intraclass polypharmacy.
10. Seeking clinical consultation at regular intervals.

Key summary points

- Psychiatric illness in persons with ID is common, but difficult to diagnose.
- Behavioral problems often coexist with psychiatric illness.
- The best psychotropic treatments are those specific to a valid psychiatric diagnosis.
- However, today many drug treatments remain symptom-based, rather than disorder- or etiology-based.
- Psychotropic medications should be only one part of combined treatment, also utilizing behavioral and psychosocial treatments.
- When psychotropic medications **are** utilized, for psychiatric disorders and/or behavioral problems, follow the WPA guidelines.

References

Agarwal, V., Sitholey, P., Kumar S., et al. (2001). Double-blind, placebo-controlled trial of clonidine in hyperactive children with mental retardation. *Mental Retardation*, 39, 259–267.

Aman, M.G., Benson, B.A., Farmer, C.A., et al. (2007). Project MED: effects of a medication education booklet series for individuals with intellectual disabilities. *Intellectual and Developmental Disabilities*, 45, 33–45.

Aman, M.G., Farmer, C.A., Hollway, J., et al. (2008). Treatment of inattention, overactivity, and impulsiveness in autism spectrum disorders. *Child and Adolescent Clinics of North America*, 17, 13–38.

Aman, M.G., Smith, T., Arnold, L.E., et al. (2014). A review of atomoxetine effects in young people with developmental disabilities. *Research in Developmental Disabilities*, 35, 1412–1424.

Antonacci, D.J. and Attiah, N. (2008). Diagnosis and treatment of mood disorders in adults with developmental disabilities. *Psychiatric Quarterly*, 79, 171–192.

Beach, S.R., Celano, C.M., Noseworthy, P.A., et al. (2013). QTc prolongation, torsades de pointes, and psychotropic medications. *Psychosomatics*, 54, 1–13.

Boada, R., Hutaff-Lee, C., Schrader, A., et al. (2012). Antagonism of NMDA receptors as a potential treatment for Down's syndrome:

a pilot randomized controlled trial. *Translational Psychiatry*, 2, e141.

Canitano R. (2014). New experimental treatments for core social domain in autism spectrum disorders. *Frontiers in Pediatrics*, 2, 61.

Costa, A.C. and Scott-McKean, J.J. (2013). Prospects for improving brain function in individuals with Down's syndrome. *CNS Drugs*, 27, 672–702.

Courtemanche, A.B., Schroeder, S.R., Sheldon, J.B. (2011). Designs and analyses of psychotropic and behavioural interventions for the treatment of problem behaviour among people with intellectual and developmental disabilities. *American Journal on Intellectual and Developmental Disabilities*, 116, 315–328.

Davis, E., Saeed, S.A., Antonacci, D.J. (2008). Anxiety disorders in persons with developmental disabilities: empirically informed diagnosis and treatment. *Psychiatric Quarterly*, 79, 249–263.

De Kuijper G., Mulder, H., Evenhuis, H., et al. (2013). Determinants of physical health parameters in individuals with intellectual disability who use long-term antipsychotics. *Research in Developmental Disabilities*, 34, 2799–2809.

De Leon, J., Greelee, B., Barber J., et al. (2009). Practical guidelines for the use of new generation antipsychotic drugs (except clozapine) in adult individuals with intellectual disabilities. *Research in Developmental Disabilities*, 30, 613–669.

Deb, S. and Unwin, G.L., (2007). Psychotropic medication for behaviour problems in people with intellectual disability: a review of the current literature. *Current Opinion in Psychiatry*, 20, 461–466.

Deb, S., Sohanpal, S.K., Soni, R., et al. (2007). The effectiveness of antipsychotic medication in the management of behaviour problems in adults with intellectual disabilities. *Journal of Intellectual Disability Research*, 51, 766–777.

Deb, S., Chaplin, R., Sohanpal, S., et al. (2008). The effectiveness of mood stabilizers and antiepileptic medications for the management of behaviour problems in adults with intellectual disability: a systematic review. *Journal of Intellectual Disability Research*, 52, 107–113.

Deb, S., Salvadoe-Carulla, J., Barnhill, J., et al. (2010). *Problem Behaviours in Adults with Intellectual Disabilities: An International Guide for Using Medication*. The World Psychiatric Association (WPA): Section Psychiatry of Intellectual Disability. At: http://www.wpanet.org/uploads/Sections/Psychiatry_Intellectual/WPA-SPID-International-Guide.pdf

Doig, J., McLennan, J.D., Gibbard, W.B. (2008). Medication effects on symptoms of attention-deficit/hyperactivity disorder in children with fetal alcohol spectrum disorder. *Journal of Child and Adolescent Psychopharmacology*, 18, 365–371.

Dykens, E. and Shah, B. (2003). Psychiatric disorders in Prader–Willi syndrome: epidemiology and management. *CNS Drugs*, 17, 167–178.

Edelsohn, G.A., Schuster, J.M., Castelnovo K., et al. (2014). Psychotropic prescribing for persons with intellectual disabilities and other psychiatric disorders. *Psychiatric Services*, 65, 201–207.

Fletcher, R., Loschen, E., Stavrakaki, C. (eds.) (2007). *Diagnostic Manual – Intellectual Disability (DM-ID): A Textbook of Diagnosis of Mental Disorders in Persons with Intellectual Disability*. Kingston, NY: NADD Press.

Frighi, V., Stephenson, M.T., Moroval, A., et al. (2011). Safety of antipsychotics in people with intellectual disability. *British Journal of Psychiatry*, 199, 289–295.

Frankel, F., Paley, B., Marquardt, R., et al. (2006). Stimulants, neuroleptics, and children's friendship training for children with fetal alcohol spectrum disorders. *Journal of Child and Adolescent Psychopharmacology*, 16, 777–789.

Ghanizadeh A., Sahraeizadeh A., Berk M., (2014). A head-to-head comparison of aripiprazole and risperidone for safety and treating autistic disorders, a randomized double blind clinical trial. *Child Psychiatry and Human Development*, 45, 185–192.

Gormez, A., Rana, F., Varghese, S. (2014). Pharmacological interventions for self-injurious behaviour in adults with intellectual disabilities: abridged republication of a Cochrane systematic review. *Journal of Psychopharmacology,* 28, 624–632

Gothelf, D., Schneider, M., Green, T., et al. (2013). Risk factors and the evolution of psychosis in 22q11.2 deletion syndrome. A longitudinal 2-site study. *Journal of the American Academy of Child and Adolescent Psychiatry,* 52, 1192–1203.

Green, T., Weinberger, R., Diamond, A., et al. (2011). The effect of methylphenidate on prefrontal cognitive functioning, inattention, and hyperactivity in velocardiofacial syndrome. *Journal of Child and Adolescent Psychopharmacology,* 21, 589–595.

Green, T., Avda, S., Dotan, I., et al. (2012). Phenotypic psychiatric characterization of children with Williams syndrome and response of those with ADHD to methylphenidate treatment. *American Journal of Medical Genetics Part B: Neuropsychiatric Genetics,* 159B, 13–20.

Hagerman, R., Des-Portes, V., Gasparini, F., et al. (2014). Translating molecular advances in Fragile X syndrome into therapy: a review. *Journal of Clinical Psychiatry,* 75, e294–e307.

Handen, B.L., Sahl, R., Hardan A.Y. (2008). Guanfacine in children with autism and/or intellectual disabilities. *Journal of Developmental and Behavioral Pediatrics,* 29, 303–308.

Hanney, M., Prasher, V., Williams, N., et al. (2012). Memantine for dementia in adults older than 40 years with Down's syndrome (MEADOWS): a randomized, double-blind, placebo-controlled trial. *Lancet,* 379, 528–536.

Harris, J.C. (2006). *Intellectual Disability.* New York, NY: Oxford University Press.

Hurwitz, R., Blackmore, R., Hazell, P., et al. (2012). Tricyclic antidepressants for autism spectrum disorder (ASD) in children and adolescents. *Cochrane Database of Systematic Reviews,* 3, CD008372.

James, S., Montgomery P., Williams, K. (2011). Omega-3 fatty acids supplementation for autism spectrum disorders (ASD) *Cochrane Database for Systematic Reviews,* 11, CD007992.

Jones, R.M., Arlidge, J., Gillham, R., et al. (2011). Efficacy of mood stabilizers in the treatment of impulsive or repetitive aggression: systematic review and meta-analysis. *British Journal of Psychiatry,* 198, 93–98.

Kalachnik, J.E. and Hanzel, T.E. (2001). Behavioral side effects of barbiturate antiepileptic drugs in individuals with mental retardation and developmental disabilities. *National Association for Dual Diagnosis Bulletin,* 4, 49–55.

Kalachnik, J.E., Hanzel, T.E., Sevenich, R., et al. (2002). Benzodiazepine behavioral side effects: review and implications for individuals with mental retardation. *American Journal on Mental Retardation,* 107, 376–410.

King, B.H (2007). Psychopharmacology in intellectual disabilities. In N. Bouras and G. Holt (eds.), *Psychiatric and Behavioural Disorders in Intellectual and Developmental Disabilities,* second edition. Cambridge: Cambridge University Press.

King, B.H., Hollander, E., Sikich, L., et al. (2009). Lack of efficacy of citalopram in children with autism spectrum disorders and high levels of repetitive behavior: citalopram ineffective in children with autism. *Archives of General Psychiatry,* 66, 583–590.

Kishnani, P.S., Sommer, B.R., Handen, B.L., et al. (2009). The efficacy, safety, and tolerability of donepezil for the treatment of young adults with Down syndrome. *American Journal of Medical Genetics Part A,* 149, 1641–1654.

Kishnani, P.S., Heller, J.H., Spiridigliozzi, G.A., et al. (2010). Donepezil for treatment of cognitive dysfunction in children with Down syndrome aged 10–17. *American Journal of Medical Genetics Part A,* 152, 3028–3035.

Kondoh, T., Kanno, A., Itoh, H., et al. (2011). Donepezil significantly improves abilities in daily lives of female Down syndrome patients with severe cognitive impairment: a 24-week randomized, double blind, placebo-controlled trial. *International Journal of Psychiatry in Medicine*, 41, 71–89.

Levitas, A. (2003). Reader response to Zarcone et al. (2001) "Effects of risperidone on aberrant behavior in persons with developmental disabilities: I. A double-blind crossover study using multiple measures." *American Journal on Mental Retardation*, 108, 212–216.

Levitas, A.S., Hurley, A.D., Pary, R. (2001). The mental status examination in patients with mental retardation and developmental disabilities. *Mental Health Aspects of Developmental Disability*, 41, 1–30.

Lott, I.T., Doran, E., Nguyen, V.Q., et al. (2011). Down syndrome and dementia: a randomized, controlled trial of antioxidant supplementation. *American Journal of Medical Genetics Part A*, 155, 1939–1948.

Martens M.A., Seyfer, D.L., Andridge, R.R., et al. (2012). Parent report of antidepressant, anxiolytic, and antipsychotic medication use in individuals with Williams syndrome: effectiveness and adverse effects. *Research in Developmental Disabilities*, 33, 2106–2121.

Matson, J.L. and Mahan, S. (2010). Antipsychotic drug side effects for persons with intellectual disability. *Research in Developmental Disabilities*, 31, 1570–1576.

McGrother, C.W., Bhaumik, S., Thorp, C.F., et al. (2006). Epilepsy in adults with intellectual disabilities: prevalence, associations, and service implications. *Seizure*, 15, 376–386.

Menolascino, F.J., Ruedrich, S.L., Golden, C.J., et al. (1985). Diagnosis and pharmacotherapy of schizophrenia in the retarded. *Psychopharmacology Bulletin*, 21, 316–322.

Oliver-Africano, P., Murphy, D., Tyrer P. (2009). Aggressive behavior in adults with intellectual disability: defining the role of drug treatment. *CNS Drugs*, 23, 903–913.

Posey, D.J., Aman M.G., McCracken J.T., et al. (2007). Positive effects of methylphenidate

on inattention and hyperactivity in pervasive developmental disorders: an analysis of secondary measures. *Biological Psychiatry*, 15, 538–544.

Reiss, S. and Aman, M.G. (eds.) (1998). *Psychotropic Medications and Developmental Disabilities: The International Consensus Handbook*. Columbus, OH: Ohio State University, Nisonger Center Press.

Rojahn, J., Matson, J.L., Naglieri, J.A., et al. (2004). Relationships between psychiatric conditions and behavior problems among adults with mental retardation. *American Journal on Mental Retardation*, 109, 21–33.

Rossignol, D.A. and Frye, R.E. (2013). Melatonin in autism spectrum disorders. *Current Clinical Pharmacology*, 8, 1–9.

Rowles, B.M. and Findling, R.L. (2010). Review of pharmacotherapy options for the treatment of attention-deficit/hyperactivity disorder (ADHD) and ADHD-like symptoms in children and adolescents with developmental disorders. *Developmental Disabilities Research Reviews*, 16, 273–282.

Roy, A., Roy, M., Deb, S., et al. (2015). Are opioid antagonists effective in attenuating the core symptoms of autism spectrum conditions in children: a systematic review. *Journal of Intellectual Disability Research*, 59(4), 293–306.

Rueda, J.R., Ballesteros, J., Tejada, M.I. (2009). Systematic review of pharmacological treatments in Fragile X syndrome. *BMC Neurology*, 9, 53.

Ruedrich, S.L. and Erhardt, L. (1999). Beta-adrenergic blockers in mental retardation and developmental disabilities. *Mental Retardation and Developmental Disabilities Research Reviews*, 5, 290–298.

Ruedrich, S.L., Hurley, A., Sovner, R. (2001). Treatment of mood disorders in mentally retarded persons. In A. Dosen and K. Day (eds.), *Treating Mental Illness and Behavior Disorders in Children and Adults with Mental Retardation*. Washington, DC: American Psychiatric Press.

Rush, A.J. and Frances, A. (eds.) (2000). The Expert Consensus Guideline Series. Treatment of psychiatric and behavioral problems in mental retardation. *American Journal on Mental Retardation*, 105 (Issue 3, Special Issue), 159–228.

Schroeder, S.R., Bouras, N., Ellis, C.R., et al. (1998). Past research on psychopharmacology of people with mental retardation and intellectual disabilities. In S. Reiss and M.G. Aman (eds.), *Psychotropic Medications and Developmental Disabilities: The International Consensus Handbook.* Columbus, OH: Ohio State University, Nisonger Center Press.

Schupf, N. and Sergievsky, G.H. (2002). Genetic and host factors for dementia in Down syndrome. *British Journal of Psychiatry*, 180, 405–410.

Shapira, N., Lessig, M., Lewis, M. et al. (2004). Effects of topiramate in adults with Prader–Willi syndrome. *American Journal on Mental Retardation*, 109, 301–309.

Simonoff, E., Taylor, E., Baird G., et al. (2013). Randomized controlled double-blind trial of optimal dose methylphenidate in children and adolescents with severe attention deficit hyperactivity disorder and intellectual disability. *Journal of Child Psychology and Psychiatry*, 54, 527–535.

Sipes, M., Matson, J.L., Belva, B., et al. (2011). The relationship among side effects associated with anti-epileptic medications in those with intellectual disability. *Research in Developmental Disabilities*, 32, 1646–1651.

Sohanpal, S.K., Deb, S., Thomas, R., et al. (2007). The effectiveness of antidepressant medication in the management of behaviour problems in adults with intellectual disabilities: a systematic review. *Journal of Intellectual Disability Research*, 51, 750–765.

Tauber, M., Mantoulan, C., Copet, P., et al. (2011). Oxytocin may be useful to increase trust in others and decrease disruptive behaviours in patients with Prader–Willi syndrome: a randomized placebo-controlled trial in 24 patients. *Orphanet Journal of Rare Diseases*, 6, 47.

Torrioli, M.G., Vermacotola, S., Peruzzi, L., et al. (2008). A double-blind, parallel, multicenter comparison of L-acetylcarnitine with placebo on the attention deficit

hyperactivity disorder in Fragile X syndrome boys. *American Journal of Medical Genetics Part A*, 146, 803–812.

Torrioli, M.G., Vemacotola, S., Setini, C., et al. (2010). Treatment with valproic acid ameliorates ADHD symptoms in Fragile X syndrome boys. *American Journal of Medical Genetics Part A*, 152, 1420–1427.

Tsiouris, J.A. (2010). Pharmacotherapy for aggressive behaviours in persons with intellectual disabilities: treatment or mistreatment? *Journal of Intellectual Disability Research*, 54, 1–16.

Tyrer, P., Oliver-Africano, P.C., Ahmed, Z., et al. (2008). Risperidone, haloperidol, and placebo in the treatment of aggressive challenging behavior in patients with intellectual disability: a randomized controlled trial. *Lancet*, 371, 57–63.

Tyrer, P., Oliver-Africano, P., Romeo, R., et al. (2009). Neuroleptics in the treatment of aggressive challenging behaviour for people with intellectual disabilities: a randomized controlled trial (NACHBID). *Health Technology Assessment*, 13, 1–54.

Unwin, G.L. and Deb, S. (2008). Use of medication for the management of behavior problems among adults with intellectual disabilities: a clinicians' consensus survey. *American Journal on Mental Retardation*, 113, 19–31.

Unwin, G.L. and Deb, S. (2011). Efficacy of atypical antipsychotic medication in the management of behaviour problems in children with intellectual disabilities and borderline intelligence: a systematic review. *Research in Developmental Disabilities*, 332, 2121–2133.

Valdovinos, M.G., Caruso, M., Roberts, C., et al. (2005). Medical and behavioral symptoms as potential medication side effects in adult with development disabilities. *American Journal on Mental Retardation*, 110, 164–170.

Ward, F., Tharian, P., Roy, M., et al. (2013). Efficacy of beta blockers in the management of problem behaviors in people with intellectual disabilities: a systematic review. *Research in Developmental Disabilities*, 34, 4293–4303.

Williams, K., Wheeler, D.M., Silove, N., et al. (2010). Selective serotonin reuptake inhibitors (SSRIs) for autism spectrum disorders (ASD). *Cochrane Database of Systematic Reviews*, 8, CD004677.

Williams, K., Wray J.A., Wheeler, D.M. (2012). Intravenous secretin for autism spectrum disorders (ASD). *Cochrane Database of Systematic Reviews*, 4, CD003495.

Wilner, P. (2015). The neurobiology of aggression: implications for the pharmacotherapy of aggressive challenging behaviour by people with intellectual disabilities. *Journal of Intellectual Disability Research*, 59(1), 82–92.

Wilson, J.G., Lott, R.S., Tsai L. (1998). Side effects: recognition and management. In S. Reiss and M.G. Aman (eds.), *Psychotropic Medications and Developmental Disabilities: The International Consensus Handbook*. Columbus, OH: Ohio State University, Nisonger Center Press.

Chapter

14

Psychodynamic psychotherapy

Nigel Beail

Introduction

People who have intellectual disabilities (ID), like anyone else, are at risk of suffering from psychological problems. Thus, like everyone else, they need access to a range of psychological therapies. The focus of this chapter is the provision of psychodynamic psychotherapy. Psychodynamic psychotherapy has its roots in the theory and practice of psychoanalysis. Psychoanalysis was considered to be unsuitable for people who have ID, and indeed it has only had a limited application (Jackson and Beail, 2013). Psychoanalysis is undertaken for 50 minutes five times a week and is not widely available outside major cities, and is mostly provided in private practice. Thus, it is outside of the economic means of most people and certainly those of people who have ID. However, psychodynamic psychotherapy has a little more flexibility and is delivered less frequently like other psychological interventions available today. In this chapter the theories which have informed the development of the practice of psychodynamic therapy with people who have ID will be elucidated along with the adaptations that have been made to ensure that it is accessible for many people who have ID.

People who have ID have only been in receipt of psychodynamic psychotherapy since about 1980, and then provision is not widespread. O'Driscoll (2009) has tried to map the history prior to this, but, unfortunately earlier published accounts of psychodynamic psychotherapy with people with ID have been ambiguous as to the nature or degree of impairment presented by clients, and further confused by a lack of consensus, consistency, and clarity in the terminology used to describe people with ID (Sinason, 1992). There were various suitability criteria applied when considering what treatment people need. Unfortunately, these served to exclude many in the general population and certainly people who have ID. These include factors such as ability to enter an intensive treatment relationship, emphasizing the importance of possessing psychological mindedness, motivation, and adequate ego strength (Brown and Pedder, 1979). As ego strength and intelligence have been associated, and a lack of them is seen as barriers to engagement in psychodynamic psychotherapy, these need to be evaluated a little more critically.

Freud (1940) described a psychical apparatus or model of the mind consisting of three parts; the id, the ego, and the super-ego. The ego functions as an intermediary between the id (which contains everything that is inherited and, in particular, the

Psychiatric and Behavioral Disorders in Intellectual and Developmental Disabilities, ed. Colin Hemmings and Nick Bouras. Published by Cambridge University Press. © Cambridge University Press 2016.

unconscious life and death drives), and the real world. In Freud's theory, the ego has the task of self-preservation and performs such tasks as becoming aware of stimuli and building memories. The ego also takes action in the service of self-preservation in the form of helping the person to avoid or adapt to situations, or through activity bring about changes to their advantage through the use of defense mechanisms (for example, denial and repression). Thus, the ego uses a range of mechanisms to enable the person to put disagreeable things out of mind, which makes them unconscious. The ego simultaneously gains control over the internal drives and decides whether to allow, deny, or postpone satisfaction. Freud also described a further internal agency called the super-ego, into which we take representations of the parents, and the parental influence is prolonged. Thus, the ego has to manage the tensions that arise between the internal world of the drives and the unconscious, reality, and the super-ego. So, if we consider here what poor ego strength may mean, then it suggests that the capacity to manage tensions and anxiety is poor. However, how this should make someone unsuitable for psychotherapy is not clear. Perhaps it makes them more in need? The definition of the ego has also changed over time. Freud's followers in the Ego Psychology School have described the ego as containing the functions of thought, perception, language, learning, memory, and rational planning (Hartmann, 1964). Thus, the ego has many of the features that make up the construct of intelligence. Thus, it is not surprising to find that some have even suggested that the person should be of at least average intelligence to undertake psychodynamic psychotherapy (Brown and Pedder, 1979). Some suitability constructs have also been consolidated into screening tools such as the Suitability for Psychotherapy Scale (Laaksonen et al., 2012). Some of the constructs contained in the scale are the same as those used in the past to affirm that people who have ID are not suitable for psychotherapy; for example, poor ego strength, poor capacity to reflect, lack of verbal fluency, and acting-out. Clearly the application of such criteria would exclude people with ID from treatment. However, such constructs would not make sense if used to assess a child's suitability for psychotherapy. Psychodynamic therapy has been adapted and developed for use with children. Thus, if it can be used with children, how can it be argued that adults, who are developmentally delayed and could be age matched with a child, are not suitable?

There is a general consensus that the earliest published account of psychodynamic therapy with someone with an ID and meeting current diagnostic criteria is Symington's (1981) case report of his work with a man with an IQ of 59. It is also notable that clinical interest in delivering this approach increased around this time followed by an increase in published accounts (Brandon, 1989; Sinason, 1992; De Groef and Heinemann, 1999). This has now evolved into the formation of the Institute for Psychotherapy and Disability (Frankish, 2009), the emergence of the concept of disability psychotherapy (Frankish, 2013), reviews of emerging practice (Jackson and Beail, 2013), and outcomes (James and Stacey, 2013).

The evidence base

Research concerning the evidence base for psychodynamic psychotherapy with people who have ID is in its early days. The main body of literature is comprised of case studies (see Jackson and Beail, 2013). The reporting of outcomes has not been a feature; if provided, it is only anecdotally. Some single case outcome data reports have been published (Newman and Beail, 2002; Kellett et al., 2009; Alim, 2010). The first attempt at reporting outcomes was a case series by Frankish (1989). She showed that improvements in behavior occurred across the course of psychodynamic psychotherapy. The next case series was reported by Newman and Beail (2005). They demonstrated progression using the Assimilation of Problematic Experiences Scale across eight recipients of eight sessions of psychodynamic psychotherapy.

Beail (1998) published the first open trial and showed reductions in problem behavior for most recipients, and this was maintained at six months follow-up. Beail (2001) reported a study on the outcomes for 18 offenders who have ID. Of the 13 who accepted treatment, all but two remained offense-free at the end of therapy and at four years follow-up. The five men who refused treatment had all reoffended within two years. Beail et al. (2005) published a pre-, post-, and follow-up study of open-ended psychodynamic psychotherapy. They found that recipients reported statistically significant reductions in psychological distress, improvements in interpersonal functioning, and self-esteem. In a further analysis, they examined the impact of different lengths of treatment – the dose effect (Beail et al., 2007). This study showed that positive effects were found across treatment lengths and that all participants made rapid gains in the first eight sessions; thus, providing preliminary evidence for the dose–effect relationship. Controlled trials are lacking; Bichard et al. (1996) evaluated the outcome of two years of psychodynamic psychotherapy for eight adults who were matched with a waiting-list group. The outcome measure was the Draw a Person test used as a projective technique. They showed scores for emotional development significantly increased, whereas those for the control group did not.

The evidence base suggests that psychodynamic psychotherapy is effective in clinical practice, but so far no efficacy studies have been attempted. The studies have also tended to include people who have a wide range of difficulties, including psychological and behavioral issues. The work of Newman and Beail (2005) suggest that psychodynamic psychotherapy seems to be effective for clients who present with difficulties that are not assimilated. This is in contrast to CBT, which tends to work from the basis that the client has an awareness of their problem and is able to give an account in response to questions about their difficulties (Willner, 2006). The Assimilation of Problematic Experiences model was developed from research with the general population (Stiles et al. 1990), which showed that most people enter therapy at what they called the "problem statement" level. Thus, the client could articulate what they thought was their problem. Using this model with people with ID, Newman and Beail (2005) found that they present for treatment at the lower levels of assimilation – such as "warded off," experiencing "unwanted thoughts," or having some "vague awareness" of the problem. However, they also demonstrated that psychodynamic psychotherapy can enable clients with ID to move towards and beyond the level of problem statement in a few sessions.

People who have ID may present with a lack of understanding of their problems and difficulties for a variety of reasons. It may be that the problem, as seen by others, is not discussed with the person, and so information provided by the referrer is needed to enable the therapist to draw the client's attention to what others are having a problem with. The psychodynamic psychotherapist may also assume that psychological factors are playing a role, notably that the client has developed a defensive structure to keep such difficulties out of conscious awareness. Defense mechanisms are mental operations that remove thoughts and feelings from conscious awareness. Individuals deal with emotional conflicts, or internal or external stressors, by keeping something out of conscious thought or altering how events are perceived.

The therapeutic frame

In their review of psychodynamic practice with people who have ID, Jackson and Beail (2013) found that therapists tended to work according to the traditional frame, in terms of frequency (once weekly), location (a private room at their place of work), and context (1 : 1) of the therapy. Beail (1989) asserted that the same therapy room should be used on the same day each week and that it should be light, warm, and comfortable, with a couch or comfortable seating, and stresses that the therapist and client should not face each other. However, Beail and Newman (2005) and Berry (2003) noted a need for flexibility around the duration of sessions. Typical sessions last for 50 minutes, but they asserted that this should be reduced to accommodate people with low tolerance for the full duration. Some therapists have also described involving staff and family members in the process of assessment and therapy, but Bungener and McCormack (1994) asserted the importance of managing the relationship with carers, and the potential threats to confidentiality, which arise in the work. Morrissey and Jackman (1998) proposed that the therapist should meet with significant others, including the clients' families, only with the permission or presence of the client. The authors propose that families be informed of the therapeutic process so that they are more able to tolerate its impact, and that, in some cases, there may be a need to have a named person other than the therapist who the families can talk to about the boundaries of the therapy.

Therapists' activities

Therapists pursue three central activities in the therapy sessions: the gathering of information; the recontextualization/formulation of the material; and the communication of potential meaning to the person.

Information gathering

Psychodynamic psychotherapy is characterized as a talking treatment and focuses on what the client says; however, when a client has ID, there needs to be as much attention to what they do in the session. The therapist is required to sit with the client and empathically engage with them to develop a relationship, which becomes the vehicle for change. The therapist attends to the client's communication without memory or desire and does not interrupt. The therapist should not disclose aspects of themselves to the client and must avoid aspects of their life and past becoming entwined with their clients. However, clients who have ID will challenge their stance. The traditional method of asking clients to say whatever comes into their minds, however silly or upsetting ("free association"), may not be productive, as some may not understand what this means. It may be more meaningful and fruitful, as Newman and Beail (2005) have found, to focus on why the person has been referred for therapy. People with ID may also say what is on their mind and ask questions such as "Have you got a boyfriend?" Here, the therapist must not disclose but also must avoid any negative response, as people who have ID have enough negativity in their lives, and they do not want to start therapy with a negative or seemingly non-empathic person. So such questions are carefully turned round to "That's an interesting question, I'm wondering why you asked that?"

Psychodynamic psychotherapy is an exploratory method and the therapist uses a number of ways to help the client to tell their story. The therapist attends to factual content, words used, and also what is unsaid, clarifying meaning where necessary, through asking open questions. Therapists have to acknowledge the often limited expressive communication skills of people with ID, and so multiple modes of communication may be needed. Equal weight needs to be given to non-verbal behaviors, and the use of expressive materials such as paper and pens and representative objects such as figures may assist. Clients may bring things to the session with them which may not be relevant; but may have some communicative function. Beail (1989) and Sinason (1992) also describe making use of phantasy and dream material in order to gain information about unconscious processes. Therapists also monitor their countertransference: their feelings, phantasies, and reactions, as these are meaningful elements in the communication between clients and therapist.

The therapist observes the client's mood, as communicated through what they say, the way they say it, but also how they behave. As well as attending to the factual content of what the person says and the words used, the therapist also considers what is not said. Hollins and Sinason (2000) identified some mutative themes or topics that many clients who have ID may not talk about and may need to be explored; these include their disability, feelings of dependency, sex and sexuality, pain and loss, and feelings of annihilation. The psychodynamic psychotherapist would also ask exploratory questions about the person's childhood, parental relationships, and about other relationships.

The therapist makes information seeking responses aimed at clarification, which helps sort out what is happening by questioning and rephrasing. Exploratory responses are generated from hypotheses about what the client might not be saying in words but could be hinting at through behavior or tone of voice. For example, a client may not talk about their sexuality but talk excessively about others. Thus, the therapist would seek more information on this and wish to explore further. So the therapist may initially reflect back to the client that they talk about the sexuality of others but not their own; this is in order to draw attention to something the client may not be aware of. The therapist observes the client's response to this; for example, the therapist's action may raise the client's anxiety and result in the use of a defense mechanism to try and reduce this. This may lead to a gentle confrontation to draw the client attention to the defense, i.e., when I said this you denied it or changed the subject. The aim of the therapist would be to reduce the defensive inhibition to enable the client to progress to explore their phantasies regarding sexuality and to feel at ease with their own. During this part of the therapeutic process the psychodynamic psychotherapist will be forming initial hypotheses, but hold them silently whilst gathering data to support or refute them.

Recontexualization

The psychodynamic model assumes that the client's communications in therapy contain latent unconscious communications concerning their conflicts and difficulties. The aim of therapy is to help the client understand these and resolve them. A general aim is described as the attempt to understand the latent unconscious meaning behind the generally assumed and consciously intended context, a process Smith (1987) called *recontexualization*. In psychodynamic psychotherapy the intention is to allow the client–therapist relationship to be therapeutic. Our verbal and non-verbal behavior, attitudes, and mannerisms are developed though relationships with parents, siblings, friends, and so on, and result in the developing interactional style and personality. Such relationships may now be in the past, or continue to take place outside of therapy, but are also internally represented. These internal representations are called the internal objects – some are good and some may be bad due to links to negative or traumatic experiences involving them. It is the internal objects that can take on different forms and relationships due to the phantasy life of the person; for example, a past relationship that was traumatic can become more so due to the persons on going thoughts and phantasies about them. These object relationships are then transferred into the relationship with the therapist – which is called transference. Freud (1912) described transference as occurring when psychological experiences are revived and instead of being located in the past are applied to dealings with a person in the present. Transference allows the therapist to identify interpersonal issues and deal with them as empirical data in the here-and-now. For example, if the client spends most of their time when with people talking about football, they are highly likely to do the same with the therapist. The therapist allows the client to do this and focuses on what it is like to be with this person. The therapist may try and focus on why the client has been referred, but the client quickly returns to telling them about football. Thus, the therapist starts to feel what it is like for others to be with this client, which in psychodynamic psychotherapy we call the counter transference.

Smith (1987) described the two stages of interpreting meaning to clients; the first step being to analyze the material and hypothesize meaning in the therapist's mind, the second to communicate the interpretation to the client. Beail and Jackson (2013) found that psychodynamic psychotherapy with people who have ID, like that with the general population, includes interpreting, whereby the therapist would state their hypothesis about what latent unconscious meaning there might be in the client's verbal and non-verbal actions. Beail and Jackson (2013) were critical of the lack of accounts of formulations on which interpretations have been based; basically there is a lack of any explanation as to their development, or the recontextualization of the material in the literature. To be fair, the aim of many writers is not to illustrate the process of formulating in psychotherapy but to illustrate different aspects of psychotherapy. However, some descriptions of this process have been given. Beail and Jackson (2009) and Beail and Newman (2005) illustrated the application of formal completeness through the framework of Malan's triangles to describe a process of understanding the material gathered (Malan, 2001). Malan's depiction of the process of psychodynamic therapy utilized two triangles (Figure 14.1) (Malan, 2001). The first of the triangles represents a framework of conflict between defensive strategies, which serve to protect the person from the anxiety they feel about a hidden (unconscious) feeling. Initially it was noted that people with ID used primitive defenses in sessions, such as splitting, projection, and projective identification, as described by Klein (1975) in her work with children. Sinason (1992) also noted the defensive strategy of secondary handicap based on Freud's concept of secondary gain; that is, the disability being used in a way such as exaggerating it to push people away. However, in a study of the defenses observed with clients who have ID in therapy, Newman and Beail (2010) found that recipients use a wide range of defenses, but with a tendency towards greater use of more primitive defenses.

In order to understand the hidden (unconscious) feelings, the therapist has to identify the defenses and the anxiety, and then draw these to the client's attention. Then they make links between stages of the conflict, and also between life stages, represented

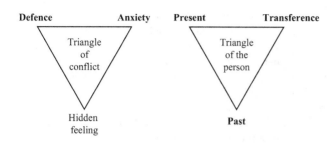

Figure 14.1 Malan's triangles of conflict and person (Malan, 2001).

by the second of Malan's triangles, the "Triangle of the Person" (Figure 14.1). This depicts the origin of the information: the setting in therapy (the transference), and a comment might be, "You feel like this when you are here with me," and then to the person's present living environment, "You feel like this towards your friend," and then the person's past (usually with parents), "You felt like this towards your mother."

When working with people who have ID, Alvarez (2012) has suggested that the therapist may need to consider different levels of interpretation. So, for a client who has ID and who is acting in an angry manner towards the therapist, this means changing the location from "you" to "others." So to extend a reflective comment, "You feel angry . . ." to make an interpretation, we go on to say, "You feel angry because . . ." However, it may be that the person with ID may not accept an interpretation with this location, i.e., "You," as the "You" may be felt as nothing but angry, which they find intolerable and so defend against this. So, for example, it may be better to say, "Part of you feels angry." However, this may also fail to be accepted, and so Alvarez (2012) suggested using the ideas of Donald Winnicott, and locating the feeling, behavior, or issue in others. So we may say something like, "Isn't it annoying when people get angry?" People who have ID also have a tendency to act-out in therapy, and sometimes the acting-out may challenge boundaries. In such situations, the interpretation may have to be put on hold and the therapist needs to bring the client back into the reality of the relationship with the therapist rather than the transferred one they are acting into. Here, Alvarez (2012) uses methods of gaining the client's attention such as saying, "Hey!" or saying the person's name clearly and firmly.

When working with clients who have ID, the therapist also needs to consider whether the client could retain the interpretation in full or does it need to be delivered in parts? Some therapists prefer to wait until the client is in a state of positive transference. However, Klein (1975) recommended making interpretations when people are at their maximal level of anxiety. As people who have ID have more difficulties in life with their memory, and also are more prone to primitive defenses such as splitting, Beail (1998) suggested, from a pragmatic point of view, that the Kleinian approach is more likely to be effective.

Conclusions

Psychodynamic psychotherapy offers people who have ID an alternative or preferred approach to the treatment of psychological distress and behavioral difficulties. Provision has grown and it can be provided as part of ID mental health service care pathways (Jackson, 2009). The therapeutic frame is virtually the same as that in general psychodynamic practice, but with some flexibility around length of sessions and the negotiated involvement of relatives and carers. The approach needs some adaptation to take account of the client's developmental needs and communication abilities. Yet Safran and Segal (1990) make the point that innovating to accommodate individual needs in therapy should not mean abandoning the therapeutic model. Instead, the therapist requires a deeper understanding of the model to ensure that innovative or creative strategies remain faithful to the underlying principles of the approach. Jackson and Beail (2013) have shown that this is proving to be the case, so far, for psychodynamic practice with people who have ID. Generally, there is a lack of accounts in the literature of the process of formulation or recontextualization of the client's communications, and this is clearly an area that needs more attention in the future to assist therapists in training. Evidence is emerging to show that this approach can be effective, but research on the model's efficacy with people who have ID have yet to be conducted, and such studies would need to make many compromises (Beail, 2010). Research is also emerging to show that recipients who have ID value it and are satisfied with it (Merriman and Beail, 2009; Khan and Beail, 2013).

Key summary points

- People who have ID need access to the same range of psychological therapies as everyone else.
- The evidence base for psychodynamic psychotherapy with people with ID is outlined; it is in its early days but evidence for effectiveness is emerging.
- Theories that have informed the development of psychodynamic psychotherapy with people with ID are elucidated.
- Adaptations to psychodynamic psychotherapy that have been made to ensure accessibility are described.

References

Alim, N. (2010). Therapeutic progressions of a client and therapist thoughout a course of psychodynamic psychotherapy with a man with mild learning disabilities and anger problems. *Advances in Mental Health and Learning Disabilities*, 4, 42–49.

Alvarez, A. (2012). *The Thinking Heart: Three Levels of Psychoanalytic Therapy with Disturbed Children*. London: Routledge.

Beail, N. (1989). Understanding emotions: the Kleinian approach explained. In D. Brandon (ed.), *Mutual Respect: Therapeutic Approaches to Working with People with Learning Difficulties*. Surbiton, Surrey, UK: Good Impressions Publishing Ltd.

Beail, N. (1998). Psychoanalytic psychotherapy with men with intellectual disabilities: a preliminary outcome study. *British Journal of Medical Psychology*, 71, 1–11.

Beail, N. (2001). Recidivism following psychodynamic psychotherapy amongst offenders with intellectual disabilities. *British Journal of Forensic Practice*, 3, 33–37.

Beail, N. (2010). The challenge of the randomized control trial to psychotherapy research with people with learning disabilities. *Advances in Mental Health and Learning Disabilities*, 4, 37–41.

Beail, N. and Jackson, T. (2009). Psychodynamic formulation. In P. Sturmey (ed.), *Varieties in Case Formulation*. New York, NY: Wiley.

Beail, N. and Jackson, T. (2013). Psychodynamic psychotherapy and people with intellectual disabilities. In J.L. Taylor, W.R. Lindsay, R.P. Hastings, C. Hatton, (eds.), *Psychological Therapies for Adults with Intellectual Disabilities*. Chichester, West Sussex, UK: Wiley.

Beail, N. and Newman, D. (2005). Psychodynamic counselling and psychotherapy for mood disorders. In P. Sturmey (ed.), *Mood Disorders in People with Mental Retardation*. Kingston, NY: NADD Press.

Beail, N., Warden, S., Morsley, K., Newman, D. (2005). Naturalistic evaluation of the effectiveness of psychodynamic psychotherapy with adults with intellectual disabilities. *Journal of Applied Research in Intellectual Disabilities*, 18(3), 245–251.

Beail, N., Kellett, S., Newman, D., Warden, S. (2007). The dose–effect relationship in psychodynamic psychotherapy with people with intellectual disabilities. *Journal of Applied Research in Intellectual Disabilities*, 20(5), 448–454.

Berry, P. (2003). Psychodynamic therapy and intellectual disabilities: dealing with challenging behaviour. *International Journal of Disability, Development and Education*, 50, 39–51.

Bichard, S.H., Sinason V., Usiskin J. (1996). Measuring change in mentally retarded clients in long term psychoanalytic psychotherapy – 1. The "draw-a-person test." *NADD Newsletter*, 13(5), 6–11.

Brandon, D., (ed.) (1989). *Mutual Respect: Therapeutic Approaches to Working with People with Learning Difficulties*. Surbiton, Surrey, UK: Good Impressions Publishing Ltd.

Brown, D. and Pedder, J. (1979). *Introduction to Psychotherapy*. London: Methuen.

Bungener, J. and McCormack, B. (1994). Psychotherapy and learning disability. In P. Clarkson and M. Pokorney (eds.), *The Handbook of Psychotherapy*. London: Routledge Publications.

De Groef, J. and Heinemann, E. (1999). *Psychoanalysis and Mental Handicap*. London: Free Association Books.

Frankish, P. (1989). Meeting the emotional needs of handicapped people: a psychodynamic approach. *Journal of Mental Deficiency Research*, 33, 407–414.

Frankish, P. (2009). History and formation of the Institute for Psychotherapy and Disability. *Advances in Mental Health and Learning Disabilities*, 3, 10–12.

Frankish, P. (2013). Thirty years of disability psychotherapy: a paradigm shift? *Advances in Mental Health and Intellectual Disabilities*, 7, 257–262.

Freud, S. (1912). The dynamics of transference. In *The Standard Edition of the Complete Psychological Works of Sigmund Freud*, Vol. 12. London: Hogarth.

Freud, S. (1940). An outline of psychoanalysis. In *The Standard Edition of the Complete Psychological Works of Sigmund Freud*, Vol. 23. London: Hogarth.

Hartmann, H. (1964). *Essays in Ego Psychology: Selected Problems in Psychoanalytic Theory*. New York, NY: International Universities Press.

Hollins, S. and Sinason, V. (2000). New perspectives: psychotherapy, learning disabilities and trauma. *British Journal of Psychiatry*, 176, 32–36.

Jackson, T. (2009). Accessibility, efficiency and effectiveness in psychological services for adults with learning disabilities. *Advances in Mental Health and Learning Disabilities*, 3, 13–18.

Jackson, T. and Beail, N. (2013). The practice of individual psychodynamic psychotherapy with people who have intellectual disabilities. *Psychoanalytic Psychotherapy*, 27, 108–123.

James, C.W. and Stacey, J.M. (2013). The effectiveness of psychodynamic interventions for people with learning disabilities: a systematic review. *Tizard Learning Disability Review*, 19, 17–24.

Kellett, S., Beail, N., Bush, A., Dyson, G., Wilbram, M. (2009). Single case experimental evaluations of psychodynamic and cognitive behavioural psychotherapy with people with learning disabilities. *Advances in Mental Health and Learning Disabilities*, 3, 36–44.

Khan, M. and Beail, N. (2013). Service user satisfaction with individual psychotherapy for people who have intellectual disabilities. *Advances in Mental Health and Intellectual Disabilities*, 7, 277–283.

Klein, M. (1975). *The Writings of Melanie Klein*, Vol. 3. London: Hogarth Press.

Laaksonen, M.A., Lindors, O., Knekt, P., Aalberg, V. (2012). Suitability for Psychotherapy Scale (SPS) and its reliability, validity, and predicition. *British Journal of Clinical Psychology*, 51, 531–537.

Malan, D.H. (2001). *Individual Psychotherapy and the Science of Psychodynamics*. London: Butterworth.

Merriman, C. and Beail, N. (2009). Service user views of long term individual psychodynamic psychotherapy. *Advances in Mental Health and Learning Disabilities*, 3, 42–47.

Morrissey, M. and Jackman, C. (1998). Psychotherapy and therapeutic environment: inside out, outside in. *Irish Journal of Child and Adolescent Psychotherapy*, 1, 49–69.

Newman, D.W. and Beail, N. (2002). Monitoring change in psychotherapy with people with intellectual disabilities. The application of the Assimilation of Problematic Experiences Scale. *Journal of Applied Research in Intellectual Disabilities*, 15, 48–60.

Newman, D.W. and Beail, N. (2005). An analysis of assimilation during psychotherapy with people who have mental retardation. *American Journal on Mental Retardation*, 110, 359–365.

Newman, D.W. and Beail, N. (2010). An exploratory study of the defence mechanisms used in psychotherapy by adults who have intellectual disabilities. *Journal of Intellectual Disability Research*, 54, 579–583.

O'Driscoll, D. (2009). Psychotherapy and intellectual disability. In T. Cottis (ed,), *Intellectual Disability, Trauma and Psychotherapy*. London: Routledge.

Safran, J. and Segal, Z. (1990). *Interpersonal Process in Cognitive Therapy*. New York, NY: Basic Books.

Sinason, V. (1992). *Mental Handicap and the Human Condition: New Approaches from the Tavistock*. London: Free Association Books.

Smith, D.L. (1987). Formulating and evaluating hypotheses in psychoanalytic psychotherapy. *British Journal of Medical Psychology*, 60, 313–316.

Stiles, W.B., Elliott, R., Llewelyn, S.P., et al. (1990). Assimilation of problematic experiences by clients in psychotherapy. *Psychotherapy*, 27, 411–420.

Symington, N. (1981). The psychotherapy of a subnormal patient. *British Journal of Medical Psychology*, 54, 187–199.

Willner, P. (2006). Readiness for cognitive therapy in people with intellectual disabilities. *Journal of Applied Research in Intellectual Disabilities*, 19, 5–16.

Chapter

15

Cognitive-behavioral therapy

Dave Dagnan

Introduction

In 1993 Lindsay and colleagues published a case study describing the application of Beck's model of cognitive-behavioral therapy (CBT) to people with intellectual disabilities (ID) and depression (Lindsay et al., 1993). Clinical and research experience has progressed considerably since then, and there have now been a number of edited reference texts (Kroese et al., 1997; Taylor et al., 2013) and systematic reviews (e.g., Sturmey, 2004; Willner, 2005; Vereenooghe and Langdon, 2013) on CBT and other psychotherapies for people with ID. For example, a recent meta-analysis of good-quality studies of psychotherapy for people with ID included 14 papers and found both a moderate between-group effect size, that individual therapy was more efficacious than group therapy, and that CBT was effective for both anger and depression (Vereenooghe and Langdon, 2013). However, the authors suggested that clinical trials need to more accurately report details of design and research process and use larger numbers of participants.

In the context of an increasing interest and sophistication of research and clinical practice in CBT with people with ID, this chapter will first consider approaches to CBT and then describe aspects of therapy that may be adapted to meet the needs of people with ID. Finally, the chapter will discuss new developments in intervention and possible future directions of clinical and research activity in the field of CBT for people with ID.

What is CBT?

There is not a single, simple identified form of therapy that is "cognitive-behavioral therapy." In categorizing cognitive therapies, Dagnan and Chadwick (1997) made an important distinction between models and interventions based on assumptions of cognitive deficit or cognitive distortion.

Models and interventions based on cognitive deficit assume that people with ID have either poor skills in cognitive mediation (e.g., they do not use self-talk/self-regulation in an efficient or skilled manner), or possibly do not use self-talk at all (Whitman, 1990). People with ID have poorer communication skills and vocabulary than people without ID and, as such, verbal processes involving self-regulation will be harder for this group (Nader-Grosbois, 2014). For example, Hebblethwaite et al. (2011) asked people with and without ID to talk about events, beliefs, and emotions around real-life examples of social conflict. People with ID offered fewer beliefs, were more evaluative, and found it harder to discuss different perspectives on the events they described. People without ID were more able to describe conflict events in more detail and with more inferential subtlety. This supports the argument that people with ID may be less effective in self-regulation and are more likely to require interventions that help them use the skills that they have more effectively, or to learn new skills to manage stress and problems in life.

Models of cognitive distortion assume that people do actively make meaning and that emotion and behaviors are cognitively mediated, but that the cognitions are in some way distorted or unhelpful and so are associated with unhelpful emotional responses (Dagnan and Chadwick, 1997). There is now evidence that negative beliefs are strongly associated with mental ill-health in people with ID (e.g., Dagnan and Sandhu, 1999). These assumptions are associated with therapies developed by clinicians and researchers such as Beck et al. (1979).

There is no assumption that intervention approaches associated with either deficit or distortion models are better. However, it is important to recognize the theoretical basis of the intervention that is being used in order to be able to link the intervention with assessment of the strengths and needs of the people with ID (Dagnan, 2008) and to enable further systematic development of the intervention approach.

The challenges of using CBT with people with ID

The following case study illustrates some of the complexities in using CBT with people with ID:

> John is a man with mild ID and a measured Full Scale IQ score of 66. He is the youngest of four children, is 38 years old, and lives with his mother and an older sister in a three-bedroomed house owned by his mother. John's father died two years ago, and his mother has increasing difficulties with her mobility, is becoming more forgetful, and has a number of health issues, which have not been discussed with John as his mother, "does not want him to be upset." John has a hemiplegia, his communication is affected by his physical disability, and he can get frustrated if people do not understand him. John was teased and bullied at school and as a young man and most of his recent social networks revolved around his father's allotment and going with his father to support his local football team. Currently John does not leave his house very often, he has lost weight, has a poor appetite, and tends to be awake into the early hours of the morning, watching television and looking at football magazines, and then sleeps to early afternoon. John has been telling his family that he is ill, that he has headaches, stomach aches, and is often tired. John is tearful at times and during these periods makes statements that suggest he is uncertain about his future, saying things such as, "No one wants to live with me," and "There are bad things happening."

In considering how to use CBT to intervene in John's case there are three areas that we will need to take into account that are pertinent to John as a person with an iID:

The social context of John's life. He has very limited life experiences and very limited social networks, and associated developmental opportunities. Therefore, we will have to consider the opportunities available in John's life to practice and build new skills and ways of solving problems. We will have to consider John's disabled appearance and physical difficulties with communication and recognize that this may change the way people interact with him and change their expectations of him in interactions.

The psychological impact of John's life experiences. John, like many people with ID, has experience of being bullied and, even within a very positive family context, has been treated as different by his family and their friends. Models of stigma suggest that people with ID may accept and "internalize" societies view of them as people with disability (Jahoda et al., 2006). Over time this may affect core self-evaluations (Dagnan and Waring, 2004) and may affect clinical processes such as formation of a therapeutic alliance (Dagnan et al., 2007).

The real impact of John's intellectual disabilities. Although John is identified as having mild ID, he is likely to have difficulties with some of the intellectual demands of CBT. This might include difficulty in identifying emotions and describing his physiological experience, and it might include difficulty in using some of the core understanding of the relationship between cognition, emotion, and behavior in CBT (Dagnan et al., 2007).

Social context

People with ID may be more likely to experience a range of developmental and social factors associated with psychological distress and mental ill-health than people without ID. For example, Kiddle and Dagnan (2011) review the evidence on developmental vulnerability for depression and link this to literature from the ID field to demonstrate that certain risk factors may be more present in the lives of adolescents with ID. For example, they note that adolescence is a time when the importance of peer relationships is coupled with greater independence from the parents, which can result in conflict between parent and child and which is, in turn, associated with depression (Sheeber et al., 1997). Achieving greater independence from parents is a very complex process for young people with ID and independence is often not fully achieved (Hollins and Sinason, 2000).

The general importance of social support in buffering the effects of negative life events is well established (Cohen, 2004) and is known to be equally important for people with ID (Reiss and Benson, 1985). However, relationships can also be a significant source of distress, and people with ID frequently experience discrimination, bullying, and harassment (Sin et al., 2010). "Social strain" has been found to be strongly associated with depression (Lunsky and Benson, 2001), and problems with social networks have been found to be a predictor of depression in this population (McGillivray and McCabe, 2007).

It is important that the social environment and its developmental implications are taken into account in formulating psychological distress for people with ID. It is also important the limitations in many people's social networks and other features of their lives are taken into account in developing cognitive-behavioral therapy; the implications for this are discussed in detail by Jahoda et al. (2009a). For example, they discuss the clinical issues in having carers take part in some of the therapy sessions with people with ID. They suggest that carers can support the use of homework, but also identify that there may be positive effects for the carer in observing the clients participation in aspects of therapy (Rose et al., 2005).

The psychological impact of life experiences

People with ID are constructed by society as different, this difference has a negative valence and, thus, they can be identified as "stigmatized" (Jahoda et al., 1988). Stigmatization has a substantial impact upon the way people with ID and their families are treated (Green et al., 2005). When people recognize that they are treated negatively and differently over long periods of time, this affects their self-image and self-evaluations (Dagnan and Sandhu, 1999; Jahoda et al., 2006). Negative core self-evaluations then influence social processes such as self-esteem and social comparison (Dagnan and Waring, 2004). These cognitive processes have been shown to be related to mental ill-health in people with ID (Dagnan and Sandhu, 1999; Dagnan and Jahoda, 2006; Hedley and Young, 2006).

A number of authors have considered how the impact of negative social construction may affect the delivery of cognitive therapy for people with ID (Jahoda et al., 2006, 2009a). For example, Jahoda et al. (2009a) discuss how a history of stigmatized experience may affect how people with ID may enter therapy, leading to processes such as negative expectations of contact with professionals or a strong tendency to acquiesce. It may be particularly important with this client group to use behavioral experimentation to challenge the client's view of themselves as a person without power in their environment, or it may be possible to use cognitive methods that use the attributional processes outlined by authors such as Corrigan and Watson (2002) to reduce the impact of stigma on self-concept. Dagnan et al. (2013) discuss how a stigmatized history may affect the formation of a therapeutic alliance. They highlight a number of activities that can serve to build the therapeutic alliance based upon an understanding of stigma. For example, they suggest that it will be important to highlight clients' strengths and positive relationships, rather than merely focusing on problem areas; it will also be important to focus on each individual achievement within therapy, and processes, such as the collaborative use of agendas (Lindsay, 1999), may create a sense of shared success, which will strengthen the alliance.

The real impact of intellectual disabilities

People with ID are likely to have difficulties with some aspects of CBT. Dagnan and colleagues have discussed the development of an assessment approach that identifies key areas of understanding that are necessary to be able to fully take part in therapy (Dagnan et al., 2007). From a consideration of basic CBT processes they suggest that:

1. A person should be able to accurately distinguish events (the activating event), thoughts (the belief), and emotions (the consequence).
2. The person should be able to identify that certain events are associated with emotional experience. It is important to recognize that not all people with mild ID immediately associate the way they feel with what is going on around them in their lives (Reed and Clements, 1989).
3. The person should be able to recognize that the emotional consequences are closely linked to beliefs. This is often one of the more complex concepts for people with ID engaging in CBT.

Dagnan and Chadwick (1997) describe the assessment process identified above in detail, and Dagnan et al. (2009) describe a detailed analysis of the types of response that people with ID may give in assessments of understanding of cognitive mediation, and discuss how such assessments may guide decisions on intervention type or may suggest the need for pretherapy work with the client. From such assessments it may be possible to suggest key areas of understanding that can be developed prior to entering therapy. For example, Bruce et al. (2010) describe a training approach that develops the understanding that people with ID have of core concepts associated with CBT.

The adaptations made to therapy to enable engagement by people with ID are broad (Whitehouse et al., 2006). Dagnan et al. (2007) describe a range of adaptations that take into account the ID of this client group. They identify the potential for shorter and more frequent sessions, the need to maintain a high level of engagement through active and "vivid" methods, such as role play, use of focused activities, and taking therapy to the environments where the issues being addressed happen. They further identify the need for accessible materials, repetition, and particular attention to breaks in therapy.

An important and developing area in the application of therapy with people with ID is that of research into therapy process. This area of research serves both to confirm that the expected processes of change are indeed present for people with ID, but also serves to identify further how adaptation in therapeutic technique might be needed. Non-specific therapy processes have been discussed for CBT with people with ID. For example, Kilbane and Jahoda (2011) discuss an important non-specific factor in therapy, that of "therapy expectation," and describe the development of the "Therapy Expectation Measure." They suggest that people with ID may be able to understand therapy as an outcome and goal-focused process, but that client and carer perceptions of therapy may be different. In further exploring these differences in perspective, Pert et al. (2008) report on the experience of CBT for people with ID, in particular it was notable that participants valued the therapeutic relationship. Stenfert Kroese et al. (2014) reported that carers have little knowledge of CBT and do not feel included in the process. Jahoda et al. (2009b) used interaction analysis of 30 transcribed therapy sessions to study whether it was possible to achieve an equal balance of power in therapy with people with ID. Their analysis suggested that therapists provided structure to therapy through asking questions whilst the clients provided the content of the interactions. This paper suggests that it is possible to maintain a collaborative relationship in CBT with people with ID.

Development of intervention

In the past 10 years intervention has developed in two areas. Firstly, there are an ongoing descriptions of single case studies of the application of cognitive therapy to specific presentations such as obsessive-compulsive disorder (Willner and Goodey, 2006; Pence et al., 2011), post-traumatic stress disorder (Kroese and Thomas, 2006; Mevissen and de Jongh, 2010), psychosis (Barrowcliff, 2008), and pain (McManus et al., 2014). Secondly, there have been a small number of controlled trials of CBT interventions structures (McGillivray et al., 2008; Hassiotis et al., 2011; Willner et al., 2013). Although some of these trials are still at the level of feasibility studies, it is notable that the field is moving towards randomized controlled trials, as the absence of such definitive trials has been identified as a significant problem in this field (Willner, 2005; Vereenooghe and Langdon, 2013). The development of definitive trials of CBT presents a number of challenges in design and implementation (Bhaumik et al., 2011); however, the systematic development of manualized approaches will make fully adapted materials and approaches widely available to clinicians working in this area.

Future directions

Dagnan (2007b) reviewed evidence for psychosocial models and interventions for people with ID. The author identified that many of the evidence-based psychosocial and cognitive interventions available for people without ID and severe mental ill-health have not been systematically described and trialed for people with ID. This remains the case, and many of the more systematic development in CBT for people with ID have been in the area of common mental health problems, such depression, anxiety, and anger. There is less systematic development of psychosocial interventions for people with ID and severe mental health problems and their families, although a few initial case studies do exist (Haddock et al. 2004; Barrowcliff, 2008). The approaches to intervention involving family systems and early-signs approaches that are within the UK's National Institute for Health and Care Excellence (NICE) guidance for severe mental illness would seem to be entirely suitable for application to people with ID (Dagnan, 2007a). It should be expected that such interventions will be more systematically developed for this population.

There is also an emerging discussion of how therapy can be delivered through mainstream services in a way that will be accessible to as many people with ID as possible. Dagnan et al. (2014) discuss training for mainstream therapists working in mental health services. There is discussion as to how such services can be made accessible to this client group (Dodd et al., 2011). However, the advantages for this approach are potentially significant in making therapy accessible to people with ID and to those who would benefit from similar adaptations but who are not formally identified as having ID (Dagnan et al., 2013). It should be expected that research describing models for the wider provision of CBT for people with ID within mainstream service structures will begin to develop.

Conclusions

This chapter has presented an overview of research and clinical developments in the application of CBT for people with ID. This is an area of intervention that now has substantial literature describing models of distress, approaches to assessment, adaptations of therapy, and therapy process. One of the previous criticisms of this area has been the lack of definitive trials of intervention (Willner, 2005); there are now a small number of published trials and a number of trials underway and in development. It should be expected that these will bring CBT for people with ID into the mainstream of clinical intervention for this population.

Key summary points

- There is no single model of therapy that can be identified as CBT, and a range of interventions concerned with enabling people to use cognitive skills more effectively, and challenging the beliefs people have about the world, have been described.
- In making adaptations to CBT for people with ID we should consider their social context, the impact of negative social construction on their well-being, and potential difficulties in understanding some therapy processes.
- There is a developing literature in therapy process for CBT with people with ID, which offers further insights into adaptation and change processes.

- There are now a number of randomized controlled trials of CBT for people with ID applied to depression, anger, and anxiety, and a recent meta-analysis suggests that CBT is effective for anger and depression.
- Future research may see development of interventions for people with ID and severe mental ill-health and a greater understanding of how to enable people with ID to use mainstream therapy services.

References

Barrowcliff, A.L. (2008). Cognitive-behavioural therapy for command hallucinations and intellectual disability: a case study. *Journal of Applied Research in Intellectual Disabilities*, 21(3), 236–245.

Beck, A.T., Ward, C.H., Shaw, B.F., Emery, G. (1979). *Cognitive Therapy of Depression*. New York, NY: Wiley.

Bhaumik, S., Gangadharan, S., Hiremath, A., Russell, P.S.S. (2011). Psychological treatments in intellectual disability: the challenges of building a good evidence base. *British Journal of Psychiatry*, 198(6), 428–430.

Bruce, M., Collins, S., Langdon, P., Powlitch, S., Reynolds, S. (2010). Does training improve understanding of core concepts in cognitive behaviour therapy by people with intellectual disabilities? A randomized experiment. *British Journal of Clinical Psychology*, 49, 1–13.

Cohen, S. (2004). Social relationships and health. *American Psychologist*, 59(8), 676.

Corrigan, P.W. and Watson, A.C. (2002). The paradox of self-stigma and mental illness. *Clinical Psychology: Science and Practice*, 9(1), 35–53.

Dagnan, D. (2007a). Psychosocial intervention for people with learning disabilities. *Advances in Mental Health and Learning Disabilities*, 1(2), 3–7.

Dagnan, D. (2007b). Psychosocial interventions for people with intellectual disabilities and mental ill-health. *Current Opinion in Psychiatry*, 20(5), 456–460.

Dagnan, D. (2008). Psychological assessment with people with learning disabilities and mental ill-health. *Advances in Mental Health and Learning Disabilities*, 2(4), 5.

Dagnan, D. and Chadwick, P. (1997). Cognitive behaviour therapy for people with learning disabilities: assessment and intervention. In B.S. Kroese, D. Dagnan, K. Loumides (eds.), *Cognitive Behaviour Therapy for People with Learning Disabilities*. London: Routledge.

Dagnan, D. and Jahoda, A. (2006). Cognitive-behavioural intervention for people with intellectual disability and anxiety disorders. *Journal of Applied Research in Intellectual Disabilities*, 19(1), 91–97.

Dagnan, D. and Sandhu, S. (1999). Social comparison, self-esteem and depression in people with intellectual disability. *Journal of Intellectual Disability Research*, 43, 372–379.

Dagnan, D. and Waring, M. (2004). Linking stigma to psychological distress: Testing a social-cognitive model of the experience of people with intellectual disabilities. *Clinical Psychology and Psychotherapy*, 11(4), 247–254.

Dagnan, D., Kroese, B., Jahoda, A. (2007). Cognitive behavioural therapy and people with intellectual disabilities. In G. O'Reilly, J. McEvoy, P. Walsh (eds.), *Handbook of Clinical Psychology and Intellectual Disability Practice*. London: Routledge.

Dagnan, D., Mellor, K., Jefferson, C. (2009). Assessment of cognitive therapy skills for people with learning disabilities. *Advances in Mental Health and Learning Disabilities*, 3(4), 25–30.

Dagnan, D., Jahoda, A.J., Kilbane, A. (2013). Preparing people with intellectual disabilities for psychological treatment. In J.L. Taylor (ed.), *Psychological Therapies for Adults with Intellectual Disabilities*. Chichester, West Sussex, UK: Wiley-Blackwell.

Dagnan, D., Masson J., Cavagin, A., Thwaites, R., Hatton, C. (2014). The development of a measure of confidence in delivering therapy to people with intellectual disabilities. *Clinical Psychology and Psychotherapy*, DOI: 10.1002/cpp.1898 (online publication ahead of issue).

Dodd, K., Joyce, T., Nixon, J., Jennison, J., Heneage, C. (2011). Improving access to psychological therapies (IAPT): are they applicable to people with intellectual disabilities? *Advances in Mental Health and Intellectual Disabilities*, 5(2), 29–34.

Green, S., Davis, C., Karshmer, E., Marsh, P., Straight, B.. (2005). Living stigma: the impact of labeling, stereotyping, separation, status loss, and discrimination in the lives of individuals with disabilities and their families. *Sociological Inquiry*, 75(2), 197–215.

Haddock, G., Lobban, F., Hatton, C., Carson, R. (2004). Cognitive-behaviour therapy for people with psychosis and mild intellectual disabilities: a case series. *Clinical Psychology and Psychotherapy*, 11(4), 282–298.

Hassiotis, A., Serfaty, M., Azam, K., et al. (2011). Cognitive behaviour therapy (CBT) for anxiety and depression in adults with mild intellectual disabilities (ID): a pilot randomised controlled trial. *Trials*, 12, 95.

Hebblethwaite, A., Jahoda, A., Dagnan, D. (2011). Talking about real-life events: an investigation into the ability of people with intellectual disabilities to make links between their beliefs and emotions within dialogue. *Journal of Applied Research in Intellectual Disabilities*, 24(6), 543–553.

Hedley, D. and Young, R. (2006). Social comparison processes and depressive symptoms in children and adolescents with Asperger syndrome. *Autism*, 10(2) 139–153.

Hollins, S. and Sinason, V. (2000). Psychotherapy, learning disabilities and trauma: new perspectives. *British Journal of Psychiatry*, 176(1), 32–36.

Jahoda, A., Markova, I., Cattermole, M. (1988). Stigma and the self-concept of people with a mild mental handicap. *Journal of Mental Deficiency Research*, 32, 103–115.

Jahoda, A., Dagnan, D., Jarvie, P., Kerr, W. (2006). Depression, social context and cognitive behavioural therapy for people who have intellectual disabilities. *Journal of Applied Research in Intellectual Disabilities*, 19(1), 81–89.

Jahoda, A., Dagnan, D., Kroese, S., et al. (2009a). Cognitive behavioural therapy: from face to face interaction to a broader contextual understanding of change. *Journal of Intellectual Disability Research*, 53, 759–771.

Jahoda, A., Selkirk, M., Trower, P., et al. (2009b). The balance of power in therapeutic interactions with individuals who have intellectual disabilities. *British Journal of Clinical Psychology*, 48, 63–77.

Kiddle, H. and Dagnan, D. (2011). Vulnerability to depression in adolescents with intellectual disabilities. *Advances in Mental Health and Intellectual Disability*, 5, 3–8.

Kilbane, A.L. and Jahoda, A. (2011). Therapy expectations: preliminary exploration and measurement in adults with intellectual disabilities. *Journal of Applied Research in Intellectual Disabilities*, 24(6), 528–542.

Kroese, B.S. and Thomas, G. (2006). Treating chronic nightmares of sexual assault survivors with an intellectual disability – two descriptive case studies. *Journal of Applied Research in Intellectual Disabilities*, 19(1), 75–80.

Kroese, B.S., Dagnan, D., Loumides, K. (eds.) (1997). *Cognitive Behaviour Therapy for People with Learning Disabilities*. London: Routledge.

Lindsay, W.R. (1999). Cognitive therapy. *Psychologist*, 12(5), 238–241.

Lindsay, W.R., Howells, L., Pitcaithly, D. (1993). Cognitive therapy for depression with individuals with intellectual disabilities. *British Journal of Medical Psychology*, 66, 135–141.

Lunsky, Y. and Benson, B.A. (2001). Association between perceived social support and strain, and positive and negative outcome for adults with mild intellectual disability. *Journal of Intellectual Disability Research*, 45(2), 106–114.

McGillivray, J.A. and McCabe, M.P. (2007). Early detection of depression and associated risk factors in adults with mild/moderate intellectual disability. *Research in Developmental Disabilities*, 28(1), 59–70.

McGillivray, J.A., McCabe, M.P., Kershaw, M.M. (2008). Depression in people with intellectual disability: an evaluation of a staff-administered treatment program. *Research in Developmental Disabilities*, 29 (6), 524–536.

McManus, S., Treacy, M., McGuire, B.E. (2014). Cognitive behavioural therapy for chronic pain in people with an intellectual disability: a case series using components of the Feeling Better programme. *Journal of Intellectual Disability Research*, 58(3), 296–306.

Mevissen, L. and de Jongh, A. (2010). PTSD and its treatment in people with intellectual disabilities: a review of the literature. *Clinical Psychology Review*, 30(3), 308–316.

Nader-Grosbois, N. (2014). Self-perception, self-regulation and metacognition in adolescents with intellectual disability. *Research in Developmental Disabilities*, 35 (6), 1334–1348.

Pence, S.L., Aldea, M.A., Sulkowski, M.L., Storch, E.A. (2011). Cognitive behavioral therapy in adults with obsessive-compulsive disorder and borderline intellectual functioning: a case series of three patients. *Journal of Developmental and Physical Disabilities*, 23(2), 71–85.

Pert, C., Jahoda, A., Trower, P., et al. (2008). Making sense of therapy: clients' views of cognitive behavioural therapy. *Journal of Intellectual Disability Research*, 52, 732.

Reed, J. and Clements, J. (1989). Assessing the understanding of emotional states in a population of adolescents and young adults with mental handicaps. *Journal of Mental Deficiency Research*, 33, 229–233.

Reiss, S. and Benson, B.A. (1985). Psychosocial correlates of depression in mentally retarded adults. I. Minimal social support and stigmatization. *American Journal of Mental Deficiency*, 89(4), 331–337.

Rose, J., Loftus, M., Flint, B., Carey, L. (2005). Factors associated with the efficacy of a

group intervention for anger in people with intellectual disabilities. *British Journal of Clinical Psychology*, 44, 305–317.

Sheeber, L., Hops, H., Alpert, A., Davis, B., Andrews J.A. (1997). Family support and conflict: prospective relations to adolescent depression. *Journal of Abnormal Child Psychology*, 25(4), 333–344.

Sin, C., Comber, N., Mguni, N., Hedges, A., Cook, C.. (2010). Targeted violence, harassment and abuse against people with learning disabilities in Great Britain. *Tizard Learning Disability Review*, 15(1), 17–27.

Stenfert Kroese, B., Jahoda, A., Pert, C., Trower, P., Dagnan, D., Selkirk, M. (2014). Staff expectations and views of cognitive behaviour therapy (CBT) for adults with intellectual disabilities. *Journal of Applied Research in Intellectual Disabilities*, 27(2), 145–153.

Sturmey, P. (2004). Cognitive therapy with people with intellectual disabilities: a selective review and critique. *Clinical Psychology and Psychotherapy*, 11(4), 222–232.

Taylor, J.L., Lindsay, W.R., Hastings, R.P., Hatton, C. (eds.) (2013). *Psychological Therapies for Adults with Intellectual Disabilities*. London: Wiley-Blackwell.

Vereenooghe, L. and Langdon, P.E. (2013). Psychological therapies for people with intellectual disabilities: a systematic review and meta-analysis. *Research in Developmental Disabilities*, 34(11), 4085–4102.

Whitehouse, R.M., Tudway, J.A., Look, R., Kroese, B.S. (2006). Adapting individual psychotherapy for adults with intellectual disabilities: a comparative review of the cognitive-behavioural and psychodynamic literature. *Journal of Applied Research in Intellectual Disabilities*, 19(1), 55–65.

Whitman, T.L. (1990). Self-regulation and mental-retardation. *American Journal on Mental Retardation*, 94(4), 347–362.

Willner, P. (2005). The effectiveness of psychotherapeutic interventions for people with learning disabilities: a critical overview. *Journal of Intellectual Disability Research*, 49, 73–85.

Willner, P. and Goodey, R. (2006). Interaction of cognitive distortions and cognitive deficits in the formulation and treatment of obsessive-compulsive behaviours in a woman with an intellectual disability. *Journal of Applied Research in Intellectual Disabilities*, 19(1), 67–73.

Willner, P., Rose, J., Jahoda, A., et al. (2013). Group-based cognitive-behavioural anger management for people with mild to moderate intellectual disabilities: cluster randomised controlled trial. *British Journal of Psychiatry*, 203(4), 288–296.

Chapter

16

Behavioral approaches

Betsey A. Benson

Introduction

The behavioral approach to assessment and intervention has had a major impact on the field of developmental disabilities. Behavioral interventions are among the most frequently used treatments and have considerable research support (Sturmey, 2012). Behavioral techniques are considered evidence-based practice for a number of challenging behaviors (Jennett and Hagopian, 2008; Carr et al., 2009; Kurtz et al., 2011) and are a first-line treatment according to professional consensus (Rush and Frances, 2000).

The behavioral approach applies the principles of learning to change behavior and is effective in teaching adaptive skills as well as in reducing maladaptive behavior. Using objective description and systematic observation, the environmental variables that influence behavior are identified and customized interventions are implemented to produce change. Data collection continues throughout intervention to document progress. Behavioral interventions are effective with individuals of all ages and levels of functioning.

Assessment

The behavioral approach to assessment includes identifying the antecedents to the behavior (A), defining the behavior of concern in specific, concrete language (B), and examining the consequent events that follow the behavior (C). The A–B–C model guides assessment and intervention. A goal of behavioral assessment is to determine the function of the behavior or what the behavior accomplishes for the individual. A behavior may result in gaining attention (social), obtaining tangibles, sensory stimulation (internal), or escape from demands. There are several methods of behavioral assessment and a combination of approaches is most often used in clinical practice.

A scatterplot is a record of the occurrence of behavior during predefined time periods throughout the day over a period of days or weeks. Data from a scatterplot is used to identify trends and patterns in the occurrence/non-occurrence of the behavior.

A–B–C charts are narrative recordings in which each occurrence of the behavior is described according to the antecedents, the behavior during that incident, and the consequences. Information from a number of occurrences is reviewed to identify common factors. A–B–C charts can be used to generate hypotheses about the function of a behavior that can be followed up with other assessment methods (Lanovaz et al., 2013).

Psychiatric and Behavioral Disorders in Intellectual and Developmental Disabilities, ed. Colin Hemmings and Nick Bouras. Published by Cambridge University Press. © Cambridge University Press 2016.

A functional analysis (FA) of behavior, or experimental FA, refers to an analog procedure in which brief, controlled sessions are arranged to present specific environmental conditions (Iwata et al., 1994). The frequency of the problem behavior and possibly the latency to the behavior are recorded. Comparisons are made across conditions to identify the likely behavioral function. For example, if a FA of self-injurious behavior, defined as fist hits to the head, indicated that a greater frequency of head hits occurred during a demand condition in which school work was presented than in either an alone condition or an attention condition in which each hit was followed by a verbal comment from an observer, then an escape function for self-injury would be hypothesized. If an FA is not conclusive in identifying a functional relationship, then follow-up sessions can be conducted to further refine the environmental variables under consideration (Tiger et al., 2009; Hagopian et al., 2013). Attention and escape are among the most commonly identified functions of challenging behavior in persons with ID (Matson et al., 2011). Interventions that are preceded by a FA are more likely to be effective (Harvey et al., 2009).

The limitations of FA are that conducting the sessions is time-consuming, requires specialized training, and is usually completed in laboratory, inpatient, or clinic settings. However, in one study, master's-level residential supervisors and assistants were trained to conduct FA sessions (Lambert et al., 2014). The appropriateness of FA to assess low-frequency challenging behavior has also been questioned, and other assessment methods, such as sequential analysis of case records, were proposed in such cases (Whitaker et al., 2004).

The functional assessment questionnaires are rating scales that focus on the probable maintaining variables of problem behavior. The two most commonly used scales are the Motivation Assessment Scale (MAS; Durand and Crimmins, 1988) and the Questions About Behavioural Function scale (QABF; Matson et al., 1999). The MAS addresses four categories of reinforcement, including attention, escape, tangible, and sensory. The QABF assesses possible maintaining variables of physical discomfort, social attention, escape, tangible, and non-social reinforcement (sensory). Both scales are intended to be completed by someone who knows the individual well. An advantage of functional assessment questionnaires is that they do not require extensive time or training and several respondents can provide input about an individual. Obtaining input from multiple respondents may improve the correspondence of the findings with other, more direct methods of assessment (Smith et al., 2012).

Another type of behavioral assessment that may be conducted is preference assessment. The goal of preference assessment is to identify potential reinforcers for an individual through interview, observation, or structured sessions in which choices are offered to the individual and selections are noted. Exercising choice is a method of expressing a preference (Cannella et al., 2005). Various methods of preference assessment have been developed, including offering a choice between stimuli, such as leisure items, activities, or edibles. A rank-ordered list of preferred items is constructed based on the selections. Preferred items can then be incorporated into an intervention program.

Interventions

Behavioral interventions are selected based on the results of the functional assessment and are chosen to match the behavioral function (Denis et al., 2011). The behavioral interventions may aim to modify the antecedent conditions that are frequently associated with the behavior, disrupt the link between the problem behavior and the consequences, or some combination of these. In recent years, there has been an increased emphasis on the use of non-aversive interventions (Harvey et al., 2009). Positive behavior support, an approach that integrates applied behavior analysis with person-centered philosophy, promotes the use of non-aversive interventions, intervening in the natural environment, incorporating the individual's choices and preferences, and using multicomponent treatment plans (McClean and Grey, 2012).

Antecedent stimuli

Antecedent factors can increase the probability that problem behavior will occur. Many procedures have been used to modify antecedent conditions, such as reducing noise or crowding, changing staffing, offering more choice of activities or sequencing of tasks, presenting tasks that are commensurate with abilities (rather than too complex), and addressing physical conditions that may be affecting behavior such as sleep deprivation, hunger, or pain. The procedures may be conceptualized as impacting the physical environment, the social environment, or the biological environment. Interventions directed at antecedent conditions aim to meet the needs of the individual in the environment and are ongoing. Greater attention is being paid to these contextual variables, sometimes referred to as setting events, and their influence on behavior (Carr et al., 2008).

Consequences

Behavioral interventions alter the consequences of problem behavior by removing reinforcement for challenging behavior (extinction) and by providing reinforcement for alternative, more acceptable behaviors. Differential reinforcement (DR) is a non-aversive intervention that aims to alter the reinforcing consequences of behavior. There are several forms of DR, all involve withholding reinforcement for a behavior and providing reinforcement for other, more acceptable behaviors. The most frequently used DR strategies are DRI, differential reinforcement of incompatible behavior, DRO, differential reinforcement of other behavior, and DRA, differential reinforcement of alternate behavior. DR strategies, when used alone or in combination with other interventions, are an effective intervention for a variety of behavioral concerns in persons with ID (Chowdhury and Benson, 2011).

Functional communication training (FCT) is a reinforcement-based intervention that develops a communication response in order to access a reinforcer that was linked with problem behavior (Tiger et al., 2008). First, an FA is completed and then an alternate behavior that is a communicative response is developed as a replacement. The alternative response is a form of communication that is recognized by others. Several different communication responses have been taught, including sign language, vocalizations, picture exchanges, and activation of a communication device. FCT is typically paired with extinction, that is, the withholding of reinforcement for problematic behavior. FCT meets the criteria to be considered a "well-established" treatment for problem behavior in children with ID and/or autism spectrum disorders and is "probably efficacious" for adults (Kurtz et al., 2011).

Non-contingent reinforcement (NCR) is a procedure in which a reinforcer that has been available contingent on problem behavior, is provided independent of the occurrence of that behavior. NCR is a function-based intervention that has been used with a number of different topographies of problem behavior, including aggression, self-injury, stereotypy, pica, and disruptive behavior (Carr et al., 2009). NCR has been administered with various schedules of reinforcement, schedules that are thinned over time, and with or without an extinction component. There is sufficient evidence to consider NCR with a fixed-time reinforcement schedule and planned thinning plus extinction as a "well-established" treatment (Carr et al., 2009).

Considerable debate has occurred about the role of aversive interventions in behavior change programs for individuals with developmental disabilities. The use of the least restrictive intervention is considered a best practice in the field. There has been a concerted effort to reduce the use of restrictive procedures and to evaluate the need for and effectiveness of the procedures when they are used.

Response cost is a punishment procedure in which reinforcement is removed contingent on an inappropriate behavior. Response cost can be implemented as a fine applied to points or tokens that were previously earned, or by withholding access to preferred items or activities. Response cost is often combined with other behavioral interventions, such as reinforcement of appropriate behavior.

Physical and mechanical restraint and timeout are aversive interventions that are used at times to manage severe challenging behavior, generally when health and safety concerns are prominent. Physical restraint, or restricting voluntary movement contingent on behavior (Luiselli, 2009), tends to be used in response to physical aggression, particularly when there is a sustained episode (Emerson et al., 2000). In extreme cases of self-injury, mechanical restraints, such as arm splints or other protective equipment, are sometimes used. Restraints can be examined according to whether they are part of a planned intervention to specific circumstances or used in unplanned situations. Planned use is a safer alternative for all involved (Matson and Boisjoli, 2009). Restraints should be used infrequently to protect the individual and others from harm, be implemented by trained people, monitored for effectiveness, and have stated criteria for discontinuation. There should also be concurrent interventions to increase appropriate behavior (Luiselli, 2009).

Timeout is a procedure that imposes a loss of access to reinforcement contingent on a behavior. When implemented in group settings, the individual may be prompted to go to a set location, sometimes a separate room. Returning to the group may require a minimum period of time without the problem behavior occurring. The safety of the individual when in a separate location must be monitored (Iwata et al., 2009).

Efforts to reduce or eliminate the use of restraint and timeout in program-wide initiatives have been successful. Timeout use was successfully withdrawn from one community residential program and replaced with alternative procedures that were less intrusive (Iwata et al., 2009). Likewise, the use of physical restraint has been reduced in organizations through staff-training programs, increased use of behavioral plans, and defining clear criteria for the use of the restraint (Gaskin et al., 2013). On an individual level, successful procedures to reduce restraint use include conducting a more precise assessment of antecedent conditions, analyzing location and activity factors that are correlated with restraint use, identifying precursor behaviors that result in restraint use, and making changes to address those factors (Luiselli, 2009).

Challenging behavior

Challenging behavior is a term that is used to refer collectively to some or all of the following behaviors: aggression; self-injury; destructive behavior; pica; and stereotypy.

Challenging behaviors are a concern because they can present a danger to the individual and/or others, and they interfere with the acquisition of and engagement in adaptive behavior. If not addressed, challenging behavior tends to persist in individuals with developmental disabilities (Murphy et al., 2005).

Aggression

Most aggressive behavior is learned and is socially mediated. The most common functions of aggression are escape, attention, and tangible (Rojahn et al., 2012). Several behavioral interventions have been used successfully to reduce or eliminate aggressive behavior. Brosnan and Healy (2011) completed a review of behavioral interventions for the treatment of aggression in children with developmental disabilities. They found that three main types of interventions were used: (i) those that changed antecedent conditions; (ii) those that were reinforcement based; and (iii) those that focused on the consequences of behavior. The antecedent conditions that were altered included offering choices among tasks and reinforcers and introducing visual schedules. The reinforcement-based interventions included FCT, DR, and NCR procedures. The interventions that altered the consequences of behavior included extinction, response cost, and overcorrection, in which an effortful behavior that has some similarity to the target behavior is required. Many interventions were used in combination.

Self-injury

Self-injury is self-harming behavior that can result in tissue damage, such as head banging, hitting self, biting self, and skin picking. Self-injury tends to co-occur with other challenging behaviors (Matson et al., 2008). Behavioral interventions for self-injury have demonstrated effectiveness, especially when preceded by a FA (Harvey et al., 2009). Changing antecedent conditions and skills training, both non-aversive interventions, are effective treatments (Denis et al., 2011).

Pica

Pica refers to repeatedly eating inedible items or non-nutritious substances (Hagopian et al., 2011). Pica can have serious and even life-threatening consequences resulting in repeated surgeries and permanent physical damage. Sensory stimulation, or automatic reinforcement, is frequently hypothesized as the function for pica, although social contingencies should also be considered. Effective interventions for pica include environmental modifications, behavioral skills training, reinforcement, or response-reduction procedures (response blocking, effort manipulation, and punishment), or a combination of these (Hagopian et al., 2011). According to Matson et al. (2013), conducting a FA followed by non-aversive interventions such as NCR is an appropriate initial course of action for pica.

Stereotypy

Stereotypy is repetitive, apparently non-functional and inappropriate behavior, such as finger twisting, hand flapping, rocking, pacing, and repetitive vocalizations (Watkins and Rapp, 2014). The behaviors are problematic because they interfere with engaging in educational programs and activities. The function of stereotypy is often determined to be sensory or escape (Rojahn et al., 2012). Environmental enrichment in the form of non-contingent access to a preferred item combined with response cost has been successful in reducing stereotypy (Watkins and Rapp, 2014).

Application to symptoms of psychiatric disorders

Phobic avoidance

The treatment of fears or phobias is among the most studied of the anxiety symptoms in persons with ID. Avoidant behavior can be operationally defined by the distance to approach the feared object or situation. Planned exposure to the feared stimulus and reinforced practice are effective interventions for persons with ID, and there is sufficient evidence to consider them "well-established" treatments for both children and adults (Jennett and Hagopian, 2008). Examples of the stimuli avoided are dogs, strangers, water, medical procedures, escalators, and climbing stairs.

Delusional statements

Bizarre speech, psychotic speech, and delusional statements are phrases used to describe verbal behavior that is generally understood by others, but is not appropriate for the situation and may be repetitive. Behavioral interventions that are successful in reducing bizarre speech and increasing appropriate speech in psychiatric settings are DR, NCR, and response-cost interventions (Travis and Sturmey, 2008).

Symptoms of depression

The symptoms of depression in individuals with developmental disabilities have been addressed with interventions focusing on verbal behavior, such as increasing positive statements about the self, and reducing negative statements. DR, modeling, and rehearsal of positive statements have been found to be successful. Interventions have also included activity monitoring (Matson, 1982).

Research to practice

The majority of the published reports of behavioral interventions with persons with ID were conducted in hospitals, clinics, and schools. The difficulties of conducting research on interventions in community settings have been well documented (Oliver et al., 2002). In a rare case of successful implementation of a randomized control trial of an intervention for challenging behavior in adults with ID in a community-based service, Hassiotis et al. (2009) compared the effectiveness of specialist behavior therapy teams to standard treatment for individuals with mild to severe ID and significant challenging behavior. The specialist team employed functional assessment and positive behavioral strategies within a multifaceted treatment plan. The standard treatment approach included inter-disciplinary treatment teams and a range of interventions. The results indicated that the specialist team service resulted in a significant decrease in challenging behavior and cost no more than standard treatment. Two years later, the specialist team service users continued to be more improved compared to the standard-care participants on a measure of challenging behavior (Hassiotis et al., 2011).

Unfortunately, although there are a number of effective behavioral interventions for problematic behavior in individuals with developmental disabilities, their application is not universal. The slow pace to transfer the findings of published research to practice has been lamented (Matson et al., 2012). The extent of the problem was brought into focus by an examination of the service plans for individuals with profound ID and serious challenging behavior in several care facilities. The findings revealed that only half of the plans had information on the individual's challenging behavior. Further, information concerning the behavioral function, frequency, setting events, and goals to reduce or prevent the behavior were also absent (Poppes et al., 2014). The staff acceptance of the behaviors over time, as well as a failure to fully appreciate the negative consequences, were factors suggested as contributing to the omissions.

One barrier to implementation of behavioral interventions is that many plans are too complicated or labor-intensive for most agencies to employ (Matson and Boisjoli, 2009). Staff training is uniformly recommended to address the need and the outcomes of some staff-training programs have been encouraging. In one program, direct care staff from community agencies were trained to perform a functional assessment, to develop and implement a behavior plan, and to monitor progress. Most staff chose to develop plans to address aggressive behavior. Significant improvement was noted for three-quarters of the individuals (McClean and Grey, 2012). This model, although requiring a significant investment, has the potential to provide long-term gains. Individuals whose behavior did not improve following the initial intervention could be referred for more professional attention, which is often in short supply. Whether or not direct care staff are responsible for the assessment and development of a behavior intervention plan, the need to ensure that they are capable and willing to implement a plan consistently is of utmost importance.

Conclusions

A number of behavioral techniques are effective with a wide range of problem behaviors in children and adults with developmental disabilities. The efficacy of specific interventions has been investigated by adapting the criteria for evidence-based practice to single-case experimental designs. The standardization of criteria to evaluate behavioral treatments lends greater weight to the claims of efficacy.

The assessment of challenging behavior is the key to developing effective intervention plans. Both functional assessment and preference assessment provide vital information that guide the selection of appropriate treatments to match the needs and the preferences of the individual.

In the current climate, there is a greater consideration of the context in which behavior occurs, the social, physical, and internal environment. Many of the interventions that focus on antecedent conditions and have proven effective in reducing problem behavior do not appear difficult to implement, such as providing choices, developing visual schedules, and alternating more and less preferred tasks. The success of these techniques and the apparent simplicity of their design naturally lead to the question, "To what extent do current school, work, and living environments support individuals with developmental disabilities?"

There continues to be an emphasis on the use of non-aversive interventions and concerted efforts to reduce or eliminate aversive interventions, especially restraint procedures. The effectiveness of techniques such as NCR, FCT, and DR suggest that they should be considered among the first-line treatments.

The implementation of behavioral techniques in practice lags far behind the research, while at the same time the training needs of professionals and staff continue unabated. Without concerted efforts to improve the training of professionals and staff in behavioral theory and practices, it is unlikely that the situation will improve. Greater support for training programs is required.

Key summary points

- The behavioral approach defines problematic behavior in concrete terms and focuses on the antecedents to the behavior and the consequences.
- Both functional assessment of behavior and preference assessment provide key input to behavioral intervention plans.
- Functional communication training, NCR, and DR are behavioral interventions that are non-aversive and effective.
- The extensive training needs of professionals and staff are a barrier to the transfer of research findings to clinical practice.

References

Brosnan, J. and Healy, O. (2011). A review of behavioural interventions for the treatment of aggression in individuals with developmental disabilities. *Research in Developmental Disabilities*, 32, 437–446.

Cannella, H.I., O'Reilly, M.F., Lancioni, G.E. (2005). Choice and preference assessment research with people with severe to profound developmental disabilities: a review of the literature. *Research in Developmental Disabilities*, 26, 1–15.

Carr, E.G., Ladd, M.V., Schulte, C.F. (2008). Validation of the Contextual Assessment Inventory for problem behaviour. *Journal of Positive Behaviour Interventions*, 10, 91–104.

Carr, J.W., Severtson, J.M., Lepper, T.L. (2009). Noncontingent reinforcement is an empirically supported treatment for problem behaviour exhibited by individuals with developmental disabilities. *Research in Developmental Disabilities*, 30, 22–57.

Chowdhury, M. and Benson, B.A. (2011). Use of differential reinforcement to reduce behaviour problems in adults with intellectual disabilities: a methodological review. *Research in Developmental Disabilities*, 32, 383–394.

Denis, J., Van den Noortgate, W., Maes, B. (2011). Self-injurious behaviour in people with profound intellectual disabilities: a meta-analysis of single-case studies. *Research in Developmental Disabilities*, 32, 911–923.

Durand, V.M. and Crimmins, D.B. (1988). Identifying the variables maintaining self-injurious behaviour. *Journal of Autism and Developmental Disorders*, 18, 99–117.

Emerson, E., Robertson, J., Gregory, N., Hatton, C., Kessissoglou, S. (2000). Treatment and management of challenging behaviours in residential settings. *Journal of Applied Research in Intellectual Disabilities*, 13, 197–215.

Gaskin, C.J., McVilly, K.R., McGillivray, J.A. (2013). Initiatives to reduce the use of seclusion and restraint on people with developmental disabilities: a systematic review and quantitative synthesis. *Research in Developmental Disabilities*, 34, 3946–3961.

Hagopian, L.P., Rooker, G.W., Rolider, N.U. (2011). Identifying empirically supported treatments for pica in individuals with intellectual disabilities. *Research in Developmental Disabilities*, 32, 2114–2120.

Hagopian, L.P. Rooker, G.W., Jessel, J., DeLeon, I.G. (2013). Initial functional analysis outcomes and modifications in pursuit of differentiation: a summary of 176 inpatient cases. *Journal of Applied Behaviour Analysis*, 46, 88–100.

Harvey, S.T., Boer, D., Meyer, L.H., Evans, I.M. (2009). Updating a meta-analysis of intervention research with challenging behaviour: treatment validity and standards of practice. *Journal of Intellectual and Developmental Disability*, 34, 67–80.

Hassiotis, A., Robotham, D., Canagasabey, A., et al. (2009). Randomized, single-blind, controlled trial of a specialist behaviour therapy team for challenging behaviour in adults with intellectual disabilities. *American Journal of Psychiatry*, 166, 1278–1285.

Hassiotis, A., Canagasabey, A., Robotham, D., et al. (2011). Applied behaviour analysis and standard treatment in intellectual disability: two-year outcomes. *British Journal of Psychiatry*, 198, 490–491.

Iwata, B.A., Dorsey, M.F., Slifer, K.J., Bauman, K.E., Richman, G.S. (1994). Towards a functional analysis of self-injury. *Journal of Applied Behaviour Analysis*, 27, 197–209.

Iwata, B.A., Rolider, N.U., Dozier, C.L. (2009). Evaluation of timeout programmes through phased withdrawal. *Journal of Applied Research in Intellectual Disabilities*, 22, 203–209.

Jennett, H.K. and Hagopian, L.P. (2008). Identifying empirically supported treatments for phobic avoidance in individuals with intellectual disabilities. *Behaviour Therapy*, 39, 151–161.

Kurtz, P.F., Boelter, E.W., Jarmolowicz, D.P., Chin, M.D., Hagopian, L.P. (2011). An analysis of functional communication training as an empirically supported treatment for problem behaviour displayed by individuals with intellectual disabilities. *Research in Developmental Disabilities*, 32, 2935–2942.

Lambert, J.M., Bloom, S.E., Clay, C.J., Kunnavatana, S.S., Collins, S.D. (2014). Training residential staff and supervisors to conduct traditional functional analyses.

Research in Developmental Disabilities, 35, 1757–1765.

Lanovaz, M.J., Argumedes, M., Roy, D., Duquette, J.R., Watkins, N. (2013). Using ABC narrative recording to identify the function of problem behaviour: a pilot study. *Research in Developmental Disabilities*, 34, 2734–2742.

Luiselli, J.K. (2009). Physical restraint of people with intellectual disability: a review of implementation reduction and elimination procedures. *Journal of Applied Research in Intellectual Disabilities*, 22, 126–134.

Matson, J.L. (1982). The treatment of behavioural characteristics of depression in the mentally retarded. *Behaviour Therapy*, 13, 209–218.

Matson, J.L. and Boisjoli, J.A. (2009). Restraint procedures and challenging behaviours in intellectual disability: an analysis of causative factors. *Journal of Applied Research in Intellectual Disabilities*, 22, 111–117.

Matson, J.L., Bamburg, J.W., Cherry, K.E., Paclawsky, T.R. (1999). A validity study on the Questions About Behavioural Function (QABF) scale: predicting treatment success for self-injury, aggression, and stereotypies. *Research in Developmental Disabilities*, 20, 163–175.

Matson, J.L., Cooper, C., Malone, C.J., Moskow, S.L. (2008). The relationship of self-injurious behaviour and other maladaptive behaviours among individuals with severe and profound intellectual disability. *Research in Developmental Disabilities*, 29, 141–148.

Matson, J.L., Kozlowski, A.M., Worley, J.A., et al. (2011). What is the evidence for environmental causes of challenging behaviours in persons with intellectual disabilities and autism spectrum disorders? *Research in Developmental Disabilities*, 32, 693–698.

Matson, J.L., Neal, D., Kozlowski, A.M. (2012). Treatment for the challenging behaviours of adults with intellectual disabilities. *Canadian Journal of Psychiatry*, 57, 587–592.

Matson, J.L., Hattier, M.A., Belva, B., Matson, M.L. (2013). Pica in persons with developmental disabilities: approaches to treatment. *Research in Developmental Disabilities*, 34, 2564–2571.

McClean, B. and Grey, I. (2012). A component analysis of positive behaviour support plans. *Journal of Intellectual and Developmental Disability*, 37, 221–231.

Murphy, G.H., Beadle-Brown, J., Wing, L., et al. (2005). Chronicity of challenging behaviours in people with severe intellectual disabilities and/or autism: a total population sample. *Journal of Autism and Developmental Disabilities*, 35, 405–418.

Oliver, P.C., Piachaud, J., Done, J., et al. (2002). Difficulties in conducting a randomized controlled trial of health service interventions in intellectual disability: implications for evidence-based practice. *Journal of Intellectual Disability Research*, 46, 340–345.

Poppes, P., Van der Putten, A.A.J., Vlaskamp, C. (2014). Addressing challenging behaviour in people with profound intellectual and multiple disabilities: analyzing the effects of daily practice. *Journal of Policy and Practice in Intellectual Disabilities*, 11, 128–136.

Rojahn, J., Zaja, R., Turygin, N., Moore, L., van Ingen, D.J. (2012). Functions of maladaptive behaviour in intellectual and developmental disabilities: behaviour categories and topographies. *Research in Developmental Disabilities*, 33, 2020–2027.

Rush, A.J. and Frances, A. (eds.) (2000). The Expert Consensus Guideline Series. Treatment of psychiatric and behavioral problems in mental retardation. *American Journal on Mental Retardation*, 105 (Issue 3, Special Issue), 156–228.

Smith, C.M., Smith, R.G., Dracobly, J.D., Pace, A.P. (2012). Multiple-respondent anecdotal assessment: an analysis of interrater agreement and correspondence with analogue assessment outcomes. *Journal of Applied Behaviour Analysis*, 45, 779–795.

Sturmey, P. (2012). Treatment of psychopathology in people with intellectual and developmental disabilities. *Canadian Journal of Psychiatry*, 57, 593–600.

Tiger, J., Hanley, G.P., Bruzek, J. (2008). Functional communication training: a review and practical guide. *Behaviour Analysis in Practice*, 1, 16–23.

Tiger, J., Fisher, W.W., Toussaint, K.A., Kodak, T. (2009). Progressing from initially ambiguous functional analyses: three case examples. *Research in Developmental Disabilities*, 30, 910–926.

Travis, R. and Sturmey, P. (2008). A review of behavioural interventions for psychotic verbal behaviour in people with intellectual disabilities. *Journal of Mental Health Research in Intellectual Disabilities*, 1, 19–33.

Watkins, N. and Rapp, J.T. (2014). Environmental enrichment and response cost: immediate and subsequent effects on stereotypy. *Journal of Applied Behaviour Analysis*, 47, 186–191.

Whitaker, S., Walker, T., McNally, C. (2004). The use of time base lag sequential analysis to look at the relationship between environmental events and challenging behaviour in people with learning disabilities. *Behavioural and Cognitive Psychotherapy*, 32, 67–76.

Psychopathology of children with intellectual disabilities

Bruce Tonge

Introduction

Emotional and behavioral problems are a significant extra dimension that burdens the lives of many children with intellectual disabilities (ID) and their families and carers. This psychopathology is a major barrier to community and educational participation and inclusion and is associated with high levels of family stress, parental mental health problems, and reduced family quality of life (Tonge and Einfeld, 2003; Gardiner and Iarocci, 2012). Young people with ID have about three to four times as much psychiatric disturbance as children of average intelligence. Rutter et al. (1970), in their Isle-of-Wight population study, found that 50% of children with ID with an IQ below 70 had a psychiatric disorder, compared with 6.8% of children with an IQ above 70. Corbett (1979), in a study of the urban area of South-East London, found a prevalence rate of psychiatric disorder of 47% in children aged up to 15 years with an IQ below 50.

A longitudinal epidemiological study of intellectually disabled Australian children aged between 4 and 18 years found that 41% had a clinically significant emotional or behavioral disorder (Einfeld and Tonge, 1996). The study also found that disruptive and antisocial behaviors were more common in young people with ID, and that self-absorbed and social-relating problem behaviors were more common in young people with more severe ID. In contrast to general childhood psychopathology, age and sex did not affect prevalence, probably due to the salience of neurobiological influences, particularly for those with more severe ID. Over time into adult life, levels of psychopathology, although remaining substantial, decreased more in males than females and more for young people with mild ID (Einfeld et al., 2006). Of concern was that fewer than 10% of these children with ID had received any specialist mental health services.

An epidemiological study of a national survey of mental health information on more than 10 000 children aged 5–15 years in Great Britain revealed that 39% of children with ID met DSM-IV and ICD-10 criteria for at least one psychiatric disorder, compared to 8.1% of children without ID (Emerson, 2003). Emerson et al. (2009) demonstrated an association between psychopathology in children with ID and family socioeconomic hardship and disadvantage, but this association might not apply to families of children with ID and autism (Gray et al. 2012).

Psychiatric and Behavioral Disorders in Intellectual and Developmental Disabilities, ed. Colin Hemmings and Nick Bouras. Published by Cambridge University Press. © Cambridge University Press 2016.

Phenomenology

Children with ID can suffer from the full range of psychopathological disorders experienced by children of normal intelligence. Although the diagnosis of psychiatric disorders is unlikely in preschool children, there is evidence that by age three, developmentally delayed children are three times more likely to have a clinically significant level of emotional and behavioral disturbance that persists to age four (Baker et al. 2002, 2003). Anxiety disorders, depression and bipolar affective disorders, attention-deficit/hyperactivity disorder (ADHD), schizophrenia, and psychotic disorders have all been described in young people with ID (Matson and Barrett, 1982). Children with ID, compared to children without ID, are at greater risk for ADHD, conduct disorders, depression, anxiety disorders (including separation anxiety and phobias), and autistic disorder (Stromme and Diseth, 2000; Emerson, 2003; Tonge and Einfeld, 2003). ID is present in at least 70% of cases of autism (Volkmar and Klin, 2005). The types of psychopathological disorders in children with mild ID are more likely to resemble those found in the general population. It is increasingly difficult for the clinician to apply the criteria of existing diagnostic classifications in young people with more severe levels of ID who do not have the ability to share with others the content of their thinking and emotional experience. In these circumstances, a diagnosis must be made on the basis of observed behaviors and change in patterns of behavior, daily living skills, interests, social interaction, and interpersonal relationships.

There are some patterns of disturbed emotions and behaviors in young people with ID that cannot be adequately described by current psychiatric diagnostic systems such as the ICD-10 (World Health Organization, 1992) and the DSM-5 (American Psychiatric Association, 2013). The validity of these two major systems of psychiatric diagnosis is yet to be demonstrated when applied to young people with ID.

Another approach to the description of emotional and behavioral problems is the quantitative taxonometric model based on the statistical analysis of symptom questionnaires collected on defined populations of individuals with ID (Aman, 1991). An example of this approach in children are studies using the Developmental Behavior Checklist (DBC), a reliable and valid 96-item questionnaire of emotional and behavioral problems in young people with ID that is completed by parents, or carers, or teachers (Einfeld and Tonge, 2002). Since 1990, these studies have followed the mental health of a representative sample of 578 Australian young people with ID who were initially aged between 4 and 18 years (Tonge et al., 1996; Tonge and Einfeld, 2003; Einfeld et al., 2006). At the beginning of this study, 45% of the children had clinically significant levels of emotional and behavioral disorder. Symptoms of ADHD manifest as poor concentration, distractibility, impulsiveness, and hyperactivity, and were present in 32% of the children. The symptoms were not related to gender, in contrast to the general population where ADHD is more prevalent in males. The prevalence of ADHD symptoms was significantly reduced to 14% over 14 years as the young people moved into late adolescence and early adult life, suggesting a maturational effect. This happened at a faster rate for girls (decreasing to 9%) than for boys (decreasing to 17%). A total of 9% of the children were reported by their parents to have persistent symptoms of depression, tearfulness, irritability, and low self-esteem. This prevalence of depression did not change over 14 years and was not related to gender, in contrast to the general population where depression increases through adolescence and is more common in females. These symptoms of depression were less prevalent (3%) among those with severe or profound ID.

Initially, 8% of the children suffered from anxiety and phobias and there was no significant gender difference. Over the next 14 years, the prevalence of anxiety disorders did not change among boys, but increased among girls to 20%. In the general population of young people, females are twice as likely as males to suffer from anxiety disorders (Tonge, 1988). Those with severe or profound ID had a lower prevalence of anxiety disorders. These findings indicate that psychopathological disorders of childhood such as ADHD, depression, and anxiety were at least 4–5 times more prevalent in children with ID than in other children. Comorbidity was also common, with 19% of the children with ADHD also suffering from depression and 12% from anxiety. For children with depression, 70% also had ADHD and 30% had anxiety. This burden of specific psychopathological disorders in young people with ID (Tonge and Einfeld, 2003) highlights the imperative for better assessment and treatment services for this at-risk group of children.

Clinical assessment

The clinical interview is the essential component in diagnosis and assessment and is, therefore, necessary in the process of deciding on a rational management and treatment plan. The presence and severity of ID in the child necessitates some modification of a routine child psychiatric assessment and mental state examination. Information from the parents or carers and teachers and direct observation of the child, preferably in a variety of settings, such as at school as well as at the clinician's office, are essential. There is usually a range of contextual problems and factors that influence and complicate the presentation of emotional and behavioral problems in young people with ID, which need to be taken into account in order to achieve a satisfactory assessment diagnosis and a rational treatment plan (Tonge and Einfeld, 1991).

Cox and Rutter (1985) have demonstrated that the combined use of non-directive interview techniques together with more directive and structured questions, supplemented by parent- and teacher-completed checklists, provides the most comprehensive information and significantly improves assessment and diagnosis. This combined, unstructured and structured approach is still effective in promoting rapport and the expression of affect.

This approach to assessment and diagnosis has been replicated in an analysis of 70 psychiatric assessments of children with ID (Einfeld and Tonge, 1993). The non-directive interview component of the assessment revealed parental concern regarding an average of nine symptoms; compared to an average of 35 symptoms scored by the parents on a DBC they had previously completed (Einfeld and Tonge, 1993). The use of a parent- or carer-completed checklist, such as the DBC, clearly enriches the clinical assessment process, and parents reported that they felt the problems they faced had been fully explored and understood.

It is useful during part of the assessment to interview the parents or carers and the child together, and if the child can manage the separation, it is essential to see the child individually. Information from others, such as teachers, provides a broader perspective as well as information on contextual elements of the child's emotional or behavioral problems, and more resilient and adaptive behavior. A comprehensive cognitive assessment is also necessary in order to place the child's behavior into a developmental perspective and to understand the influence and impact of any cognitive impairments or specific pattern of cognitive performance on behavior, communication, and comprehension. For example, children with autism usually have better visual and performance skills than verbal and social comprehension skills, which can account for some of their frustration and difficult behavior, and has implications for education and management. Developmentally excessive problems with inattention during the cognitive testing may point to ADHD or anxiety, and deficits detected in working memory might account for disruptive and oppositional behavior in the classroom.

Assessments of communication and motor skills can also add considerable information to the overall picture. To date, there are no standardized general psychiatric assessment interviews validated for use with young people with ID. The parent's version of the Anxiety Disorders Interview Schedule (Albano and Silverman, 1996), which provides an algorithm for DSM-IV diagnoses, is being used in some clinical studies of anxiety disorders in children with moderate or less severe levels of ID. In the specific area of autism spectrum disorders, Lord et al. (1994) have developed the Autism Diagnostic Instrument (ADI), which comprises a structured parental interview. The ADI is supplemented by a clinician-led, structured play–task interaction with the child; the Autism Diagnostic Observation Schedule (ADOS) (Lord et al. 1999; Gray, et al. 2008). The ADI/ADOS provides a reliable and valid diagnosis of pervasive developmental disorders (Hus and Lord, 2014). It requires a skilled clinician to administer and is appropriately time-consuming, given the complexity and the serious implications of this diagnosis.

It is evident that the psychiatric assessment of young people with ID is complex, and requires information from all those involved in their care, as well as detailed mental state, psychological, developmental, and physical assessment of the child, together with any special investigations that may be indicated, such as genetic or imaging studies. This process is usually of necessity a multidisciplinary one, requiring contributions from psychiatrists, psychologists, pediatricians, and, when appropriate, others such as speech pathologists, occupational therapists, physiotherapists, and special teachers. To be effective, this multidisciplinary assessment requires coordination, usually through a case conference in which one of the specialist clinicians is designated as the case manager.

Developmental level and cognitive ability

The diagnosis of many psychiatric disorders requires an assessment of the person's thought processes and content. This may be possible in a child with mild ID and some communication skills, but becomes progressively more difficult as the level of ID becomes more severe (Forster et al., 2011). The clinician must often rely on observation of behavior and signs such as adverse changes in play interests, social participation, appetite, sleep, and activity level, as well as observed mood, to make a presumptive diagnosis of mental disorder (Costello, 1982; Sovner, 1986).

The developmental level of a child must also be taken into account when assessing the significance of problem behaviors. Normal behaviors in young children, such as separation anxiety or short attention span, may be seen in a much older child with ID who is still functioning at that younger developmental level. This necessity to take a developmental perspective is required by some diagnoses. For example, the DSM-5 (American Psychiatric Association, 2013) and the ICD-10 (World Health Organization, 1992) require that to make a diagnosis of attention-deficit/hyperactivity disorder (hyperkinetic disorder), the behavioral symptoms must be developmentally excessive for a child of the same mental age and developmental level. The assessment of antisocial, aggressive, and defiant behavior should take into account the child's developmental level and capacity to understand social rules and right from wrong when making a diagnosis of conduct disorder. A consideration of this capacity usually excludes children with autism or more severe levels of ID from the diagnosis of conduct disorder. In some children, organic deterioration of cognitive ability, the effects of some medications on the brain, the consequences of fetal alcohol or other substance spectrum disorder on the function of the frontal lobe, or the behavioral consequences of puberty and hormonal changes may also cause psychopathological symptoms and complicate or alter response to treatment.

Multiple disabilities and medical illness

Children in the general population with chronic illness that affects the brain have a higher prevalence of associated psychiatric disorder (Tonge, 1991). Children and adolescents with ID are more likely than the general population to have a range of physical and sensory impairments and medical illness, which further increases the risk of emotional and behavioral problems (Sovner and Hurley, 1989). For example, deafness may lead to behavior that is seen in autistic children or children with conduct disorder. Hearing impairment may also aggravate psychiatric disorders such as separation anxiety. Children with ID, particularly those with more severe ID, are much more likely to have medical illnesses or abnormalities of the brain, such as epilepsy, where the risk is even higher (Amiet et al., 2008). Epilepsy can cause disturbed behavior and aggravate existing emotional and behavioral problems, particularly if the epilepsy is poorly controlled (Lewis et al., 2000). The onset of depression and a loss of interest in usual activities during adolescence might herald this decline (Einfeld and Tonge, 2000). Autism is associated with a range of medical conditions, such as tuberous sclerosis, and other psychiatric conditions, such as Tourette syndrome (Volkmar and Klin, 2005). Specific patterns of behavior are also evident as the behavioral phenotypic expression of some genetic disorders (see also Chapter 18). Intellectually disabled children may also not be able to communicate effectively that they are suffering from pain or the symptoms of a fever or physical illness. Instead, they may exhibit disturbed behavior such as irritability, restlessness, or withdrawal, which may be misunderstood as being due to a psychiatric disorder.

Psychosocial and family factors

Children and adolescents with ID are more likely than the general population to experience a range of psychosocial stresses and environmental experiences that adversely affect their personality development, emotional adjustment, and attachment behavior, and can result in impoverished or distorted and inappropriate social behavior (Sovner, 1986; Aman and Schroeder, 1990). The families of children living in alternative residential or foster care may not be available for interview to provide reliable developmental and family histories. Institutional records often give an unreliable and inadequate account of the person's history. Observation and assessment of the child's interaction with their family, or with foster parents or staff and residents of an alternative care environment, are essential in order to understand the behavior in its psychosocial context and the contribution that these interactions make to the psychopathology. For example, in response to environmental stress, some children with ID may experience a regression and disintegration of their already impaired cognition, resulting in bizarre and psychotic-like behavior that can be misdiagnosed as schizophrenia. Another child might be withdrawn, listless, and apathetic in response to parental overprotection and lack of stimulation. Environmental deprivation and abuse, and a lack of stimulation and opportunity for play, activity, and socialization, aggravate ID, prevent children from reaching their full potential, and lead to a range of attachment, personality, emotional, and behavioral problems, and handicaps.

Although some parents have a positive and life-enriching experience caring for a child with ID, for many there is an increased risk that they may suffer from mental health problems and stress, particularly when the child also has emotional and behavioral problems (Baker et al., 2003; Blacher et al., 2007; Lloyd and Hastings, 2008). Therefore, the effective management of emotional and behavioral disorder in a child with ID may also require parent education and skills training and support, and management of any parent mental health problems, such as maternal depression or paternal alcohol abuse.

Management principles

Successful management begins with the establishment of a positive relationship with the parents and carers, and, if possible, the child during the assessment process. A working diagnosis that takes into account the biological, psychological, and social contributing factors, and context provides the key to a rational management plan. Treatment is usually multimodal, requiring a combination of parent support and skills training, behavioral interventions, modifications to the social and educational environment, modified psychological treatments, and, as a second line of treatment in combination with psychological and supported management, the use of psychoactive medication when indicated.

Some young people with moderate or less severe levels of ID have sufficient communication skills and understanding of consequences to be able to benefit from a modified form of cognitive-behavioral therapy. This involves a combination of relaxation training, modeling and reinforcement of confident and pro-social behaviors, formulating positive self-thoughts and statements instead of negative attributions, and providing a structured experience of rewarding educational and social activities and skills.

There is no evidence that family therapy has a direct effect, but it does reduce family dysfunction and conflict, and modifies problematic family interactional patterns, such as parental overprotection, which contribute to psychopathology in the child. The provision to the parents of educational information on ID in general, and on the nature of the ID and the psychopathological disorder in their child in particular, helps the parents generate their own adaptive responses and cooperate as partners with a range of services in the management of their child. A cooperative working relationship with the parents makes it more likely that they will feel encouraged to share their grief regarding their child's disability, and this in itself is also therapeutic. Structured parent education and skills training to manage problems such as disruptive behavior, anxiety, and communication difficulties in children with ID leads to sustained improvements in parental mental health, child behavior, and family life (Roux et al. 2013; Tonge et al. 2014). Counseling and the provision of psychological and educational interventions for siblings may also be necessary to promote family functioning.

Behavior management using operant conditioning techniques can be an effective strategy for managing difficult behaviors. The design of an effective behavior-modification program requires a detailed behavioral analysis regarding the context, the communication intent of the behavior, consequences that reinforce the behavior, the response by others to the behavior, and the longer term consequences of the behavior.

There is a secondary role of medication, but it should form part of a broader psychotherapeutic and supportive management plan. Most research on the use of pharmacotherapy in children with ID is focused on aggression and self-injurious behaviors. Controlled trials of haloperidol and, more recently, risperidone have shown that they are effective in the treatment of aggression, hyperactivity, and stereotypic behaviors, particularly in intellectually disabled children with autism, although these medications are associated with extra-pyramidal symptoms and other adverse side effects, such as weight gain and its metabolic consequences, and cardiac dysfunction with prolongation of the electrocardiograph QTc interval (Campbell et al., 1993; Lindsay and Aman, 2003). Lithium, carbamazepine, beta-blockers, such as propranolol, and the alpha-2 antagonist clonidine have been shown (mostly in open trials) to reduce aggressive, disruptive, and agitated behavior. Opiate agonists and antagonists (e.g., naloxone and naltrexone) may have some role in reducing self-injurious behaviors (Botteron and Geller, 1993). Stimulant medications such as dexamphetamine and methylphenidate may be useful in the treatment of unequivocal ADHD (Birmaher et al., 1988; Dulcan, 1990), but the efficacy of the more recent atomoxetine in children with ID has not yet been established. A favorable response to stimulant medication in developmentally disabled children and those with autism who also have ADHD may not be as marked as in children with ADHD who do not have ID. In young people with more severe ID, stimulant drugs may even exacerbate stereotypic and disturbed behavior. Anxious and obsessional behavior in intellectually disabled young people, particularly those with autism, may respond to treatment with selective serotonin reuptake inhibitors (SSRIs), such as fluoxetine, and the older tricyclic antidepressants, such as clomipramine and imipramine, but firm evidence from controlled trials is still required, and it is not clear if these reported therapeutic effects are due to specific effects on serotonin metabolism. Medication treatment requires regular follow-up and monitoring for compliance, the development of side effects, and therapeutic response. It is preferable to document the therapeutic response through the repeated use of behavioral observations and a symptom checklist.

Case examples
The application of the clinical principles outlined in this chapter is highlighted in the following four case studies.

Susan, aged seven years
Susan was reported by the school psychologist to have a severe degree of ID and little functional language. She was integrated into a rural primary school. She did not participate in educational or social activities, and sat at the back of the class on a rubber mat because she was incontinent. Susan spent most of her time rocking, being withdrawn, and "nodding off to sleep." Both the teacher and the school psychologist were concerned that she might have autism or a degenerative condition. Her parents reported that her behavior was similar at home. Her birth was a complicated forceps delivery due

to failure to progress in labour, and there was associated perinatal cerebral anoxia. She was an irritable baby with delayed developmental milestones, but did form a reciprocal attachment with her parents and showed emerging play and social skills. She had a series of grand mal epileptic seizures between 18 months and 2 years of age, and was placed on anticonvulsant medication. The family then moved to a small country town, and although she remained on a low dose of anticonvulsant medication, a specialist neurologist did not review her epilepsy again. When this was finally reviewed as part of this assessment, it was found on electroencephalogram (EEG) that she was having frequent epileptic activity and complex partial seizures, which were associated with incontinence, cognitive impairment, and behavioral withdrawal and disturbance. The reintroduction of a therapeutic level of anticonvulsant medication produced a dramatic therapeutic response, with improvements in her cognitive ability, communication and social skills, mood and behavior, and capacity to enjoy life. Her teacher even jokingly complained that she had become assertive in pushing to join in all the classroom activities. Subsequent cognitive assessment revealed that the level of her ID was in the moderate range.

The next two examples are teenage boys who were referred with the same problem behavior, that of masturbating in public.

Bill, aged 13 years

Bill had a moderate degree of ID, with some basic language skills, and attended a special school. He lived with his mother and father and two younger siblings. The cause of his ID was not known and there was no genetic abnormality detected, although he had some dysmorphic features and was a tall, ungainly, and clumsy boy for his age. The school and his parents referred him because he was masturbating in public. This activity was solitary and in the context of general social withdrawal, but occurred in public places, such as an isolated corner of the school grounds and the back corner of a supermarket.

The parents completed the DBC, which provided a score of 50 (above the clinical cutoff score of 45) with 38 problem items checked. These comprised 22 emotional disturbance items (internalizing symptoms), 1 social-relating problem item, and 14 disturbed behavior items (externalizing problems). The items that received the highest score – of 2, being very true or often true – related to Bill appearing depressed and unhappy, crying easily, being irritable, lacking self-confidence with poor self-esteem, and loss of appetite (with weight loss of around 2 kg over the past six months). Bill also had frequent temper tantrums and the questionnaire revealed that he was generally distressed and anxious, had some nightmares, and had become fearful about going to school and leaving the house, and becoming separated from his mother. These behaviors had been getting worse over the preceding 18 months.

Bill presented as a dejected and depressed-looking boy, who was listless and appeared to have no energy. He was generally withdrawn and showed no interest in toys or play activity. He became distressed and anxious when separated from his parents and spent some time crying. His parents claimed that he had told them he wished he was dead, although it was not possible during the assessment to get him to communicate verbally, other than with some occasional monosyllabic answers. He was, however, able to indicate by pencil on visual scales that showed sad/happy and worried/calm faces that he was "very unhappy" and "very worried and anxious." He was not able to complete the irritable/calm scale.

His symptoms and presentation fulfilled the DSM-5 diagnostic criteria for a Dysthymia associated with a Separation Anxiety disorder. There were some contributing family factors. His paternal grandmother and a paternal uncle had both been treated for depressive illness. Bill's emotional disorder began about 18 months earlier, at about the time of onset of puberty. Growth and hormonal changes of puberty may have contributed to his depression, but at that time his parents also began to have increasing unresolved parental conflict about a number of interpersonal and financial problems. This marital conflict had led to brief marital separation on two occasions. Therefore, Bill's depressive illness and anxiety had occurred in the context of a probable genetic predisposition, but was also influenced by the biological and psychological impact of puberty and significant interactional distress, consequent upon parental marital conflict.

Treatment involved the use of a tricyclic antidepressant (imipramine), chosen also for its anxiolytic effects, participation in a social skills training group, and a behavioral program at school and at home aimed at building self-esteem through setting achievable tasks and rewarding and positively commenting on all achievements, no matter how small. The parents were also keen to seek help for their marital difficulties and were able to resolve these after a few sessions of marital therapy. Bill made a good response to these treatments and within four weeks, was more cheerful and positive, had regained his appetite and was sleeping well, had more energy and was interested in social relationships. He no longer engaged in self-preoccupied masturbation in public.

Brian, aged 15 years

Brian had a moderate level of ID and simple language skills. He lived with his parents and attended a special school. His mother suffered toxaemia during the pregnancy. His birth was prolonged and complicated and he may have suffered some degree of cerebral anoxia.

His parents completed the DBC, which revealed a total score of 62. A total of 35 behavioral problems (externalizing) were identified, and two emotional problems (internalizing) and eight social-relating problem behaviors were described. Most of the disturbed behavior items related to disruptive overactive behavior with associated distractibility and limited attention span. He was noisy and boisterous, particularly in the family meeting, interrupting his parents with a mixture of sounds and simple phrases. He was also aggressive, uncooperative, and generally very difficult to manage by both his parents and teachers. His masturbatory behavior, which led to the referral, was not frequent but occurred as a provocative and threatening act towards his female teacher and also a party of young girls having a picnic in a park near the family home, from which he had run away. Both the parents and the school believed that it might be better for Brian to be cared for in a community residential unit. Brian presented as a wiry boy for his age, who acted as if he was driven by a motor. He could not sit still and focus on any task, particularly when he was together with his parents in a room that contained many toys and other items of interest. In a small, confined room, bare except for table and chairs, he was able to focus better on items such as a form board when these were individually shown to him, although he generally remained easily distracted. Neurological examination revealed some soft neurological signs and clumsiness, more marked on the right side of his body. Further detailed neurological assessment failed to find any specific neurological disorder. He had entered puberty 9–12 months earlier.

Brian was the youngest child in the family, with two older brothers in their early twenties who had not experienced any developmental difficulty. There was no family history of any physical or psychiatric illnesses. His parents had a good and effective relationship and there were no significant interactional difficulties in the family. Brian had always been an overactive and easily distracted boy, but since entering puberty this behavior had become significantly worse and, with his larger body size, he was more difficult to manage.

Taking his moderate degree of ID into account, his symptoms were still excessive for a child of his mental age, and therefore a DSM-V diagnosis of ADHD could be made. It is possible that hormonal and other biological changes of puberty had produced a worsening of his behavior. Increase in body size and new behavioral problems of a sexual nature made him more difficult to manage at home and school, and created anxiety for both parents and teachers, who had previously been able to contain and manage him. On the basis of this assessment, he received a trial of a stimulant medication (methylphenidate). He became less active and his attention span improved, particularly in one-to-one or small-group teaching situations in which there was a focused activity and no distractions in the surrounding environment. He had no adverse drug side effects. A behavior-modification program, based on a combination of reducing environmental stimulation and providing a range of separate enjoyable tasks for which his performance was rewarded, was instituted. His father also involved Brian in a daily exercise program of swimming in a private pool, where there were no other distractions, and bicycle riding in a quiet park. These activities were undertaken in consultation with a physiotherapist, who also provided a remedial gymnasium program at the school. All of these interventions combined to create a significant improvement in Brian's behavior, which could be contained by his parents and teachers. The use of stimulant medication was kept under review and its effectiveness was tested by occasional periods off the medication.

Darren, aged 16 years

Darren was referred because of disruptive behavior, particularly in the environment of the residential unit in which he lived. Over the past year, he increasingly had arguments with the other residents and, when reprimanded by the staff and put into his bedroom for timeout, he would become angry and lose control, smashing furniture, breaking windows, kicking doors and walls. After up to an hour of rage, he would calm down and then usually become remorseful and emotionally upset about the episode. He had a mild degree of ID and attended a special school. His educational progress was not as good as might be expected, given his relatively mild degree of ID documented on psychological assessment. He was socially confident, at times beyond the level of his social competence and skill, and this led to problems. For example, he would abscond and take public transport, claiming he was looking for a relative, but end up getting lost. His father and three younger siblings lived in another state.

The care staff of the residential unit completed the DBC. This revealed a score of 69, with 18 problems in the emotional (internalizing) problem area and 22 items of disturbed behavior (externalizing) being identified. The major behaviors identified were that he was often downcast and unhappy, with poor self-esteem, and showed frequent mood changes, and that he also frequently had tempers and was irritable. Staff had heard him talk on several occasions about killing himself, after angry outbursts. He was reported to make up stories about what he had been doing and was regarded as untrustworthy by the staff. The record of his past history was inadequate. The record revealed that he had a mild degree of developmental delay and was rather overactive during childhood, but was otherwise no problem for his parents. His mother died in a car accident when Darren was aged nine. His behavior began to deteriorate in early secondary school and his father requested alternative care for Darren when he was 13. At that time he was reported to be irritable and aggressive, frequently absconded from home, and was threatening towards the young children of the woman with whom his father was living and subsequently married. His father, stepmother, and all the other children in the family moved to another state shortly after Darren was placed in a residential unit. Since then, he had only occasional contact with his father and had not been given his telephone number or address.

Darren presented as a tall, rather thin young man. He was initially inappropriately overfriendly, demonstrating clumsy social skills. He embellished accounts of events and it was obvious that at times he made up stories to put himself in a favorable light. He had few, if any, friends, although he was very keen to visit places where young people gathered, such as a local shopping center, and observe and try to participate in the activities of these young people. He became upset when talking of his father, and it became clear that he could not understand why his father had gone to live in another state without taking him with the family. When asked to draw a picture of a bad dream, he described it as, "I'm in mum's car on the way from her work. A truck was out of the lane. There was crash. Mum died." (Tonge, 1982). He spoke with increasing distress about the car accident in which his mother died. He was also in the car, but was lucky to escape uninjured. He observed his mother being covered by a sheet and taken away in the ambulance, never to see her again. He was not allowed to go to the funeral. He claimed that often he would go out to try to look for the cemetery where his mother is buried, although he had no idea where that is. He was asked to draw a picture of himself, showing how he still felt about his mother's death. He drew a picture of himself crying, with a puddle of tears at his feet, saying that he was "very unhappy 100 percent."

Darren presented with a depressive disorder that fulfilled the DSM-V criteria for Dysthymia. This was in the setting of prolonged psychosocial stress, beginning with the death of his mother. He had not been able to resolve his loss satisfactorily and the process of grief and mourning had been further complicated by rejection from his family and his placement in a residential unit that had frequently changing staff. A number of different treatment approaches was needed in order to help him recover from this complex psychological disorder, from which he had suffered for seven years of his life. A morning dose of a SSRI antidepressant (fluoxetine) was prescribed. A behavioral program was provided that focused on relaxation skills and training for anger management, which included some aspects of cognitive therapy that taught him to say positive things about himself. It was realized that Darren's superficial social confidence covered some significant deficits in social skills, so arrangements were made for him to attend a social skills training group at his school. He attended every two weeks for some brief psychotherapy aimed at helping him ventilate his grief, anger, and distress about events in his life such as his mother's death and his father moving away. Arrangements were made for him to visit his mother's grave. The supervisor of the residential unit went to considerable effort to contact the father and, after some initial difficulty, managed to get the father to contact Darren on a regular basis by telephone. Finally, regular holidays with his father were arranged. This treatment process took about 12 months, but at the end of that time Darren had become a cooperative and helpful member of the residential unit, was making significant educational progress at school, and was exhibiting social behavior more appropriate to a young adolescent.

Conclusions

There is no doubt that psychiatric disorder is a major source of distress, extra handicap, and burden for young people with ID and their families, carers, and teachers. Considerable research is required to understand further the epidemiology, phenomenology, classification, etiology, and treatment of this psychopathology. However, by taking a comprehensive biopsychosocial approach to the assessment of these often complex emotional and behavioral problems, a diagnosis and multidimensional formulation become possible, which then provide the basis for a rational treatment and management plan.

Key summary points

- The prevalence of psychopathology in children with ID is 3–4 times that of other children. Comorbidity is common.
- Assessment requires a combined non-directive and structured clinical interview of parents and child together and separately, supplemented by psychometric behavior questionnaires completed by parents and teachers and, if indicated, laboratory and imaging investigations.
- Diagnosis is increasingly difficult with more severe ID, but the use of modified forms of ICD or DSM categorical diagnoses and a quantitative checklist description of behavioral symptoms provides a useful formulation on which to base a treatment plan.
- The behavior and mental state of the child is a reflection of the complex interaction of genetic influences, intellectual level and profile of cognitive skills, any physical disabilities and medical illness, parental mental health and family functioning, educational opportunity, and social context.
- Evidence-based treatment is multimodal and family-focused, including parent education and skills training, special education, psychological therapy, such as behavioral training and modified cognitive-behavioral therapy, and, if indicated, pharmacotherapy targeted at specific diagnostic symptoms for which there is evidence of efficacy.
- Follow-up response to treatment using a symptom checklist.

References

Albano, A.M. and Silverman, W.K. (1996). *Anxiety Disorders Interview Schedule for DSM4V: Clinicians Manual*. San Antonio, TX: The Psychological Corporation, Harcourt Brace and Company.

Aman, M.G. (1991). Review and evaluation of instruments for assessing emotional and behavioural disorders. *Australian and New Zealand Journal of Developmental Disabilities*, 17, 127–145.

Aman, M.G. and Schroeder, S.R. (1990). Specific learning disorders and mental retardation. In B.J. Tonge, G.D. Burrows, J. Werry (eds.), *Handbook of Studies on Child Psychiatry*. Amsterdam: Elsevier.

American Psychiatric Association. (2013). *Diagnostic and Statistical Manual of Mental*

Disorders, Fifth Edition. Washington, DC: American Psychiatric Association.

Amiet, C., Gourfinkel-An, I., Bouzamondo, A., et al. (2008). Epilepsy in autism is associated with intellectual disability and gender: evidence from a meta-analysis. *Biological Psychiatry*, 64(7), 577–582.

Baker, B.L., Blacker, J., Crnic, K.A., Edelbrock, C. (2002). Behaviour problems and parenting stress in families of three-year-old children with and without developmental delay. *American Journal on Mental Retardation*, 107, 433–444.

Baker, B.L., McIntyre, L.L., Blacker, J., et al. (2003). Preschool children with and without developmental delay: behaviour problems and parenting stress over time. *Journal of Intellectual Disability Research*, 47, 217–230.

Birmaher, B., Quintana, H., Greenville, L.L. (1988). Methylphenidate treatment of hyperactive autistic children. *Journal of the American Academy of Child and Adolescent Psychiatry*, 27, 248–251.

Blacher, J., Baker, B., MacLean, W. (2007) Positive impact of intellectual disability on families. *American Journal on Mental Retardation*, 112(5), 330–348.

Botteron, K. and Geller, B. (1993). Disorders, symptoms and their pharmacotherapy. In J. Werry and M. Aman (eds.), *Practitioner's Guide to Psychoactive Drugs for Children and Adolescents*. New York, NY: Plenum Medical.

Campbell, N., Gonzales, N.M., Bernst N., Silva R.R., Werry J.S. (1993). Antipsychotics (neuroleptics). In J. Werry and M. Aman (eds.), *Practitioner's Guide to Psychoactive Drugs for Children and Adolescents*. New York, NY: Plenum Medical.

Corbett, J.A. (1979). Psychiatric morbidity and mental retardation. In F.E. James and R.P. Snaith (eds.), *Psychotherapy in the Mentally Retarded*. New York, NY: Grune and Stratton.

Costello, A. (1982). Assessment and diagnosis of psychopathology. In J.L. Matson and R.P. Barrett (eds.), *Psychopathology in the Mentally Retarded*, second edition. New York, NY: Grune and Stratton.

Cox, A. and Rutter, M. (1985). Diagnostic appraisal and interviewing. In M. Rutter and L. Hersov (eds.), *Child and Adolescent Psychiatry: Modern Approaches*, second edition. Oxford: Blackwell Scientific Publications.

Dulcan, M.K. (1990). Using psycho-stimulants to treat behavioural disorders of children and adolescents. *Journal of Child and Adolescent Psychopharmacology*, 1, 7–20.

Einfeld, S.L. and Tonge, B.J. (1993). *Manual for the Developmental Behaviour Checklist*. Sydney and Melbourne: University of New South Wales and Monash University.

Einfeld, S.L. and Tonge, B.J. (1996). Population prevalence of behavioural and emotional disturbance in children and adolescents with mental retardation: II. Epidemiological findings. *Journal of Intellectual Disability Research*, 40(2), 99–109.

Einfeld, S.L., and Tonge, B.J. (2000). Observations on the use of the ICD-10 guide for mental retardation. *Journal of Intellectual Disability Research*, 44(3–4), 273.

Einfeld, S.L. and Tonge, B.J. (2002). *Manual for the Developmental Behaviour Checklist*, second edition. Melbourne: Monash University Centre for Developmental Psychiatry and Psychology.

Einfeld, S.L., Piccinin, A.M., Mackinnon, A., et al. (2006). Psychopathology in young people with intellectual disability. *Journal of the American Medical Association*, 296(16), 1981–1989.

Emerson, E. (2003). Prevalence of psychiatric disorders in children and adolescents with and without intellectual disability. *Journal of Intellectual Disability Research*, 47, 51–58.

Emerson, E., Einfeld, S.L., Stancliffe, R.J. (2009). The mental health of young children with intellectual disabilities or borderline intellectual functioning. *Social Psychiatry and Psychiatric Epidemiology*, 45, 579–587.

Forster, S., Gray, K.M., Taffe, J., Einfeld, S.L., Tonge, B.J. (2011). Behavioural and emotional problems in people with severe and profound intellectual disability. *Journal of Intellectual Disability Research*, 55, 190–198.

Gardiner, E. & Iarocci, G. (2012). Unhappy (and happy) in their own way: a developmental psychopathology perspective on quality of life for families living with developmental disability with and without autism. *Research in Developmental Disabilities*, 33, 2177–2192.

Gray, K., Tonge, B.J., Sweeney, D.J. (2008). Using the autism diagnostic interview-revised and the autism diagnostic observation schedule with young children with developmental delay: evaluating diagnostic validity. *Journal of Autism and Developmental Disorders*, 38, 657–667.

Gray, K., Keating, C., Taffe, J., et al. (2012). Trajectory of behavioural and emotional problems in autism. *American Journal on Intellectual and Developmental Disabilities*, 117(2), 121–133.

Hus, V. and Lord, C. (2014). The autism diagnostic observation schedule, module 4: revised algorithm and standardized severity scores. *Journal of Autism and Developmental Disorders*, 44, 1996–2012.

Lewis, J.N., Tonge, B.J., Mowat, D.R., et al. (2000). Epilepsy and associated psychopathology in young people with intellectual disability. *Journal of Paediatrics and Child Health*, 36(2), 172–175.

Lindsay, R.L., and Aman, M.G. (2003). Pharmacologic therapies aid treatment for autism. *Paediatric Annals*, 32(10), 671–676.

Lloyd, T. and Hastings, R.P. (2008). Psychological variables as correlates of adjustment in mothers of children with intellectual disabilities: cross-sectional and longitudinal relationships. *Journal of Intellectual Disability Research*, 52(1), 37–48.

Lord, C., Rutter, M., Le Couteur, A. (1994). Autism Diagnostic Interview – Revised: a revised version of a diagnostic interview for caregivers of individuals with possible pervasive developmental disorders. *Journal of Autism and Developmental Disorders*, 24(5), 659–685.

Lord, C., Rutter, M., DiLavore, P., and Risi, S. (1999). *Autism Diagnostic Observation Schedule (ADOS) Manual*. Los Angeles, CA: Western Psychological Services.

Matson, J. and Barrett, R.P. (eds.) (1982). *Psychopathology in the Mentally Retarded*, second edition. New York, NY: Grune and Stratton.

Roux, G., Sofronoff, K., Sanders, M. (2013). A randomised controlled trial of group Stepping Stones Triple P: a mixed-disability trial. *Family Process*, 52, 411–424.

Rutter, M., Tizard, J., Whitmore, K. (1970). *Education Health and Behaviour*. London: Longman.

Sovner, R. (1986). Limiting factors in the use of DSM III criteria with mentally ill/mentally retarded persons. *Psychopharmacology Bulletin*, 22, 1055–1059.

Sovner, R. and Hurley, A.D. (1989). Ten diagnostic principles for recognizing psychiatric disorder in mentally retarded persons. *Psychiatric Aspects of Mental Retardation Reviews*, 8, 9–13.

Stromme, P. and Diseth, T.H. (2000). Prevalence of psychiatric diagnoses in children with mental retardation: data from a population-based study. *Developmental Medicine and Child Neurology*, 42, 266–270.

Tonge, B.J. (1982). Draw a dream: an intervention promoting change in families in conflict. In E.W. Kaslow (eds.), *The International Book of Family Therapy*. New York, NY: Brunnel/Mazel.

Tonge, B.J. (1988). Anxiety in adolescence. In R. Noyes, M. Roth, G.D. Burrows (eds.), *Handbook of Anxiety Vol. 1.2. Classification, Etiological Factors and Associated Disturbances*. Amsterdam: Elsevier.

Tonge. B.J. (1991). Children with physical impairments. In F.K. Judd, G.D. Burrows, D.R. Lipsitt (eds.), *Handbook of Studies on General Hospital Psychiatry*. Amsterdam: Elsevier.

Tonge, B.J. and Einfeld, S. (1991). Intellectual disability and psychopathology in Australian children. *Australia and*

New Zealand Journal of Developmental Disabilities, 17(2), 155–167.

Tonge, B.J., and Einfeld, S. (2003). Psychopathology and intellectual disability: the Australian child to adult longitudinal study. In L.M. Glidden (ed.), *International Review of Research in Mental Retardation*. San Diego, CA: Academic Press.

Tonge, B.J., Einfeld, S.L., Krupinski J., et al. (1996). The use of factor analysis for ascertaining patterns of psychopathology in children with intellectual disability. *Journal of Intellectual Disability Research*, 40(3), 198–207.

Tonge, B.J., Bull, K., Brereton, A.V., Wilson, R. (2014). A review of evidence-based early intervention for behavioural problems in children with autism spectrum disorder: the core components of effective programs, child-focused interventions and comprehensive treatment models. *Current Opinion in Psychiatry*, 27, 158–165.

Volkmar, F. and Klin, A. (2005). Issues in the classification of autism and related conditions. In F. Volkmar, R. Paul, A. Klin, D. Cohen (eds.), *Handbook of Autism and Pervasive Developmental Disorders*, Vol. 1. Hoboken, NJ: John Wiley and Sons.

World Health Organization (1992). *International Classification of Diseases (ICD-10)*. Geneva: World Health Organization.

Chapter 18

Behavioral phenotypes/genetic syndromes

Robert M. Hodapp, Nathan A. Dankner, and Elisabeth M. Dykens

Introduction

As we update this chapter we face a very different landscape, one that again can be characterized by both advances and challenges. Some advances have become almost commonplace. Consider cross-disciplinary research. When we originally described etiology-based approaches in the 1990s (Hodapp and Dykens, 1994; Dykens et al., 2000), we noted that there existed "two cultures" of behavioral research in intellectual disabilities (ID). One culture, consisting mostly of psychologists (of various types) and special educators, possessed expertise on various aspects of behavior, even as they did not much consider differences in those behaviors across etiological groups. The other, consisting of pediatricians, geneticists, and other (mostly biomedical) professionals, knew much about genetic conditions, less about behavior. But by the present decade, such distinctions between the two cultures were lessening (Hodapp and Dykens, 2012). By now, the two cultures have mostly come together, with multidisciplinary research teams and perspectives ubiquitous in behavioral research in ID.

Still, some problems persist. We continue to need more studies of individuals with many genetic conditions. Such research needs to be more targeted to individuals of specific ages and genders and more often focused on specific cognitive, linguistic, adaptive, or maladaptive behavior. A wider set of genetic conditions needs to be examined; at the current time, we have active research into barely 15–20 of the 1000+ genetic conditions associated with ID. We need more research on psychopathology in all of these conditions.

Tenets of behavioral phenotypes

At its most basic meaning, the term "behavioral phenotype" highlights the outcome (i.e., phenotype) – in this case concerning behavior – that results from a particular genotype. We propose that a behavioral phenotype involves "the heightened probability or likelihood that people with a given syndrome will exhibit certain behavioral and developmental sequelae relative to those without the syndrome" (Dykens, 1995). This more probabilistic definition highlights four basic facts as outlined below.

Within-syndrome variability

Behavioral phenotypes are probabilistic. Thus, among individuals with most genetic conditions, many but not all will show the syndrome's "characteristic" behaviors. Indeed,

---

Psychiatric and Behavioral Disorders in Intellectual and Developmental Disabilities, ed. Colin Hemmings and Nick Bouras. Published by Cambridge University Press. © Cambridge University Press 2016.

rarely are etiology-related behaviors found in every person with a particular syndrome. Consider hyperphagia (or over eating), the behavior that most would identify as Prader–Willi syndrome (PWS)'s hallmark psychiatric symptom. Yet even this behavior does not occur in every child or adult with PWS. In a study of 4–19-year-old children, Dykens and Kasari (1997) showed that parents rated the item "overeats" for 80% of children with PWS. While issues of increasing chronological age and genetic subtypes all enter in, within-syndrome variability remains important to consider.

Total versus partial specificity

Total specificity means that a particular behavior is unique to a single syndrome; partial specificity means that two or more etiological groups show a higher-than-normal risk to have the same psychiatric behavior or behavioral profile (Hodapp, 1997). In the first, unique pattern, a genetic syndrome results in a particular outcome that is simply not seen in other genetic disorders. At present, the following behaviors seem unique to one and only one syndrome:

- the "cat-cry" in 5p-syndrome (Sigafoos et al., 2009);
- extreme self-mutilation in Lesch–Nyhan syndrome (Schretlen et al., 2005);
- stereotypic "hand washing" or "hand wringing" in Rett syndrome (Van Acker, 1991); and
- body "self-hugging" and putting objects into bodily orifices in Smith–Magenis syndrome (Finucane and Haas-Givler, 2009).

In contrast to this relatively short list, more instances occur in which partial specificity is operating. Within psychiatric symptoms (and compared to groups with ID in general), hyperactivity is more frequently found in children with 5p-syndrome (Dykens and Clarke, 1997) and in boys with Fragile X syndrome (Baumgardner et al., 1995). In a few genetic disorders, then, the same type of maladaptive behavior–psychopathology is found in higher percentages of individuals than is commonly noted among others with ID.

Finally, partially specific behavioral effects seem more in line with many areas of genetics, child psychiatry, and psychiatry. Across these different disciplines, researchers are now discussing the many pathways – both genetic and environmental – by which one comes to have one or another psychiatric disorder. As the clinical geneticist John Opitz (1985) noted, "The causes are many, but the common developmental pathways are few."

Multiple domains, complex interactions

Behavioral phenotypes are not limited to maladaptive behavior or psychopathology; instead, they are also found across many different domains. Individuals with Down syndrome show particular deficits in grammar, articulation, and expressive (as opposed to receptive) language (Abbeduto et al., 2007). In terms of cognitive processing styles, patterns of "simultaneous over sequential processing" on the Kaufman Assessment Battery for Children (K-ABC) have been noted for most individuals with PWS (Dykens et al., 1992) and for boys with fragile X syndrome (Dykens et al., 1987; Kemper et al., 1988).

It is also the case that various etiology-related characteristics themselves inter-relate. To give some obvious examples, researchers in Down syndrome are increasingly appreciating the ways in which these children's high levels of hearing problems (estimated at from 35% to 70%; Porter and Tharpe, 2010) tie to decreased levels of language, or even that the articulation levels of these individuals might be associated with the characteristic structure of the tongue (thickness, size, placement in mouth; Bunton and Leddy, 2011). Within the area of psychopathology, researchers have long discussed the connection between aggression and the inability to make one's needs known verbally – there may also be more "etiology-linked" examples of such ties of physical, medical, and cognitive-linguistic characteristics and behavioral sequelae.

Development, context, and families

Just as behavioral phenotypes are seen in many areas and different behavioral and physical characteristics inter-relate, so too do other considerations enter in. One prominent issue concerns development, the ways in which etiology-related behaviors, profiles, or symptoms present differently in individuals who are of diverse ages. Fidler (2011) examined development in young children with Down syndrome, Fragile X syndrome, and Williams syndrome. In each case, developments in cognitive–linguistic profiles were described over the first few years of life, eventually producing in most children the etiology-related strengths and weaknesses found by the adult years. Age-related differences are also shown in maladaptive behavior–psychopathology. Comparing four age groups of children and adults with PWS, Dykens (2004) found a general mellowing as these individuals reached their 20s, 30s, and 40s, with externalizing problems decreasing across age groups. For other behaviors – including hoarding – the peak age-period was the 20s, with lower average scores before and after that period. Even when a particular behavior or symptom shows itself in most persons with a syndrome, the frequency and intensity of such symptoms often vary by age.

Genetic conditions also need to be embedded in a social and familial context, a context that often greatly affects the amount, type, and effectiveness of the services that individuals receive. Compared to other groups, for example, mothers of children with Down syndrome are more likely to be older (Grosse, 2010), and such mothers are more often highly educated, married, and have had prior children (Hodapp and Urbano, 2008). As such, mothers of children with Down syndrome may (as a group) be more skillful in knowing about their children's development, as well as in locating, contacting, and effectively utilizing most every type of service (Hodapp et al., 2012).

By the time that the individual with Down syndrome has reached their mid 40s, however, having older parents (and experiencing earlier aging oneself) is detrimental and may lead to earlier and more complicated old-age care. Compared to same-aged adults with other forms of ID, 40–49-year-old adults with Down syndrome disproportionately showed that either they or their parents were experiencing health and/or functional declines, necessitating the increased caregiving roles (including legal guardianship) from one or more of the family's non-disabled siblings. Something as simple as parental age, then, may greatly affect the care received by children or adults with Down syndrome.

Three examples

Anxiety in Williams syndrome

Williams syndrome is a salient example of a genetic syndrome whose behavioral phenotype reflects increased propensity for the development of psychopathology. Individuals with Williams syndrome are at high risk for anxiety, both compared to typically developing populations and compared to ID groups of mixed etiology (Dankner and Dykens, 2012). This anxiety is largely manifest as fears and phobias, as well as generalized anxiety (Dykens, 2003; Cherniske et al., 2004; Leyfer et al., 2006).

Unlike in typically developing populations, in Williams syndrome the fears and phobias that appear in early childhood do not decline over age (Leyfer et al., 2006). Instead, phobias tend to cluster into a few discrete domains, as many of these individuals fear heights, uncertainty, loss, and loud noises, such as thunderstorms (Dykens, 2003). Generalized anxiety also appears to be a persistent aspect of the Williams syndrome phenotype. Cross-sectional work indicates that the risk for generalized anxiety problems in Williams syndrome begins to increase as children reach age 7–10 years (Leyfer et al., 2006). Longitudinal studies indicate that risk and severity remain stable across adolescence and young adulthood, although generalized anxiety may begin to decline in later adulthood (Einfeld et al., 2001; Woodruff-Borden et al., 2010).

Although problems with anxiety characterize Williams syndrome, they are not unique to the syndrome. Increased risk for anxiety is seen in other genetic syndromes and neurodevelopmental disorders, though often in different forms. Social anxiety is common in Fragile X syndrome (Cordeiro et al., 2011), while anxiety related to restricted interests and compulsions is often observed in PWS (Dykens et al., 1996). Anxiety and obsessions and restricted, repetitive, compulsive-like behaviors are also common features of autism spectrum disorders (ASD) (Moskowitz et al., 2013).

Moreover, anxiety is among the most common forms of psychopathology in the general population, and one of the best researched with regards to phenomenology and treatment. On one hand, then, this lack of specificity regarding anxiety in Williams syndrome makes it more difficult for professionals to use this phenotypic trait to glean information regarding the mechanisms or etiology of anxiety. On the other, the presence of anxiety across populations allows knowledge gained from typically developing individuals to improve outcomes in Williams syndrome and other high-risk populations.

Severe, adverse behavioral changes in Down syndrome

Although children with Down syndrome may less frequently show severe psychopathology, a small subset of children and young adults experience episodes of severe adverse behavioral changes. Such episodes, which Prasher (2002) described as Young Adults with a Disintegrative Disorder, have more recently been characterized as autistic regression (Worley et al., 2013), childhood depression (Stein et al., 2013), psychosis (Dykens et al., 2015), or young adult depression (Myers and Pueschel, 1991; Dykens, 2007).

Although we continue to know little about such adverse behavioral changes, several studies have begun to provide some basic information. Reviewing the medical records of 14 youths with Down syndrome who had experienced such adverse behavioral changes, Devenny and Matthews (2011) noted that about half experienced their first episode from age 4 to 12 years, half from age 18 to 21 years. In a larger, web-based parent survey examining 72 additional youths, Hodapp et al. (pers. comm.) found that half of all episodes began from when the child was age 4–9 years and most episodes lasted 3 years or less (about 20% lasted 4+ years).

Recent studies have also begun to describe the nature of and reactions to such events. For almost 90% of these youths and young adults, their episodes featured both substantial losses of adaptive–functional skills (e.g., regressions in their ability to communicate and in academic skills), as well as new or intensified problem behaviors. The most common problem behaviors – which either arose for the first time or increased greatly in either frequency or intensity – included anxiety; bizarre, inappropriate behaviors; attention seeking; obsessive-compulsive behaviors; aggressiveness; and depression. In response to the onset of such events, parents consulted a variety of professionals, usually beginning 2–6 months after the episode's onset. These youths then mostly received a variety of behavioral and pharmacological treatments, usually for more than 18 months. Parents judged half of all treatments to be somewhat or very effective (Hodapp et al., pers. comm.).

Obviously, such studies barely scratch the surface of this rare but severe phenomenon. Why such changes occur remains a mystery, although risk factors may include major transitions or changes in the environment (Devenny and Matthews, 2011; Hodapp et al., pers. comm.), as well as co-occurring medical or neurological vulnerabilities (Hodapp et al., pers. comm.). Further studies are needed on this subgroup of atypical children with Down syndrome.

Hyperphagia, psychosis, and ASD in PWS

Prader–Willi syndrome is caused by a lack of paternally derived imprinted material in the 15q11–q13 region, either through a deletion in the genetic material contributed by the father (i.e., paternal deletion) or by having two chromosome 15s from the mother (i.e., maternal uniparental disomy, or mUPD). The syndrome is well known for its complex phenotype, with diverse medical, cognitive, emotional, and behavioral problems that do not cleanly fit into traditional psychiatric nosologies. Psychiatric problems in PWS are further complicated by developmental changes over time, the genetic subtypes associated with PWS, and (similar to the general population) a family history of psychiatric disorders and environmental stressors and supports. We here focus on three aspects of the PWS psychiatric phenotype: hyperphagia, severe psychiatric illness, and ASD.

Hyperphagia. As a salient feature of PWS, hyperphagia leads to high risks for morbid obesity. As a result, individuals with PWS need physical activities and strict dietary and food supervision in order to avoid life-threatening complications of obesity and early mortality (Dykens and Roof, 2008). In addition, as hyperphagia onsets in early childhood, many emotional and behavioral problems worsen (Dimitropoulos et al., 2001), including tantrums, aggression, rigidity, irritability, sadness, skin picking, low tolerance for change or different perspectives, insistence on sameness, arranging and rearranging, and hoarding. These problems may wax and wane over time, and lessen in some individuals in middle to late adulthood (Dykens and Roof, 2008).

Severe psychiatric illness. People with PWS have been variably described as being at high risk for obsessive-compulsive disorder; compulsivity that reflects arrested development; affective illness; bipolar illness with or without psychosis; mood disorder with or without a psychotic component; psychotic illness; and bipolar affective disorder (e.g., Dykens et al., 1996; Boer et al., 2002; Clarke et al., 2002; Descheemaeker et al., 2002; Dykens and Shah, 2003; Soni et al., 2007). Although those with mUPD are more prone to mood disorders or psychotic illness, especially as they transition into young adulthood, severe problems can also found in those with deletions, including those with positive family histories of psychiatric illness (Soni et al., 2007).

Unfortunately, psychiatric studies in PWS have relied solely on diagnostic labels, leaving specific psychiatric symptoms unclear or poorly described (Dykens and Shah, 2003). It remains unknown, for example, whether psychosis in PWS is best characterized by such positive symptoms as auditory or visual hallucinations, or delusional thinking, or by such negative symptoms as affective blunting, anhedonia, or withdrawal. Psychosis in PWS may shed light on genetic risks for psychosis in the general population, with recent work implicating the duplication and increased expression of maternally imprinted genes, especially *UBE3A*, in mUPD, as well as a differentially methylated region within the *GABRA* receptor genes located in the PWS 15q11–q13 region. Although two studies (Webb et al., 2008; Sharp et al., 2010) have implicated this locus or variation as a promising candidate for psychosis in mUPD, more targeted treatments and future genotype-phenotype research will require a precise characterization of specific psychotic symptoms.

Autism spectrum disorders. Studies find that approximately 40% of children with the mUPD subtype of PWS have co-occurring ASD, compared to 18% of deletion cases (e.g., Veltman et al., 2005; Descheemaeker et al., 2006). Even so, social communicative deficits are core features of ASD, yet remarkably little is known about social communicative functioning in PWS during infancy or early childhood (Dykens et al., 2011). Although the15q11–q13 region has been deemed an epigenetic "hotspot" for associations to ASD (Schanen, 2006; Hogart et al., 2010), the lack of detailed data on social or communicative functioning in PWS limits its usefulness as a genetic model for ASD. In addition, despite similarities across PWS and ASD in, for example, insistence on sameness or restricted interests, individuals with PWS also display hoarding and skin picking, whereas in ASD there may be increased instances of stereotypies and more diverse and severe self-injurious behaviors (Dykens et al., 2011). Thus, further work is needed on these different profiles of repetitive behaviors across PWS, ASD, and related 15q disorders (e.g., Angelman syndrome; maternal interstitial duplications of chromosome 15).

Finally, more studies are needed to explore the impact of hyperphagia on the types or severity of psychiatric symptoms in PWS. With impaired satiety, people with PWS are, as the motto of the PWS Association-US (PWSA-US) states, "always hungry, never full." More formally, Holland et al. (2003) have described these individuals as being in states of "starvation that manifests as obesity in a food-rich environment." Previously, Dykens et al. (2007) found that, compared to individuals with PWS who were overweight or obese, those who were lean and with a lower body mass index (BMI) exhibited greater levels of distress, disorganized thinking, sadness, and irritability. This finding, though counterintuitive, can perhaps be attributed to the psychological effort and stress of maintaining a low weight, to hormonal changes that come with weight loss, or to the distressed feelings we all sometimes experience when we are very, very hungry and in need of food.

Future directions: using specific genetic conditions as models for psychiatric disorders

The continuing, as yet unrealized hope of etiology-oriented researchers has been that individuals with a specific genetic condition might shed light on why a specific psychiatric disorder occurs. If, for example, the risks of anxiety are much higher among individuals with Williams syndrome, or of hyperphagia in PWS, or of other conditions in different genetic conditions (e.g., Alzheimer's disease in adults with Down syndrome), then maybe these conditions can teach us about the causes of such problems. Indeed, the field is replete with discussions of model systems, pathways, epigenetic changes, genomics, and gene–brain–behavior relations.

Although researchers across a variety of fields are gradually making connections between genetic etiologies and psychiatric disorders, we are only at the earliest stages of such research. Several complications must also be noted. First, to date the field has examined in depth only 15–20 of the 1000+ genetic conditions associated with ID (Hodapp and Dykens, 2012). These conditions include Down syndrome, Fragile X syndrome, PWS, Williams syndrome, Rett syndrome, velo cardio facial syndrome, Lesch–Nyhan syndrome, and Angelman syndrome, along with 10 or so other genetic conditions. Although these conditions have been subject to anywhere from a few to hundreds of behavioral studies, the remaining 1000 genetic etiologies have not. For these other conditions, a few general studies exist, often focused mostly on genetics and physical features, with a short section on behavior.

Second, even for those genetic conditions noted above, we do not have anything approaching a comprehensive understanding about a wide range of behavior. One wants to know about the specifics of early development of language, cognition, social, and other skills; about cognitive and academic strengths and weaknesses; and about those psychiatric conditions for which individuals with a specific genetic condition are at particular risk – and then, about the onset, course, characteristics, predisposing factors, and treatment of these psychiatric conditions. As noted above for Down syndrome, the syndrome's characteristic physical features (e.g., mouth structure for articulation) and common health problems all enter in, as do issues related to physical and cognitive-functional aging and to family history and context. Even for the small number of "known" conditions of ID, then, we are only partway along in developing such a comprehensive base of knowledge.

Third, some genetic conditions have been aided greatly by animal models. Such models have been developed in Down syndrome (Ts65Dn mouse), as well as using knock-out, knock-in, and other animal models in PWS, Angelman syndrome, and other conditions. Many such models are "partial" models, with, for instance, only some of the relevant Down syndrome genes in triplicate (e.g., the Ts65Dn mouse model in Down syndrome; Patterson, 2009). Still, when used in conjunction with detailed human studies, such models promise to inform us about the mechanisms underlying such complex conditions as anxiety, hyperphagia, Alzheimer's disease, or schizophrenia.

Finally, it remains unclear the degree to which the psychiatric problems exhibited by those with specific genetic conditions of ID map onto traditional psychiatric nosologies. Although efforts have been made to address this issue (Fletcher et al., 2007), many maladaptive behaviors seem difficult to classify. Note, for instance, the various terms that have been applied to children experiencing severe, adverse behavioral changes in Down syndrome, or to those young adults with the severe psychopathologies seen in the mUPD subtype of PWS. In these and other cases, clinicians and researchers struggle to fit specific psychiatric symptoms into traditional classificatory systems.

Conclusions

Over the past few decades, great progress has been made in how we understand the connections between genetic etiology and psychiatric problems. Surveying three editions of this volume, we see the movement from a basic argument, to beginning findings showing such connections, to more sophisticated findings, often related to either smaller subsets of individuals with a specific condition (e.g., youths with Down syndrome who experience adverse behavioral changes), or to certain variants of the genetic syndrome (e.g., PWS due to mUPD). At the same time, many gaps remain. We continue to need more studies of maladaptive behavior–psychopathology within those with specific genetic conditions, studies that examine issues related to onset age, course, predisposing factors, and treatment.

Key summary points

- Genetic syndromes put individuals at risk for particular forms of maladaptive behavior and psychopathology.
- Although research activity continues to increase, the field has thus far focused only on a small percentage of genetic syndromes.
- Ongoing studies demonstrate the complexities of such problems as anxiety disorders in Williams syndrome; severe, adverse behavioral changes in a small subset of youths with Down syndrome; and hyperphagia, psychosis, and ASD in persons with PWS.
- Next steps include improved characterization of maladaptive behavior–psychopathology in persons with specific genetic conditions.
- Next steps also include increased use of animal models and greater appreciation of developmental, familial, and contextual influences on etiology-related psychiatric conditions.
- Next steps also include the development of treatment models of high-risk psychiatric disorders in genetic syndromes, including anxiety in Williams syndrome, as well as of OCD and hyperphagia in PWS.

References

Abbeduto, L., Warren, S.F., Conners, F.A. (2007). Language development in Down syndrome: from the prelinguistic period to the acquisition of literacy. *Mental Retardation and Developmental Disabilities Research Reviews*, 13, 247–261.

Baumgardner, T.L., Reiss, A.L., Freund, L.S., Abrams, M.T. (1995). Specification of the neurobehavioral phenotype in males with Fragile X syndrome. *Pediatrics*, 95, 744–752.

Boer, H., Holland, A., Whittington, J., et al. (2002). Psychotic illness in people with PWS due to chromosome 15 maternal uniparental disomy. *Lancet*, 359, 135.

Bunton, K. and Leddy, M. (2011). An evaluation of articulatory working space area in vowel production of adults with Down syndrome. *Clinical Linguistics and Phonetics*, 25, 321–334.

Cherniske, E.M. Carpenter, T.O., Klaiman, C., et al. (2004). Multisystem study of 20 older adults with Williams syndrome. *American Journal of Medical Genetics Part A*, 131, 255–264.

Clarke, D.J., Boer, H., Whittington, J., et al. (2002). Prader–Willi syndrome, compulsive and ritualistic behaviors: the first population-based study. *British Journal of Psychiatry*, 180, 358–362.

Cordeiro, L., Ballinger, E., Hagerman, R., Hessl, D. (2011). Clinical assessment of DSM-IV anxiety disorders in Fragile X syndrome: prevalence and characterization. *Journal of Neurodevelopmental Disorders*, 3(1), 57–67.

Dankner, N. and Dykens, E.M. (2012). Anxiety in intellectual disabilities:

challenges and next steps. *International Review of Research in Developmental Disabilities*, 42, 57–84.

Descheemaeker, M.J., Vogels, A, Govers, V., et al. (2002). Prader–Willi syndrome: new insights in the behavioural and psychiatric spectrum. *Journal of Intellectual Disability Research*, 46, 41–50.

Descheemaeker, M.J., Govers, V., Vermeulen, P., Fryns, J.-P. (2006). Pervasive developmental disorders in Prader–Willi syndrome: the Leuven experience in 59 subjects and controls. *American Journal of Medical Genetics Part A*, 140, 1136–1142.

Devenny, D. and Matthews, A. (2011). Regression: atypical loss of attained functioning in children and adolescents with Down syndrome. *International Review of Research in Developmental Disabilities*, 41, 233–264.

Dimitropoulos, A., Feurer, I.D., Butler, M.G., Thompson, T. (2001). Emergence of compulsive behavior and tantrums in children with Prader–Willi syndrome. *American Journal on Mental Retardation*, 106, 39–51.

Dykens, E.M. (1995). Measuring behavioral phenotypes: provocations from the "new genetics." *American Journal on Mental Retardation*, 99, 522–532.

Dykens, E.M. (2003). Anxiety, fears, and phobias in persons with Williams syndrome. *Developmental Neuropsychology*, 23, 291–316.

Dykens, E.M. (2004). Maladaptive and compulsive behavior in Prader–Willi syndrome: new insights from older adults. *American Journal on Mental Retardation*, 109, 142–153.

Dykens, E.M. (2007). Psychiatric and behavioral disorders in persons with Down syndrome. *Mental Retardation and Developmental Disabilities Research Reviews*, 13, 272–278.

Dykens, E.M. and Clarke, D.J. (1997). Correlates of maladaptive behavior in individuals with 5p-(cri-du-chat) syndrome. *Developmental Medicine and Child Neurology*, 39, 752–756.

Dykens, E.M. and Kasari, C. (1997). Maladaptive behavior in children with Prader–Willi syndrome, Down syndrome, and non-specific mental retardation. *American Journal on Mental Retardation*, 102, 228–237.

Dykens, E.M. and Roof, E. (2008). Behavior in Prader–Willi syndrome: relationship to genetic subtypes and age. *Journal of Child Psychology and Psychiatry*, 49, 1001–1008.

Dykens, E.M. and Shah, B. (2003). Psychiatric disorders in Prader–Willi syndrome: epidemiology and treatment. *CNS Drugs*, 17, 167–178.

Dykens, E.M., Hodapp, R.M., Leckman, J.F. (1987). Strengths and weaknesses in intellectual functioning of males with Fragile X syndrome. *American Journal of Mental Deficiency*, 92, 234–236.

Dykens, E.M., Hodapp, R.M., Walsh, K.K., Nash, L. (1992). Adaptive and maladaptive behavior in Prader–Willi syndrome. *Journal of the American Academy of Child and Adolescent Psychiatry*, 31, 1131–1136.

Dykens, E.M., Leckman, J.F., Cassidy, S.B. (1996). Obsessions and compulsions in Prader–Willi syndrome. *Journal of Child Psychology and Psychiatry*, 37, 995–1002.

Dykens, E.M., Hodapp, R.M., Finucane, B. (2000). *Genetics and Mental Retardation Syndromes: A New Look at Behavior and Treatments*. Baltimore, MD: Paul H. Brookes Publishing Company.

Dykens, E.M., Maxwell, M.A., Pantino, E., Kossler, R., Roof, E. (2007). Assessment of hyperphagia in Prader–Willi syndrome. *Obesity*, 15, 1816–1826.

Dykens, E.M., Lee, E., Roof, E. (2011). Prader–Willi syndrome and autism spectrum disorders: an evolving story. *Journal of Neurodevelopmental Disorders*, 3, 225–237.

Dykens, E.M., Shah, B., Davis, B., Baker, C., Fife, T., Fitzpatrick, J. (2015). Psychiatric disorders in adolescents and young adults with Down syndrome and other intellectual disabilities. *Journal of Neurodevelopmental Disorders*, 7, 9.

Einfeld, S.L., Tonge, B.J., Rees, V.W. (2001). Longitudinal course of behavioral and emotional problems in Williams syndrome.

American Journal on Mental Retardation, 106(1), 73–81.

Fidler, D.J. (ed.) (2011). Early development in neurogenetic disorders. *International Review of Research in Developmental Disorders,* 40, 1–318.

Finucane, B.R. and Haas-Givler, B. (2009). Smith–Magenis syndrome: genetic basis and clinical implications. *Journal of Mental Health Research in Intellectual Disabilities,* 2, 134–148.

Fletcher, R., Loschen, E., Stavrakaki, C. (eds.) (2007). *Diagnostic Manual – Intellectual Disability (DM-ID): A Textbook of Diagnosis of Mental Disorders in Persons with Intellectual Disability.* Kingston, NY: NADD Press.

Grosse, S.D. (2010). Sociodemographic characteristics of families of children with Down syndrome and the economic impacts of child disability on families. *International Review of Research on Mental Retardation,* 39, 257–294.

Hodapp, R.M. (1997). Direct and indirect behavioral effects of different genetic disorders of mental retardation. *American Journal on Mental Retardation,* 102, 67–79.

Hodapp, R.M. and Dykens, E.M. (1994). Mental retardation's two cultures of behavioral research. *American Journal on Mental Retardation,* 98, 675–687.

Hodapp, R.M. and Dykens, E.M. (2012). Genetic disorders of intellectual disability: expanding our concepts of phenotypes and of family outcomes. *Journal of Genetic Counseling,* 21, 761–769.

Hodapp, R.M. and Urbano, R.C. (2008). Demographics of African-American and European-American mothers of newborns with Down syndrome. *Journal of Policy and Practice in Intellectual Disabilities,* 5, 187–193.

Hodapp, R.M., Burke, M.M., Urbano, R.C. (2012). What's age got to do with it? Implications of maternal age on families of offspring with Down syndrome. *International Review of Research in Developmental Disabilities,* 42, 109–145.

Hogart, A., Wu, D., LaSalle, J.M., Schanen, C. (2010). The comorbidity of autism with the genomic disorders of chromosome 15q11.2-q13. *Neurobiology of Disease,* 38, 181–191.

Holland, A, Whittington, J, Hitton, E, (2003). The paradox of Prader–Willi syndrome: a genetic model of starvation. *Lancet,* 362, 989–991.

Kemper, M.B., Hagerman, R.J., Altshul-Stark, D. (1988). Cognitive profiles of boys with Fragile X syndrome. *American Journal of Medical Genetics,* 30, 191–200.

Leyfer, O.T., Woodruff-Borden, J., Klein-Tasman, B.P., Fricke, J.S., Mervis, C.B. (2006). Prevalence of psychiatric disorders in 4 to 16-year-olds with Williams syndrome. *American Journal of Medical Genetics Part B: Neuropsychiatric Genetics,* 141, 615–622.

Moskowitz, L.J., Mulder, E., Walsh, C.E., et al. (2013). A multimethod assessment of anxiety and problem behavior in children with autism spectrum disorders and intellectual disability. *American Journal on Intellectual and Developmental Disabilities,* 116, 419–434.

Myers, B.A. and Pueschel, S.M. (1991). Psychiatric disorders in persons with Down syndrome. *Journal of Nervous and Mental Disease,* 179(10), 609–613.

Opitz, J.M. (1985). The developmental field concept. *American Journal of Medical Genetics,* 21(1), 1.

Patterson, D. (2009). Molecular genetic analysis of Down syndrome. *Human Genetics,* 126, 195–214.

Porter, H. and Tharpe, A.M. (2010). Hearing loss among persons with Down syndrome. *International Review of Research in Mental Retardation,* 39, 195–220.

Prasher, V.P. (2002). Disintegrative syndrome in young adults. *Irish Journal of Psychological Medicine,* 19(3), 101.

Schanen, N.C. (2006). Epigenetics of autism spectrum disorder. *Human Molecular Genetics,* 15, R138–R150.

Sharp, A.J., Migliavacca, E., Dupre, Y., et al. (2010). Methylation profiling in individuals with uniparental disomy identifies novel differentially methylated regions on chromosome 15. *Genome Research*, 20, 1271–1278.

Schretlen, D.J., Ward, J., Yun, J., et al. (2005). Behavioral aspects of Lesch–Nyhan disease and its variants. *Developmental Medicine and Child Neurology*, 47, 673–677.

Sigafoos, J., O'Reilly, M.F., Lancioni, G.E. (2009). Editorial: cri-du-chat. *Developmental Neurorehabilitation*, 12, 119–121.

Soni, S., Whittington, J., Holland, A.J., et al. (2007). The course and outcome of psychiatric illness in people with Prader–Willi syndrome: implications for management and treatment. *Journal of Intellectual Disability Research*, 51, 32–42.

Stein, D.S., Munir, K.M., Karweck, A.J., Davidson, E.J., Stein, M.T. (2013). Developmental regression, depression, and psychosocial stress in an adolescent with Down syndrome. *Journal of Developmental and Behavioral Pediatrics*, 34, 216–218.

Van Acker, R. (1991). Rett syndrome: a review of current knowledge. *Journal of Autism and Developmental Disorders*, 21, 381–406.

Veltman, M.W., Craig, E.E., Bolton, P.F. (2005). Autism spectrum disorders in Prader–Willi and Angelman syndromes: a systematic review. *Psychiatric Genetics*, 15, 243–254.

Webb, T., Maina, E.N., Soni, S., et al. (2008). In search of the psychosis gene in people with Prader–Willi syndrome. *American Journal of Medical Genetics Part A*, 146, 843–853.

Woodruff-Borden, J., Kistler, D.J., Henderson, D.R., Crawford, N.A., Mervis, C.B. (2010). Longitudinal course of anxiety in children and adolescents with Williams syndrome. *American Journal of Medical Genetics Part C: Seminars in Medical Genetics*, 154, 277–290.

Worley, G., Crissman, B., Cardogan, E., Kishnani, P. (2013). *New onset autistic regression, cognitive decline and insomnia in older children and adolescents with Down syndrome*. Presentation to the Down Syndrome Medical Interest Group–USA, Denver, CO.

Offending behavior

19

John L. Taylor and William R. Lindsay

Introduction

It is not clear whether people with intellectual disabilities (ID) commit more crime than those without ID, or, in fact, whether the nature and frequency of offending by people with ID differs from that committed by offenders in the general population. The ambiguity concerning these issues is due in large part to methodological problems in prevalence studies in this area (Lindsay and Taylor, 2010). One source of variation in prevalence of offending reported across studies is the location of the study (community, prison–remand, prison–sentenced, hospital–high/medium/low-secure), which can result in sampling bias and filtering effects. Frequently, the inclusion criteria used in prevalence studies vary or are not clear and this can affect the rates obtained – particularly if people with borderline intelligence are included. Also, the method used to identify ID (standardized vs. screening IQ tests, educational history, clinical assessment) can have a significant impact.

These methodological issues are well illustrated in the research literature concerning the prevalence of offenders with ID in prisons. MacEachron (1979) reviewed the literature for prevalence of offenders with ID in prisons in the USA and found a range of 2.6–39.6%. Fazel et al. (2008) reviewed 10 well-conducted studies of prevalence of ID in prisons (remand and sentenced) conducted between 1988 and 1997 in five common law countries and reported rates between 0% and 2.9%.

More recently, Crocker et al. (2007) assessed 281 pretrial prisoners in Montreal, Canada using three subscales of a standardized ability scale and reported that 18.9% were in the ID range. Søndenaa et al. (2008) used an IQ screening assessment with 143 prisoners in Norway and found that 10.8% fell in the ID range. Contrast these findings with a study of prisoners in Victoria, Australia in which Holland and Persson (2011) found a prevalence of less than 1.3% using the Wechsler Adult Intelligence Scale; and the results of a study of 389 remand prisoners in Scotland that indicated that less than 0.5% of those assessed had ID (Davidson et al., 1995). It is difficult to reconcile these findings without concluding that the location, assessment, and sampling methods account for the variance in large part.

Recidivism

Studies of recidivism rates for offenders with ID are also affected by similar methodological problems. Reported rates tend to be high but vary considerably depending on research setting, procedures, and definitions of reoffending used (Linhorst et al., 2003). For example, Lund (1990) found a reoffending rate of 67–72% in a follow-up study involving 155 Danish offenders with ID who had been detained on statutory orders – while Klimecki et al. (1994) reported a reoffending rate of 41.3% for 75 released prisoners with ID in Victoria, Australia. More recently, Linhorst et al. (2003) reported that 25% of 252 offenders with developmental disabilities who completed a case management community program were rearrested within a six-month period following case closure; 43% of those who dropped out of the program were rearrested during the same period.

Due to the lack of controlled studies involving ID and non-intellectual disabilities offenders, it is difficult to make direct comparisons of recidivism rates. It would appear, however, that recidivism rates for offenders with ID are no higher than those for populations of general offenders. Gray et al. (2007) conducted a two-year follow-up of 145 offenders with ID and 996 offenders without ID, all discharged from independent sector hospitals in the UK. The ID group had a lower rate of reconviction for violent offenses after two years (4.8%) than the non-ID group (11.2%). This trend held true for general offenses also (9.7% and 18.7% for the respective groups).

Intellectual functioning and offending

Historically, low intellectual functioning was viewed as a determinant of criminal behavior. Scheerenberger (1983) described in detail the historical association between low intelligence and crime in the late 19th and early 20th centuries. Famously, Terman (1911) stated that "There is no investigator who denies the fearful role of mental deficiency in the production of vice, crime and delinquency . . .." Goddard (1921) suggested that up to 50% of people in prisons were "mentally defective," and later still Sutherland (1937) concluded that 50% of delinquents residing in prisons were "feeble-minded." People with lower levels of intellectual functioning were often considered a threat to society up to the middle of the last century.

In fact, the research evidence supporting the relationship between IQ and offending is robust (West and Farrington, 1973; Hirschi and Hindelang, 1977; Goodman et al., 1995), with those in lower IQ groups having greater rates of offending than those in higher functioning groups. Even when socioeconomic status is controlled for, offending behavior has been found to be significantly related to IQ (e.g., Moffit et al., 1991; Farrington, 1995). However, most studies involve participants with IQs in the 80–120 range and there is some evidence that when participants with IQs around 1–2 standard deviations below the mean (<80) are included, the relationship with offending is less straightforward. For example, McCord and McCord (1959) found that, while the offending rate for those in the low-average IQ group (81–90) was higher than that for those with above average IQ, those in the lowest IQ group (<80) had an offending rate lower than that for the low-average group. More recently, Mears and Cochran (2013) reported data from the National Longitudinal Survey of Youth project in the USA that indicated that the relationship between IQ and offending is curvilinear, with lower IQs (<85) associated with lower levels of offending. Thus, while there would seem to be a clear relationship between offending rates and intellectual functioning, when studies are extended to include people with IQs below 80–85, the relationship does not appear to be simple or linear.

Nature of offending behavior

A policy of deinstitutionalization has been implemented across the Western world since the mid 1970s and has had a significant effect on services for people with ID who offend or engage in offending-type behavior. Such people are now more likely to be living in community settings where their offending and offending-type behavior is more visible and subject to scrutiny by the criminal justice system. This phenomenon is demonstrated by Lund (1990) in a study of 123 offenders with ID on statutory care orders in Denmark, which found a 2–3 times increase in the incidence of sex, violence, and arson offenses when comparing sentencing in 1973 and 1983. Lund suggested that these increases were less to do with an increase in offending per se in this population, but a result of deinstitutionaliza-tion policies during this period, whereby people with ID were no longer detained in hospital for indeterminate lengths of time, but living in the community where their offending behavior was more likely to be subject to normal legal processes.

In the Northgate, Cambridge, and Abertay Pathways (NCAP) project, O'Brien et al. (2010) reported on the offense characteristics of 477 adults with ID referred to ID services in three regions of the UK during a 12-month period because of antisocial or offending behavior. They found that aggression (physical and verbal) accounted for over 80% of the antisocial and offending behavior referred, with sex offenses (contact and non-contact) making up almost 30%. Just 4% of referrals concerned firesetting, whilst 19% were related to property damage. Despite the majority of those referred having significant histories of offending behavior, just under a third were found to have any kind of structured care plan.

Since most ID institutions in the UK have now closed, or reduced in capacity significantly, people with ID who offend and require secure provision are often sent to out-of-area facilities, with a consequent drain on the resources available to local ID services (Crossland et al., 2005). This is an important issue, as Carson et al. (2010) found in the NCAP study that 50% of referrals for offending behavior were to generic ID community services, and these were received mainly from primary and secondary healthcare and social services. Compared to referrals to specialist forensic ID services (including secure services), referrals to community ID services included significantly more women, were slightly older, and included significantly more people with IQ levels below 50. In contrast, those referred to specialist forensic ID services were more often referred by the courts, offender management, and tertiary healthcare services, had committed contact sex offenses, had been charged in connection with their index offenses, and had significantly higher levels of mental illness (psychoses, personality disorder, attention-deficit/hyperactivity disorder, and conduct disorder).

The early findings from service referrals and pathways research suggest that ID offenders require a range of community and specialist inpatient services available to meet their needs, and to manage the risks they present to others and to themselves. In particular, resources need to be invested in helping community services staff to develop their knowledge and skills in managing these clients using structured care plans informed by risk needs assessments.

Interventions for offenders with ID

Risk assessment

Whilst not a therapeutic intervention in the traditional sense, risk assessment is the cornerstone of therapeutic endeavor aimed at reducing offending behavior and is the foundation for clinical formulations of treatment need. Significant advances in the development of measures designed to accurately predict future violence and sexual aggression have now been extended to include offenders with ID. For example, Quinsey et al. (2004) demonstrated that the Violence Risk Appraisal Guide (VRAG), one of the best-established actuarial risk measures in the general offender literature, has good predictive accuracy when used with ID offenders. Gray et al. (2007) conducted a more extensive investigation into the VRAG. They compared 145 patients with ID and 996 mainstream patients all discharged from hospital having been admitted due to serious offending-type behavior. They found that the VRAG predicted reconviction rates in the ID sample with an effect size as large as that for the non-ID sample.

This important research on the assessment and management of risk in offenders with ID has continued in a study (the "212 Multi-Centre Risk Study") involving 212 clients across a range of security settings: hospital high, medium and low-security, and community forensic ID services (Hogue et al., 2006). The most complex presentations, in particular comorbid personality disorder, were found in the more secure samples. Lindsay et al. (2008) combined the total cohort of offenders with ID from the 212 risk study to evaluate the predictive validity of a range of static and dynamic risk assessments. They found that the VRAG, the Historical, Clinical, Risk Management-20 (HCR-20) (Webster et al., 1997), the Short Dynamic Risk Scale (SDRS; Quinsey, 2004), and the Emotional Problems Scale (Prout and Strohmer, 1991) all showed significant "areas-under-the-curve" (AUC) (using receiver-operator characteristics (ROC) analyses) in relation to the prediction of violent incidents. The Static-99 sex offender risk assessment instrument (Hanson and Thornton, 1999) also showed a significant area-under-the-curve in relation to the prediction of sexual incidents.

Dynamic risk assessments (e.g., the SDRS) contrast with static risk assessments (e.g., the VRAG) in that the variables are amenable to change through treatment and management of the individual. As there seemed to be strong relationships between dynamic risk factors and future incidents for this client group, Lofthouse et al. (2014) reanalyzed the risk assessment data published by Lindsay et al. (2008) that showed that both the VRAG (an actuarial assessment) and the SDRS (an easy and-quick-to-complete dynamic risk assessment) had equivalent risk predictive values of AUC = 0.71 and 0.72, respectively. They investigated the functional relationships between VRAG and SDRS items to determine whether they were independent, mediating/moderating, or acting as a proxy and found that the dynamic variables on the SDRS acted as a proxy for the VRAG variables. They concluded that since these risk factors captured elements of the same underlying risk construct associated with violence, and as dynamic variables are more accessible and clinically meaningful, dynamic assessment, in the form of the SDRS, could provide more immediate and clinically relevant information to manage patients' risk needs.

An alternative approach to understanding forensic risk has been advanced by Wheeler et al. (2014) in a study examining the impact of social and environmental variables on offending behavior by people with ID. Lack of work or routine activity, serious problems with family relationships, and exposure to antisocial or abusive friends were found to be strongest predictors of offending behavior in people with ID referred to community ID teams. This approach echoes Willis and Grace's (2009) work on non-ID sexual offenders that showed that discharge planning, including organization (or lack of it) of accommodation, employment, and social support, predicted recidivism equally as well as established criminogenic variables.

This research has demonstrated that there are several well-established actuarial, dynamic, and clinical instruments, some of which have been developed specifically for this client group, that have good reliability, discriminative validity, and predictive validity with offenders with ID. If we can confirm that proximal dynamic indicators of risk not only have more clinical utility but are also as predictive as established static risk indicators, this could have a significant impact on developing practice to help offenders with ID to access better services in the least restrictive environments.

Anger and aggression

Research on several continents has found high rates of aggression amongst people with ID – with much higher rates for those living in institutional and secure forensic facilities than for those residing in community settings (Taylor and Novaco, 2013).

While it is neither necessary nor sufficient for aggression to occur, anger has been shown to be strongly associated with and predictive of violence in men with ID and offending histories (Novaco and Taylor, 2004). Thus, anger has become a legitimate therapeutic target. The treatment of anger and aggression using cognitive-behavioral therapy (CBT) has been extensively evaluated with a range of clinical populations (see Taylor and Novaco, 2005 for a review). One potential advantage of CBT anger treatment over interventions based on applied behavior analysis, is that self-actualization through the promotion of portable and internalized control of behavior is intrinsic to the skills-training components of these approaches (Taylor et al., 2002b). Further, there is evidence from studies in non-disability fields that for a range of psychological problems the effects of CBT are maintained and increase over time compared to control conditions (Taylor and Novaco, 2005).

Willner (2007) reviewed nine controlled studies involving people with ID that compared CBT for anger control problems with wait-list control conditions. Most of these interventions were based on the treatment approach developed by Novaco (1975) that incorporates Meichenbaum's (1985) stress inoculation paradigm. All of these studies reported significant improvements on outcome measures for those in treatment conditions that were maintained at 3–12-month follow-up. Nicoll et al. (2013) systematically reviewed 12 studies of CBT for anger in adults with ID published between 1999 and 2011. Nine studies were included in a meta-analysis that yielded a large uncontrolled effect size (ES) (average ES = 0.84).

Taylor and colleagues have evaluated individual CBT anger treatment with detained male patients with mild–borderline ID and significant histories of violence in a linked series of studies (Taylor et al., 2002a, 2004a, 2005). The 18-session treatment package included a 6-session broadly psychoeducational and motivational preparatory phase; followed by a 12-session treatment phase based on individual formulation of each participant's anger problems and needs, following the classical CBT stages of cognitive preparation, skills acquisition, skills rehearsal, and then practice *in vivo*. These studies showed significant improvements on self-reported measures of anger disposition, reactivity, and imaginal provocation following intervention in the treatment groups compared with scores for the control groups, and these differences were maintained for up to four months following treatment.

The impact of these anger interventions on aggressive behavior, including physical violence, has been investigated empirically on only a few occasions. Allan et al. (2001) and Lindsay et al. (2003) reported reductions in violence following a group intervention in a case series of six women and six men with violent convictions living in the community. In a larger study involving 47 people with ID and histories of aggression, Lindsay et al. (2004a) showed that, following a community-group anger intervention, 14% of participants had been aggressive during follow-up, compared with 45% of people in a control condition.

Novaco and Taylor (2015) described an evaluation of the impact of the cognitive-behavioral anger treatment described earlier (e.g., Taylor et al., 2005) on violent behavior by offenders with ID living in secure forensic hospital settings. The participants in this study were 44 men and six women referred by their clinical teams for anger treatment on the basis of their histories of aggression and/or current presentation. The total number of physical attacks against staff and patients fell from 319 in the12-months before treatment to 153 in the 12-month period following treatment. This represents a reduction after treatment of 52%. Importantly, the reduction in physical assaults was associated with measured reductions in anger over the course of treatment as indexed by several anger measures validated for use with this population.

In summary, there is an emerging research evidence base that CBT anger interventions can be effective in the treatment of offenders with ID and histories of aggression and violence in terms of improvements on self-report and informant anger-dependent measures that are associated with significant reductions in the number of violent incidents recorded following treatment.

Sexually aggressive behavior

Psychological treatment interventions for sex offenders with ID were reviewed by Courtney and Rose (2004). Nineteen studies published post 1990 were reviewed. These included drug treatment, problem solving, psychoeducational, and cognitive-behavioral approaches. Eleven studies were single case or small case series designs – four involved drug therapy and seven involved psychological interventions. The reported outcomes in these studies were generally positive. Eight "larger" studies, including one drug therapy, three service/management interventions, and five psychological treatments, were also reviewed. In terms of outcomes, psychological interventions appeared to be marginally superior. Eight of the studies involved group therapy interventions which were found to yield mixed outcomes, with reported recidivism rates ranging between 0% and 40%. Based on this review, and that by Lindsay (2002), it appears that most treatment approaches show some promise, but the studies were quite limited – involving small, heterogeneous samples, utilizing measures with limited reliability and validity, using poorly defined outcomes, and incorporating treatment interventions that were often described poorly. The main methodological shortcoming, however, is the absence of any controlled studies. This is due primarily to the ethical difficulty in withholding a potentially beneficial treatment given the social and legal issues involved.

More recently there has been some support for the use of cognitive and problem solving techniques in therapy for sex offenders with ID that have been shown to be effective in reducing reoffending rates in the mainstream sex offender field (see Hanson et al., 2002). Support for the centrality of cognitive distortions in the sex offending perpetrated by people with ID came from a qualitative study of nine male sex offenders by Courtney et al. (2006). They concluded that all aspects of the offense process were linked to offender attitudes and beliefs, such as denial of the offense, blaming others, and seeing themselves as the victim. Lindsay et al. (1998a–c) reported on a series of case studies with offenders with ID using CBT in which various forms of denial and mitigation of the offense were challenged over treatment periods of up to three years. Strategies for relapse prevention and the promotion of self-regulation were also component parts of the treatment. Across these studies, participants consistently reported positive changes in cognitions during treatment as assessed using the Questionnaire on Attitudes Consistent with Sexual Offenses (QACSO; Lindsay et al. 2007). More importantly, lengthy follow-up of these cases over 4–7 years showed that none had reoffended following initial conviction.

Rose et al. (2012) reported on a six-month treatment group for 12 sex offenders with ID who were living in community settings. Efforts were made to involve aspects of the offender's broader social life into treatment by inviting carers to accompany participants. They found significant improvements on the QACSO, locus of control, and sexual knowledge and attitudes. One participant committed a sexual offense during an 18-month follow-up period.

Murphy et al. (2010) conducted a multisite study of group sex offender therapy with 46 men living in community and secure hospital settings. Following the 12-month weekly treatment schedule, significant improvements were found on the QACSO and other measures, sexual attitudes, knowledge, and victim empathy. Improvements on the QACSO and sexual knowledge were maintained at six-month follow-up. Three patients (6.5%) reoffended during the treatment program and four patients (8.7%) reoffended by carrying out 11 offenses during the six-month follow-up period. Thirty-four participants from this study were followed up for an extended period of between 15 and 106 months (Heaton and Murphy, 2013). Significant improvements on the QACSO, sexual knowledge, and victim empathy were maintained at follow-up in this study; however, eight participants (24%) reoffended during the follow-up period.

There have been a number of sex-offender treatment studies involving comparison groups with ID, although they all fall well short of adequate experimental standards, and it is important to consider the study results in light of their methodological shortcomings. Lindsay and Smith (1998) compared seven patients who had been in treatment for two or more years with another group of seven patients who had been in treatment for less than one year. Participants in the group that had been in treatment for less than one year showed significantly poorer progress and were more likely to reoffend than those treated for at least two years. Despite the small numbers involved, this study suggested that shorter treatment periods might be of limited value for this client group. This was supported by the results of a study by Rose et al. (2002) involving five men with ID living in community settings who underwent a relatively short 16-week group sex offender treatment program. No significant pre–post intervention differences were found on the QACSO or victim empathy measures.

In a further series of comparison studies involving larger groups, Lindsay and colleagues have compared individuals with ID who have committed sexual offenses with those who have committed other types of offenses. Lindsay et al. (2004b) compared 106 men who had committed sexual offenses or sexually abusive incidents with 78 men who had committed other types of offenses or serious incidents. There was a significantly higher reoffending rate in the non-sex offender cohort (51%) when compared to the sex offender cohort (19%). In a subsequent, more comprehensive evaluation, Lindsay et al. (2006) compared 121 sex offenders with 105 other types of male offenders. Reoffending rates were reported for up to 12 years after the index offense. The difference in reoffending rates between the groups was highly significant, with rates of 23.9% for male sex offenders and 59% for other types of offenders. The same authors also investigated harm reduction by examining the number of offenses committed by recidivists. They found that for those participants who reoffended, the number of offenses at up to 12 years follow-up was a quarter to a third of those recorded before treatment. This indicated a considerable harm-reduction effect following the intervention.

In a follow-up of community forensic service clients, Lindsay et al. (2013b) followed up 156 sex offenders and 126 non-sex offenders for up to 20 years. All but 15 of the study participants continued to have some access to the wider community throughout the follow-up period. Sixteen percent of sex offender participants reoffended during this lengthy follow-up period. Analyses showed that approximately 50% of the reoffending in the sex offender group occurred within the first 12 months following treatment. Some participants continued to reoffend for up to nine years post treatment; however, after that point there was no further reoffending recorded in the sex offender group up to 20 years post treatment. Comparing the number of sex offenses committed prior to referral with the offenses recorded during the 20-year follow-up period, a 95% harm-reduction effect was calculated.

Based on the limited evidence available, it is possible to conclude, albeit tentatively, that psychologically informed and well-structured interventions appear to yield reasonable outcomes in the treatment of sex offenders with ID. CBT appears to have a positive effect on offense-related attitudes and cognitions, sexual knowledge, and victim empathy. Longer periods of treatment may result in better outcomes that are maintained for longer periods. Comparison studies, although limited methodologically, indicate that psychological interventions may significantly reduce recidivism rates in sex offenders with ID – and where recidivism does occur, treatment may result in significant harm-reduction effects.

Firesetting behavior

It has been suggested that arson is over-represented in offenders with ID (e.g., Raesaenen et al., 1994). However, there is no clear research evidence to suggest that firesetting behavior is more prevalent amongst people with ID than in the general population, or whether people with ID are over-represented in the arson offender population.

Despite the alarm that firesetting behavior causes in society, there are limited published studies concerning therapeutic interventions for adults who set fires in general, and the research literature involving firesetters with ID is even sparser. Rice and Chaplin (1979) delivered a social-skills training intervention to two groups of five firesetters in a high-security psychiatric facility in North America. One of the groups was reported to be functioning in the mild–borderline ID range. Following treatment, both groups were reported to have improved, and following discharge none of the treated patients had been reconvicted or suspected of setting fires at 12 months follow-up. Clare et al. (1992) reported a case study involving a British man with mild ID who had prior convictions for arson and making nuisance telephone calls to the emergency services. Significant clinical improvements were reported following a multifaceted self-control and skills-training intervention. The client was discharged to a community placing and did not engage in any fire-related offending behavior at 30 months follow-up.

Hall et al. (2005) described the delivery of 16-session group CBT to six male patients with ID and histories of firesetting detained in a hospital medium-secure unit in the UK. Unfortunately, outcome data were not provided, although most group participants were reported to have responded positively to the intervention in terms of their clinical presentations, and two patients were successfully transferred to less secure placements following completion of the program.

Taylor et al. (2004b) reported on a case series of four detained men with ID and convictions for arson offenses. They received a broadly CBT, 40-session, group-based intervention that involved work on offense cycles, education about the costs associated with setting fires, training of skills to enhance future coping with emotional problems associated with previous firesetting behavior, and work on personalized plans to prevent relapse. The treatment successfully engaged these patients, all of whom completed the program delivered over a period of four months. Despite their intellectual and cognitive limitations, all participants showed high levels of motivation and commitment, which was reflected in generally improved attitudes with regard to personal responsibility, victim issues, and awareness of risk factors associated with their firesetting behavior. In a further series of case studies on six women with mild–borderline ID and histories of firesetting, Taylor et al. (2006) also employed the same group intervention to successfully engage participants in the therapy process. All participants completed the program and scores on measures related to fire-treatment targets generally improved following the intervention. All but one of the treatment group participants had been discharged to community placements at two-year follow-up and there had been no reports of participants setting any fires or engaging in fire risk-related behavior.

Using the same assessment and treatment approach as that used by Taylor and colleagues above, Taylor et al. (2002b) investigated the outcomes for 14 men and women with ID and arson convictions. Study participants were assessed pre and post treatment on a number of fire-specific, anger, self-esteem, and depression measures. Following treatment, significant improvements were found in all areas assessed, except for depression. Taylor (2014) reported on a follow-up of 24 firesetters with ID who had completed a specialist group treatment program. The follow-up period ranged between 4 and 13 years post treatment, at which point there had been no further arrests or convictions for arson in this cohort. File data available for 17 study participants showed that prior to treatment that subgroup had been responsible for setting a total of 425 fires. This suggests that the group-firesetters intervention used by Taylor et al. above is associated with a significant harm-reduction effect.

The results of these small and methodologically weak pilot studies do provide some limited encouragement and guidance to practitioners concerning the utility of group-based interventions for firesetting behavior by people with ID. These CBT-orientated approaches are associated with significant improvements on firesetter-specific and clinically relevant measures and reductions in firesetter behavior following treatment.

Interventions for other offense-related problems
Alcohol misuse
In general, studies have found that alcohol misuse in people with ID is at a lower rate when compared to the mainstream population. In a study involving 329 people with ID, Rimmer et al. (1995) found that less than 5% of individuals used alcohol at all. McGillicuddy and Blane (1999) reported on a sample of 122 people with ID and found that, although the majority did not use alcohol, around 50% of those who did drink did so to problematic levels. The problems experienced by people with ID who misuse alcohol are similar to the medical, social, family, and occupational problems experienced by people in the general population (Westermeyer et al., 1996).

McGillivray and Moore (2001) compared 30 offenders and 30 non-offenders, both groups with ID, in Australia. The offender group reported greater use of alcohol, and a third had used alcohol prior to their index offenses. In a study of 212 offenders with ID in a range of security settings in the UK, Hogue et al. (2006) found that 18.4% had a history of alcohol misuse and alcohol was involved in the index offense of 13.7% of cases. In a study involving 477 people with ID referred to forensic services, Lindsay et al. (2013a) found that 20.8% had a history of alcohol abuse and that alcohol was involved in the index offense in 5.9% of cases (3.8% in community and 13.2% in low/medium-secure service referrals).

Given the relevance of alcohol use/misuse amongst offenders with ID, there is virtually no literature concerning alcohol-focused interventions in this client group. This is despite there being a strong evidence base for the effectiveness of psychosocial interventions for alcohol-related problems in non-disabled offenders (see McMurran, 2013 for a review). Lindsay et al. (2014) reported positive outcomes for a pilot 13-session program for alcohol-related violence run with four offenders with ID. The alcohol-focused program was run concurrently with an anger treatment or emotional control program and comprised of sessions on knowledge and awareness of alcohol and its effects, management of alcohol use, including skills in bars and other environments, a detailed analysis of the role of alcohol in the individual's offending cycle, and development of a relapse prevention plan to better manage alcohol use in the future. The results from this case series were promising in terms of increased knowledge and awareness of alcohol-related issues and reductions in self-reported anger, anxiety, and depression.

In a similar development involving detained male offenders with ID, Gillmer (2013) described the development of a skills-training program aimed at helping patients better manage alcohol-related violence as part of their predischarge preparations. This approach takes into account the neurodevelopmental problems experienced by many people in this population that are often expressed as impulse-control difficulties. Using motivational techniques the group program comprises *in vivo* skills training concerning how to conduct oneself in bars and similar environments, and a reflective group component where participants discuss their difficulties in managing their thoughts and feelings in environments where alcohol is available. This and the Lindsay et al. (2014) study represent the first attempts at dealing with this important area in the treatment and management of offenders with ID who use or misuse alcohol.

Cognitive skills training

An important development in offender rehabilitation over the last 15 years has been the introduction of programs to improve cognitive skills in relation to social and offense-related problem situations. Cognitive skills programs aim to change beliefs and attitudes that support offending behaviors. The purpose of these programs is to equip offenders with thinking skills that promote alternative, pro-social approaches to situations, particularly those situations in which the person is at risk of offending. In a wider context, such alternative-thinking skills help offenders to move away from lifestyles that are associated with offending, and which may have been reinforced by criminal-thinking styles.

Reviews of the effectiveness of cognitive skills programs such as "Reasoning and Rehabilitation" ("R and R"; Ross and Fabiano, 1985) have concluded that there is reasonable evidence for significant reductions in offending following program completion (e.g., Joy Tong and Farrington, 2006). Given the difficulties that offenders with ID are likely to have with moral development and self-regulation, it is surprising that these programs have not been applied in this field other than some pilot investigations (e.g., Doyle and Hamilton, 2006). Recently, Lindsay et al. (2011) conducted a study reviewing the effectiveness of an adapted cognitive skills program for offenders with ID. The program draws heavily on the "Stop and Think!" program (McMurran, et al., 2001), which is an offense-related problem solving program for offenders with personality disorders. In an evaluation of 10 participants with ID who had completed the program, reductions in measures of impulsiveness and increases in social problem solving skills were reported. This provides some initial, limited evidence that interventions aimed at changing criminal-thinking styles may be feasible with offenders with ID.

Conclusions

It remains unclear whether people with ID are over- or under-represented in offender populations, or whether offending is more prevalent among people with ID than the general population. There is a need for controlled studies involving offenders with ID versus non-ID offenders versus non-offenders with ID in order to make direct comparisons of prevalence. This same requirement applies to recidivism studies, although some limited comparative research indicates that rates of reoffending are no higher, and may be lower, amongst offenders with ID compared with non-ID offender groups.

Recent political, health, and social care policies, such as deinstitutionalization and resettlement, have had a significant impact on offenders with ID who are now more visible in the wider community than before. This, in turn, has meant that more people with ID who engage in antisocial or offending behavior are being dealt with by the criminal justice system, and local generic ID services are managing more complex and forensically riskier cases. To date, developments in the design and delivery of services for offenders with ID have not been informed by good-quality research. This is beginning to change with service-pathway research indicating an urgent need for services for these clients to be based on structured care plans underpinned by robust risk assessment procedures.

This situation could be improved in the future given the significant advances in the identification of risk factors for this client group and the results of studies investigating the effectiveness of risk assessments for violence and sexual offending. In general, the data from these studies of actuarial, dynamic, and clinical risk assessment tools suggest that they are generally as effective for offenders with ID as they are for mainstream offenders.

There have been some significant developments in the treatment of offenders with ID based on interventions using cognitive-behavioral approaches. The most significant treatment innovations have been in the field of anger treatment where programs have been evaluated in a number of controlled studies. Although these studies have generally involved wait-list control rather than randomized designs, the raft of positive outcomes indicate that anger treatment programs can be incorporated into the general management of violent and aggressive offenders with ID with some confidence.

The second main development in treatment has been in cognitive-behavioral approaches for sexual offenders with ID. There have been a number of single case reports producing encouraging results and, more importantly, employing lengthy follow-up periods. Comparisons of convenience samples have produced positive outcomes. Given the methodological weaknesses of these studies, the results should be treated cautiously but with optimism.

There have been a small number of studies concerning cognitive-behaviorally framed interventions for firesetters with ID that have provided promising outcomes and guidance for practitioners. However, controlled evaluations of these interventions are certainly required. Similarly, there are some early indications that alcohol-misuse and cognitive-skills training interventions adapted from mainstream-offender practice may have value in work with offenders with ID.

For the future, more research and evaluation is required on the application and inclusion of valid risk assessments into care-planning procedures designed to manage offenders with ID. Larger, more powerful and better-designed controlled trials (and small n studies) are needed to show if the effects of treatment interventions obtained to date can be replicated, and longer term follow-up would help to evaluate the impact of psychological treatment gains on reducing future offending behavior. A range of process issues including optimum length of treatment, the systematic involvement of carers, and relative costs require further investigation also.

Key summary points

- The evidence that people with ID commit more crime than others is highly equivocal.
- Reported recidivism rates for offenders with ID are high but vary widely depending on methodology.
- Risk assessments used in the non-ID population have now been successfully evaluated in offenders with ID.
- Cognitive-behavioral therapy has been effective in small-scale studies in the treatment of anger and aggression in offenders with ID.
- More evidence has emerged regarding the treatments, including group therapy, of sexual offenders with ID.
- Evidence regarding firesetting in people with ID remains sparser.

References

Allan, R., Lindsay, W.R., Macleod, F., Smith, A.H.W. (2001). Treatment of women with intellectual disabilities who have been involved with the criminal justice system for reasons of aggression. *Journal of Applied Research in Intellectual Disabilities*, 14, 340–347.

Carson, D., Lindsay, W.R., O'Brien, G, et al. (2010). Referrals into services for offenders with intellectual disabilities: variables predicting community or secure provision. *Criminal Behaviour and Mental Health*, 20, 39–50.

Clare, I.C.H., Murphy, G.H., Cox, D., Chaplin, E.H. (1992). Assessment and treatment of firesetting: a single case investigation using a cognitive behavioural model. *Criminal Behaviour and Mental Health*, 2, 253–268.

Courtney, J. and Rose, J. (2004). The effectiveness of treatment for male sex offenders with learning disabilities: a review of the literature. *Journal of Sexual Aggression*, 10, 215–236.

Courtney, J., Rose, J., Mason, O. (2006). The offence process of sex offenders with intellectual disabilities: a qualitative study. *Sexual Abuse: A Journal of Research and Treatment*, 18, 169–191.

Crocker, A.J., Cote, G., Toupin, J., St-Onge, B. (2007). Rate and characteristics of men with an intellectual disability in pre-trial detention. *Journal of Intellectual and Developmental Disabilities*, 32, 143–152.

Crossland, S., Burns, M., Leach, C., Quinn, P. (2005). Needs assessment in forensic learning disability. *Medicine, Science and the Law*, 45, 147–153.

Davidson M., Humphreys, M.S., Johnstone, E.C., Owens, D.G. (1995). Prevalence of psychiatric morbidity among remand prisoners in Scotland. *British Journal of Psychiatry*, 167, 548–554.

Doyle, M.C. and Hamilton, C. (2006). An evaluation of a social problem solving group work programme for offenders with intellectual disabilities. *Journal of Applied Research in Intellectual Disabilities*, 19, 257.

Farrington, D.P. (1995). The development of offending and antisocial behaviour from childhood: key findings from the Cambridge study in delinquent development. *Journal of Child Psychology and Psychiatry*, 36, 929–964.

Fazel, S, Xenitidis, K. and Powell, J. (2008). The prevalence of intellectual disabilities among 12,000 prisoners: a systematic review. *International Journal of Law and Psychiatry*, 31, 369–373.

Gillmer, B.T. (2013). *Intellectual and developmental disability, alcohol misuse and risk for violence.* Paper presented at the 8th European Conference on Violence in Clinical Psychiatry, Ghent, Belgium, October, 2013.

Goddard, H.H. (1921). *Juvenile Delinquency.* New York, NY: Dodd, Mead and Company.

Goodman, R., Simonoff, E., Stevenson, J. (1995). The impact of child IQ, parent IQ and sibling IQ on child and behaviour deviance scores. *Journal of Child Psychology and Psychiatry*, 36, 409–425.

Gray, N.S., Fitzgerald, S., Taylor, J., MacCulloch, M., Snowden, R. (2007). Predicting future reconviction in offenders with intellectual disabilities: the predictive efficacy of the VRAG, PCL-SV and the HCR-20. *Psychological Assessment*, 19, 474–79.

Hall, I., Clayton, P., Johnson, P. (2005). Arson and learning disability. In T. Riding, C. Swann, B. Swann (eds.), *The Handbook of Forensic Learning Disabilities*. Oxford: Radcliffe Publishing.

Hanson, R.K. and Thornton, D. (1999). *Static-99: Improving Actuarial Risk Assessments for Sex Offenders.* (User report 1999–02). Ottowa, ON: Department of the Solicitor General of Canada.

Hanson, R.K., Gordon, A., Harris, A.J.R., et al. (2002). First report of the collaborative outcome data project on the effectiveness of psychological treatment for sex offenders. *Sexual Abuse: A Journal of Research and Treatment*, 14, 169–194.

Heaton, K.M. and Murphy, G.M. (2013). Men with intellectual disabilities who have attended sex offender treatment groups:

a follow-up. *Journal of Applied Research in Intellectual Disabilities*, 26, 489–500.

Hirschi, T. and Hindelang, M.J. (1977). Intelligence and delinquency: a revisionist view. *American Sociological Review*, 42, 571–587.

Hogue, T., Steptoe, L., Taylor, J.L., et al. (2006). A comparison of offenders with intellectual disability across three levels of security. *Criminal Behaviour and Mental Health*, 16, 13–28.

Holland, S. and Persson, P. (2011). Intellectual disability in the Victorian prison system: characteristics of prisoners with an intellectual disability released from prison in 2003–2006. *Psychology, Crime and Law*, 17, 25–41.

Joy Tong, L.S. and Farrington, D.P. (2006). How effective is the "Reasoning and Rehabilitation" programme in reducing offending? A meta-analysis of evaluations in four countries. *Psychology, Crime and Law*, 12, 3–24.

Klimecki, M.R., Jenkinson, J., Wilson, L. (1994). A study of recidivism among offenders with intellectual disability. *Australia and New Zealand Journal of Developmental Disabilities*, 19, 209–219.

Lindsay, W.R. (2002). Research and literature on sex offenders with intellectual and developmental disabilities. *Journal of Intellectual Disability Research*, 46(Suppl. 1), 74–85.

Lindsay, W.R. and Smith, A.H.W. (1998). Responses to treatment for sex offenders with intellectual disability: a comparison of men with one and two year probation sentences. *Journal of Intellectual Disability Research*, 42, 346–353.

Lindsay, W.R. and Taylor, J.L. (2010). Mentally disordered offenders: intellectual disability. In G.J. Towl and D.A. Crighton (eds.), *Forensic Psychology*. Chichester, West Sussex, UK: BPS Blackwell.

Lindsay, W.R., Marshall, I., Neilson, C.Q., Quinn, K., Smith, A.H.W. (1998a). The treatment of men with a learning disability convicted of exhibitionism. *Research in Developmental Disabilities*, 19, 295–316.

Lindsay, W.R., Neilson, C.Q., Morrison, F., Smith, A.H.W. (1998b). The treatment of six men with a learning disability convicted of sex offences with children. *British Journal of Clinical Psychology*, 37, 83–98.

Lindsay, W.R., Olley, S., Jack, C., Morrison, F., Smith, A.H.W. (1998c). The treatment of two stalkers with intellectual disabilities using a cognitive approach. *Journal of Applied Research in Intellectual Disabilities*, 11, 333–344.

Lindsay, W.R., Allan, R., Macleod, F., Smart, N., Smith, A.H.W. (2003). Long term treatment and management of violent tendencies of men with intellectual disabilities convicted of assault. *Mental Retardation*, 41, 47–56.

Lindsay, W.R., Allan, R., Parry, C., et al. (2004a). Anger and aggression in people with intellectual disabilities: treatment and follow-up of consecutive referrals and a waiting list comparison. *Clinical Psychology and Psychotherapy*, 11, 225–264.

Lindsay, W.R., Elliot, S.F., Astell, A. (2004b). Predictors of sexual offence recidivism in offenders with intellectual disabilities. *Journal of Applied Research in Intellectual Disabilities*, 17, 267–274.

Lindsay, W.R., Steele, L., Smith, A.H.W., Quinn, K., Allan, R. (2006). A community forensic intellectual disability service: twelve year follow-up of referrals, analysis of referral patterns and assessment of harm reduction. *Legal and Criminological Psychology*, 11, 113–130.

Lindsay, W.R., Whitefield, E., Carson, D. (2007). An assessment for attitudes consistent with sexual offending for use with offenders with intellectual disability. *Legal and Criminological Psychology*, 12, 55–68.

Lindsay, W.R., Hogue, T.E., Taylor, J.L., et al. (2008). Risk assessment in offenders with intellectual disability: a comparison across three levels of security. *International Journal of Offender Therapy and Comparative Criminology*, 52, 90–111.

Lindsay, W.R., Hamilton, C., Moulton, S., et al. (2011). Assessment and treatment of social problem solving in offenders with intellectual disability. *Psychology, Crime and Law*, 17, 181–197.

Lindsay, W.R., Carson, D., Holland, A.J., et al. (2013a). Alcohol and its relationship to offence variables in a cohort of offenders with intellectual disabilities. *Journal of Intellectual and Developmental Disability*, 38, 325–231.

Lindsay, W.R., Steptoe, L., Wallace, L., Haut, F., Brewster, E. (2013b). An evaluation and 20 year follow up of recidivism in a community intellectual disability service. *Criminal Behaviour and Mental Health*, 23, 138–149.

Lindsay, W.R., Smith, J.S., Tinsley, S., Macer, J., Miller, S. (2014). A programme for alcohol related violence with offenders with intellectual disability. *Journal of Intellectual Disabilities and Offending Behaviour*, 5, 107–119.

Linhorst, D.M., McCutchen, T.A., Bennett, L. (2003). Recidivism among offenders with developmental disabilities participating in a case management programme. *Research in Developmental Disabilities*, 24, 210–230.

Lofthouse, R.E., Totsika, V., Hastings, R.P., et al. (2014). How do static and dynamic risk factors work together to predict violence amongst offenders with an intellectual disability? *Journal of Intellectual Disability Research*, 58, 125–133.

Lund, J. (1990). Mentally retarded criminal offenders in Denmark. *British Journal of Psychiatry*, 156, 726–731.

MacEachron, A.E. (1979). Mentally retarded offenders prevalence and characteristics. *American Journal of Mental Deficiency*, 84, 165–176.

McCord, W. and McCord, J. (1959). *Origins of Crime: A New Evaluation of the Cambridge-Somerville Study*. New York, NY: Columbia Press.

McGillicuddy, N.B. and Blane, H.T. (1999). Substance use in individuals with mental retardation. *Addictive Behaviours*, 24, 869–878.

McGillivray, J. and Moore, M.R. (2001). Substance abuse by offenders with mild intellectual disability. *Journal of Intellectual and Developmental Disability*, 26, 279–310.

McMurran, M. (2013). Treatments for offenders in prison and the community. In M. McMurran (ed.), *Alcohol Related Violence: Prevention and Treatment*. Chichester, West Sussex, UK: Wiley-Blackwell.

McMurran, M., Fyffe, S., McCarthy, L., Duggan, C., Latham, A. (2001). Stop and think! Social problem solving therapy with personality disordered offenders. *Criminal Behaviour and Mental Health*, 11, 273–285.

Mears, D.P. and Cochran, J.C. (2013). What is the effect of IQ on offending? *Criminal Justice and Behavior*, 40, 1280–1300.

Meichenbaum, D. (1985). *Stress Inoculation Training*. Oxford: Pergamon Press.

Moffit, T.E., Gabrielli, W.F., Mednick, S.A., Schulsinger, F. (1991). Socio-economic status, IQ and delinquency. *Journal of Abnormal Psychology*, 90, 152–157.

Murphy, G.H., Sinclair, N., Hays, S-J., et al. (2010). Effectiveness of group cognitive-behavioural treatment for men with intellectual disabilities at risk of sexual offending. *Journal of Applied Research in Intellectual Disabilities*, 23, 537–551.

Nicoll, M., Beail, N., Saxon, D. (2013). Cognitive behavioural treatment for anger in adults with intellectual disabilities: a systematic review and meta-analysis. *Journal of Applied Research in Intellectual Disabilities*, 26, 47–62.

Novaco, R.W. (1975). *Anger Control: The Development and Evaluation of an Experimental Treatment*. Lexington, MA: Heath.

Novaco, R.W. and Taylor, J.L. (2004). Assessment of anger and aggression in male offenders with developmental disabilities. *Psychological Assessment*, 16, 42–50.

Novaco, R.W. and Taylor, J.L. (2015). Reduction of assaultive behaviour following anger treatment of forensic hospital patients with intellectual disabilities. *Behaviour Research and Therapy*, 65, 52–59.

O'Brien, G., Taylor, J.L., Lindsay, W.R., et al. (2010). A multi-centre study of adults with learning disabilities referred to services for antisocial or offending behaviour: demographic, individual, offending and service characteristics. *Journal of Learning Disabilities and Offending Behaviour*, 1(2), 5–15.

Prout, H.T. and Strohmer, D.C. (1991). *Emotional Problems Scales*. Odessa, FL: Psychological Assessment Resources.

Quinsey, V.L. (2004). Risk assessment and management in community settings. In W.R. Lindsay, J.L. Taylor, P. Sturmey (eds.), *Offenders with Developmental Disabilities*. Chichester, West Sussex, UK: John Wiley and Sons.

Quinsey, V.L., Book, A., Skilling, T.A. (2004). A follow-up of deinstitutionalised developmentally handicapped men with histories of antisocial behaviour. *Journal of Applied Research in Intellectual Disabilities*, 17, 243–254.

Raesaenen, P., Hirvenoj, A., Hakko, H., Vaeisaenen, E. (1994). Cognitive functioning ability of arsonists. *Journal of Forensic Psychiatry*, 5, 615–620.

Rice, M.E. and Chaplin, T.C. (1979). Social skills training for hospitalised male arsonists. *Journal of Behaviour Therapy and Experimental Psychiatry*, 10, 105–108.

Rimmer, J.H., Braddock, D., Marks, B. (1995). Health characteristics and behaviors of adults with mental retardation residing in three living arrangements. *Research in Developmental Disabilities*, 16, 489–499.

Rose, J., Jenkins, R., O'Conner, C., Jones, C., Felce, D. (2002). A group treatment for men with intellectual disabilities who sexually offend or abuse. *Journal of Applied Research in Intellectual Disabilities*, 15, 138–150.

Rose, J., Rose, D., Hawkins, C., Anderson, C. (2012). A sex offender treatment group for men with intellectual disabilities in a community setting. *British Journal of Forensic Practice*, 14, 21–28.

Ross, R.R. and Fabiano, E.A. (1985). *Time to Think: A Cognitive Model on Delinquency Prevention and Offender Rehabilitation*.

Johnson City, TN: Institute of Social Sciences and Arts.

Scheerenberger, R.C. (1983). *A History of Mental Retardation*. London: Brooks Publishing Company.

Søndenaa, E., Rasmussen, K., Palmstierna, T., Nøttestad, J. (2008) The prevalence and nature of intellectual disability in Norwegian prisons. *Journal of Research in Intellectual Disabilities*, 53, 1129–1137.

Sutherland, E.H. (1937). *The Professional Thief*. Chicago, IL: Chicago University Press.

Taylor, J.L. (2002). A review of assessment and treatment of anger and aggression in offenders with intellectual disability. *Journal of Intellectual Disability Research*, 46(Suppl. 1), 57–73.

Taylor, J.L. (2014). *Roots, referrals, risks and remedies for offenders with intellectual disabilities*. Paper presented to "A Risky Business" BPS conference, University of Manchester, UK, October, 2014.

Taylor, J.L. and Novaco, R.W. (2005). *Anger Treatment for People with Developmental Disabilities: A Theory, Evidence and Manual Based Approach*. Chichester, West Sussex, UK: Wiley.

Taylor, J.L. and Novaco, R.W. (2013). Anger control problems. In J.L. Taylor, W.R. Lindsay, R. Hastings, C. Hatton (eds.), *Psychological Therapies for Adults with Intellectual Disabilities*. Chichester, West Sussex, UK: Wiley.

Taylor, J.L., Novaco, R.W., Gillmer, B., Thorne, I. (2002a). Cognitive-behavioural treatment of anger intensity among offenders with intellectual disabilities. *Journal of Applied Research in Intellectual Disabilities*, 15, 151–165.

Taylor, J.L., Thorne, I., Robertson, A., Avery, G. (2002b). Evaluation of a group intervention for convicted arsonists with mild and borderline intellectual disabilities. *Criminal Behaviour and Mental Health*, 12, 282–293.

Taylor, J.L., Novaco, R.W., Guinan, C., Street, N. (2004a). Development of an imaginal provocation test to evaluate treatment for anger problems in people with intellectual disabilities. *Clinical Psychology and Psychotherapy*, 11, 233–246.

Taylor, J.L., Thorne, I., Slavkin, M. (2004b). Treatment of firesetters. In W.R. Lindsay, J.L. Taylor, P. Sturmey (eds.), *Offenders with Developmental Disabilities*. Chichester, West Sussex, UK: Wiley.

Taylor, J.L., Novaco, R.W., Gillmer, B.T., Robertson, A., Thorne, I. (2005). Individual cognitive-behavioural anger treatment for people with mild–borderline intellectual disabilities and histories of aggression: a controlled trial. *British Journal of Clinical Psychology*, 44, 367–382.

Taylor, J.L., Robertson, A., Thorne, I., Belshaw, T., Watson, A. (2006). Responses of female firesetters with mild and borderline intellectual disabilities to a group-based intervention. *Journal of Applied Research in Intellectual Disabilities*, 19, 179–190.

Terman, L. (1911). *The Measurement of Intelligence*. Boston, MA: Houghton Mifflin.

Webster, C.D., Eaves, D., Douglas, K.S., Wintrup, A. (1997). *The HCR-20: The Assessment of Dangerousness and Risk. Version 2*. Vancouver, BC: Simon Fraser University and British Colombia Forensic Psychiatric Services Commission.

West, D.J. and Farrington, D.P. (1973). *Who Becomes Delinquent?* London: Heinemann.

Westermeyer, J., Kemp, K., Nugent, S. (1996). Substance disorder among persons with mental retardation: a comparative study. *American Journal on Addiction*, 5, 23–31.

Wheeler, J.R., Clare, I.C.H., Holland, A.J. (2014). What can social and environmental factors tell us about the risk of offending by people with intellectual disabilities? *Psychology, Crime and Law*, 20, 635–658.

Willis, G.M., and Grace, R.C. (2009). Assessment of community reintegration planning for sex offenders: poor planning predicts recidivism. *Criminal Justice and Behavior*, 36, 494–512.

Willner, P. (2007). Cognitive behaviour therapy for people with learning disabilities: focus on anger. *Advances in Mental Health and Learning Disabilities*, 1(2), 14–21.

Problem behaviors and the interface with psychiatric disorders

Sally-Ann Cooper

Introduction

Problem behaviors are common amongst people with intellectual disabilities (ID), and typically have a negative impact on their quality of life. The interface between problem behaviors and mental disorders has been a topic of debate for some time, with consideration, for example, of whether problem behaviors are "behavioral equivalents" for other disorders, such as depression, or are symptoms of such disorders. Current classifications of psychopathology do little to throw any light on this. This may be due to the limited research in this area, despite its importance.

Problem (or "challenging") behaviors

Problem behaviors are of clinical and societal significance, having implications for the person, including restricting their opportunities for community participation and even where they live, impacting on quality of life, with implications also for family and paid carers, and a financial cost to the state providing care. They are also common amongst people with ID. Prevalence has been reported to range from 1.7% (Rojahn, 1986) to 41% (Salovita, 2000) for self-injurious behavior, and from 7.0% (Emerson et al., 2001) to 51.8% (Crocker et al., 2006) for aggressive behavior. These wide ranges are accounted for by methodological differences and limitations in studies, particularly the type of sample studied (for example institutional or community), age ranges, methods of data collection, time period included, and definitions/criteria. Hemmings et al. (2013) provide a solid review of studies, particularly with regards to adults with ID. A recent population-based study of 1023 adults with ID reported a point prevalence of 22.5% for all problem behaviors (Jones et al., 2008), and, specifically, 4.9% for self-injurious behavior (Cooper et al., 2009a) and 9.8% for aggressive behavior (6.3% for physically aggressive behavior to others, 3.0% for destructiveness, and 7.5% for verbally aggressive behavior) (Cooper et al., 2009b), with Emerson et al. (2001) providing similar rates. Within the same population, mental ill-health of any type, excluding problem behaviors, had a point prevalence of 28.1% (Cooper et al., 2007). Clearly then, given that both problem behaviors and mental ill-health are so common, they will coexist in some individuals. This itself is important, and additionally it has been suggested that there may be a more intimate relationship, with problem behaviors presenting sometimes as a symptom of

Psychiatric and Behavioral Disorders in Intellectual and Developmental Disabilities, ed. Colin Hemmings and Nick Bouras. Published by Cambridge University Press. © Cambridge University Press 2016.

another mental disorder. Additionally, other mental disorders may occur more commonly in people with problem behaviors. Figure 20.1 shows the overlap between mental ill-health, problem behaviors, and epilepsy (another common neuropsychiatric disorder in this population), taken from the same cohort of 1023 adults.

Despite the variation in reported prevalences, it is apparent that problem behaviors are common, so it is perhaps suprising that the relationship with mental ill-health has been so little examined. There is still considerable controversy as to whether problem behaviors should be considered as a type of mental disorder at all. Some clinicians point to the fact that environmental factors can play such a strong role in determining whether or not a person challenges services (hence coining the term "challenging behavior" with the focus on the service adapting to ameliorate the challenge). Yet clearly there is strong evidence for some problem behaviors being biologically driven in some people, as seen, for example, in the behavioral phenotypes of some of the syndromes that cause ID such as Smith–Magenis syndrome, Angelman syndrome, and Prader–Willi syndrome. It seems likely that for many people with problem behaviors, both these views are over-simplistic, and an interaction between biological, psychological, social, environmental, and developmental factors are etiological to the onset and continuation or remission of problem behaviors.

Some studies suggest that problem behaviors have much in common with other types of mental ill-health. For example, one study of 651 community-based adults with ID used logistic regression analyses and found that the independant predictors for onset of problem behaviors were divorce of parents in childhood, not living with a family carer, lower ability level, and preceding life events (Smiley et al., 2007). Indeed, several studies have reported associations between life events and problem behaviors (Wigham et al.,

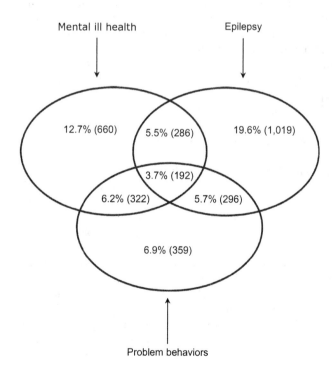

Figure 20.1 Coexistence of problem behaviors, mental ill-health, and epilepsy in 1023 adults with intellectual disabilities.

Mental ill health

Epilepsy

12.7% (660)

5.5% (286)

19.6% (1,019)

3.7% (192)

6.2% (322)

5.7% (296)

6.9% (359)

Problem behaviors

2011), and between severity of ID and problem behaviors (Collacott et al., 1998; Emerson et al., 2001; Tyrer et al., 2006; Lowe et al., 2007). These findings are similar to other types of common mental disorders that are often triggered by life events, showing a gradient across ability levels extending not just in the ID range but into average and high intellectual ability.

Large-scale investigation of the course of problem behaviors over time has also received little attention, and in view of methodological differences and study limitations, published research shows high variations. Self-injurious behavior has been reported to remit in between 3.7% and 96% of people (Schroeder et al., 1978, 1986; Murphy et al., 1993), with Emerson et al. (2001) suggesting a 29% remission rate at eight-year follow-up, and Cooper et al. (2009a) demonstrating a 38.2% remission rate after two years. Aggression has been shown to follow a remitting–relapsing course (Cooper et al., 2009b) with a 27.7% remission after two years, and another study of a cohort over 11 years also showed that some people improved (Totsika et al., 2008). Parallels can be drawn with other types of mental ill-health, some of which can show relapsing–remitting courses, such as depressive illness and schizophrenia.

Current nosological status of problem behaviors is reflected in current classifications. Classifications should have face validity, descriptive validity whereby categories do not overlap, and predictive validity. Initially, classificatory systems merely describe the symptoms and signs within disorders; then, as evidence increases, they should gradually integrate scientific characteristics to classify disorders of structure, function, and etiology, and so become increasingly sophisticated and evidence based. Inspection of the main classifications in use today show how little progress has been made towards this goal. The *International Classification of Diseases and Related Health Problems, Tenth Revision* (ICD-10) (World Health Organization, 1992) classified various problem behaviors, including conduct disorder in children (which does not quite encapsulate the problem behaviors seen so commonly in people with ID), pica of infancy and childhood, and various other behaviors that seem less relevant to most people with ID (Table 20.1). The specifier, "significant impairment of behavior," which is available on the main codes for ID, does not actually report whether this refers to adaptive behavior or maladaptive behavior, and provides no description or operational rules for its use. It is, at the time of writing, still unclear as to the extent to which problem behaviors as experienced by people with ID will be included in the *International Classification of Diseases, Eleventh Edition* (ICD-11), which is currently underway. The *Diagnostic and Statistical Manual of Mental Disorders, Fifth Edition* (DSM-5) (American Psychiatric Association, 2013), includes a section on disruptive, impulse-control, and conduct disorders, which includes oppositional defiant disorder (which requires the presence of deliberate intent, so is less relevant to most people with ID who have problem behaviors), intermittent explosive disorder, conduct disorder (which also requires the presence of deliberate intent), pyromania, and kleptomania. The differences between the two manuals and their failures to encapsulate even a description of problem behaviors as experienced by people with ID is rather revealing in terms of how advanced existing evidence is.

There have been some studies that have gone back to the starting point and attempted to statistically analyze the relationship between mental ill-health and problem behaviors. Sixteen studies were identified by Melville (2010) as using factor analysis to identify the factors/dimensions of psychopathology that do occur in adults with ID, rather than presuming which disorders exist and how they present. This is an interesting way

Table 20.1 Problem behaviors specified in ICD-10

Mental retardation – significant impairment of behavior (*ICD-10 Guide for Mental Retardation*; WHO, 1996) (F70–79.x)	Overeating associated with other psychological disturbances (F50.4)
Conduct disorder (F91)	Vomiting associated with other psychological disturbances (F50.5)
Oppositional defiant disorder (F91.3)	Abuse of non-dependence-producing substances (F55)
Personality and behavioral disorders due to brain disease, damage, and dysfunction (F07)	Other specified disorders of adult personality and behavior (F68.8)
Trichotillomania (F63.3)	Elective mutism (F94.0)
Pyromania (F63.1)	Non-organic enuresis (F98.0)
Pathological stealing (F63.3)	Non-organic encopresis (F98.1)
Other habit and impulse disorders (F63.8)	Feeding disorder of infancy or childhood (F98.2)
Other specified behavioral disorders, with onset in childhood and adolescence (F98.8)	Pica of infancy and childhood (F98.3)

forward to investigate the nature of problem behaviors within the context of other psychopathology. However, several of these studies have not included problem behaviors in their datasets in view of the instruments they used, and some have not used best practice guidelines for factor analysis as described by Costello and Osborne, 2005. Only three studies were identified which have included problem behaviors as well as other types of psychopathology (Sturmey et al., 2010; Tsiouris et al., 2011; Melville et al., 2014).

With improvements in methodology over time, Melville et al.'s (2014) study is one of the more informative. They followed best practice guidelines and conducted both exploratory and confirmatory factor analysis using two discrete clinical datasets ($N = 457$; $N = 274$), to examine the relationship between problem behaviors and other psychopathology. They also reported predictive validity of the dimensions they extracted using five-year longitudinal data. Five factors/dimensions were identified and then confirmed. Problem behaviors were included in a factor/dimension, which they termed "emotion dysregulation-problem behavior" and this was distinct from the depressive factor/dimension, demonstrating descriptive validity, and that problem behaviors should not be viewed as a behavioral equivalent in depressive disorders. The identified factor/ dimension had strong predictive validity in terms of severity ratings on the *Health of the Nation Outcome Scales for People with Learning Disabilities* (HoNOS-LD; Roy et al., 2002), the *Global Assessment of Functioning* (GAF; American Psychiatric Association, 2000), the *Clinical Global Impression* (CGI; Guy, 1976), and the *Camberwell Assessment of Need for Adults with Developmental and Intellectual Disabilities* (CANDID; Xenitidis et al., 2000) rating scales. It also had strong predictive validity after five years on the HoNOS-LD, the GAF, and the CGI outcome measures. The symptom profile within emotion dysregulation-problem behavior was verbal aggression, physical aggression, mood lability, irritable mood, and self-harm. This approach to better understanding the interface between problem behaviors and other psychopathology appears promising, and may be the way forward in future to improve on current classificatory systems and clinical care and supports for people with ID.

Problem behaviors may be a representation of distress experienced by adults with ID. The distinction of the emotion dysregulation-problem behavior factor/dimension from the depressive factor/dimension does not mean people with problem behaviors do not develop depression; indeed, they may be at higher risk of it, as problem behaviors can result in stress, limitations, and restrictions to the adult's life, which might predispose to depression.

Studies from developmental cognitive neuroscience are increasingly recognizing the importance of emotion regulation to developmental psychopathology (Gross and Thompson, 2007). However, such work is at only an early stage with regards to people with ID (McClure et al., 2009), though studies have now begun to investigate the relationship between emotional dysregulation, problem behaviors, and mental ill-health in adults with ID (Sappok et al., 2014).

How the existing evidence base has been translated into practice for the benefit of service users

Managing and supporting people with problem behavior is essential to improve their quality of life. There is some promising research showing that group therapies may help people with ID and aggression (Willner et al., 2013). Clinical services often provide a range of psychosocial interventions to help people, but the reality is that antipsychotic medication is often used for persons with problem behaviors (Tyrer et al., 2014). Concern over the use of such drugs has been voiced repeatedly over recent decades, yet they are still in common use, despite a lack of research demonstrating their effectiveness. This demonstrates our current poor understanding of the nature of problem behaviors and their interface with mental disorders, and highlights the need for further research; for example, into the use of mood-stabilizing drugs and interventions to enhance emotional regulation.

Conclusions

The interface between problem behaviors and other mental disorders remains poorly understood, as highlighted by current classificatory manuals for mental disorders. This is despite their common occurence, and that they are distressing for the individual, and can have wider ramifications for the individual and their family and carers. Recent research has included statistical approaches to better understand this interface, and is starting to suggest that there may be a role for the development of emotional-regulation strategies. In time, we may be better equipped to assist people with this need.

Key summary points

- Problem (or challenging) behaviors are common, and can follow a relapsing–remitting course.
- An interaction between biological, psychological, social, environmental, and developmental factors are probably etiological to the onset and continuation or remission of the majority of problem behaviors.
- Studies have now begun to investigate the relationship between emotional dysregulation, problem behaviors, and mental ill-health in adults with ID.

References

American Psychiatric Association. (2000). *Diagnostic and Statistical Manual of Mental Disorders – Text Revision, Fourth Edition.* Washington, DC: American Psychiatric Association.

American Psychiatric Association. (2013). *Diagnostic and Statistical Manual of Mental Disorders, Fifth Edition.* Washington, DC: American Psychiatric Association.

Collacott, R.A., Cooper, S-A., Branford, D., McGrother, C. (1998). Epidemiology of self injurious behavior in adults with learning disabilities. *British Journal of Psychiatry,* 173, 428–432.

Cooper, S-A., Smiley, E., Morrison, J., Allan, L., Williamson, A. (2007). Prevalence of and associations with mental ill-health in adults with intellectual disabilities. *British Journal of Psychiatry,* 190, 27–35.

Cooper, S-A., Smiley, E., Allan, L., et al. (2009a). Adults with intellectual disabilities. Prevalence, incidence and remission of self-injurious behaviour, and related factors. *Journal of Intellectual Disability Research,* 53, 200–216.

Cooper, S-A., Smiley, E., Jackson, A., et al. (2009b). Adults with intellectual disabilities. Prevalence, incidence, and remission of aggressive behaviour, and related factors. *Journal of Intellectual Disability Research,* 53, 217–232.

Costello, A.B. and Osborne, J.W. (2005). Best practices in exploratory factor analysis: four recommendations for getting the most from your analysis. *Practical Assessment, Research and Evaluation,* 10, 1–9.

Crocker, A.G., Mercier, C., Lachapelle, Y., et al. (2006). Prevalence and types of aggressive behaviour among adults with intellectual disabilities. *Journal of Intellectual Disability Research,* 50, 652–661.

Emerson, E., Kiernan, C., Alborz, A., et al. (2001). The prevalence of challenging behaviours: a total population study. *Research in Developmental Disabilities,* 22, 77–93.

Gross, J. and Thompson, R.A. (2007) Emotion regulation: conceptual foundations. In J.

Gross (ed.), *Handbook of Emotion Regulation.* New York, NY: Guilford.

Guy, W. (ed.) (1976). *ECDEU Assessment Manual for Psychopharmacology.* Rockville, MD: US Department of Heath, Education, and Welfare, Public Health Service, Alcohol, Drug Abuse, and Mental Health Administration.

Hemmings, C., Deb, S., Chaplin, E., Hardy, S., Mukherjee, R. (2013). Research for people with intellectual disabilities and mental health problems: a view from the UK. *Journal of Mental Health Research in Intellectual Disability,* 6, 127–158.

Jones, S., Cooper, S-A., Smiley, E., et al. (2008). Prevalence of, and factors associated with, problem behaviours in adults with intellectual disabilities. *Journal of Nervous and Mental Disease,* 196, 678–686.

Lowe, K., Allen, D., Jones E., et al. (2007). Challenging behaviours: prevalence and topographies. *Journal of Intellectual Disability Research,* 51, 625–636.

McClure, K.S., Halpern, J., Wolper, P.A., Donahue, J.J. (2009). Emotion regulation and intellectual disability. *Journal of Developmental Disabilities,* 15, 38–44.

Melville, C. (2010). Examining dimensional models of psychopathology experienced by adults with intellectual disabilities. MD thesis. Glasgow: University of Glasgow.

Melville, C., McConnachie, A., Simpson, N., Smiley, E., Cooper, S-A. (2014). *Developing Valid Models of Psychopathology Experienced by Adults with Learning Disabilities, Final Report.* Edinburgh: Chief Scientist Office, Scottish Government.

Murphy, G.H., Oliver, C., Corbett, J., et al. (1993). Epidemiology of self-injury: characteristics of people with severe self-injury and initial treatment outcome. In C. Kiernan (ed.), *Research to Practice? Implications of Research on the Challenging Behaviour of People with Learning Disability.* Clevedon, North Somerset, UK: BILD Publications.

Rojahn, J. (1986). Self-injurious and stereotypic behaviour of non-institutionalised mentally retarded people: prevalence and classification. *American Journal of Mental Deficiency,* 91, 268–276.

Roy, A., Matthews, H., Clifford, P., Fowler, V., Martin, D.M. (2002). Health of the Nation Outcome Scales for People with Learning Disabilities (HoNOS-LD). *British Journal of Psychiatry*, 180, 61–66.

Salovita, T. (2000). The structure and correlates of self-injurious behaviour in an institutional setting. *Research in Developmental Disabilities*, 21, 501–511.

Sappok, T., Budczies, J., Dziobek, I., et al. (2014). The missing link: delayed emotional development predicts challenging behavior in adults with intellectual disability. *Journal of Autism and Developmental Disorders*, 44, 786–800.

Schroeder, S.R., Schroeder, C.S., Smith, B., Dallorf, J. (1978). Prevalence of self-injurious behaviors in a large state facility for the retarded: a three-year follow-up study. *Journal of Autism and Childhood Schizophrenia*, 8, 261–269.

Schroeder. S.R., Bickel, W.K., Richmond, G. (1986). Primary and secondary prevention of self-injurious behaviours: a life long problem. *Advances in Learning and Behavioural Disabilities*, 5, 63–85.

Smiley, E., Cooper, S-A., Finlayson, J., et al. (2007). The incidence, and predictors of mental ill-health in adults with intellectual disabilities. Prospective study. *British Journal of Psychiatry*, 191, 313–319.

Sturmey, P., Laud, R.B., Cooper, C.L., Matson, J.L., Fodstad, J.C. (2010). Challenging behaviors should not be considered depressive equivalents in individuals with intellectual disabilities. II. A replication study. *Research in Developmental Disabilities*, 31, 1002–1007.

Totsika, V., Toogood, T., Hastings, R.P., et al. (2008). Persistence of challenging behavoiurs in adults with intellectual disability over a period of 11 years. *Journal of Intellectual Disability Research*, 52, 446–457.

Tsiouris, J.A., Kim, S.Y., Brown, W.T., Cohen, I.L. (2011). Association of aggressive behaviours with psychiatric disorders, age, sex and degree of intellectual disability: a large-scale survey. *Journal of Intellectual Disability Research*, 55, 636–649.

Tyrer, F., McGrother, C.W., Thorp, C.F., et al. (2006). Physical aggression towards others in adults with learning disabilities: prevalence and associated factors. *Journal of Intellectual Disability Research*, 50, 294–304.

Tyrer, P., Cooper, S-A., Hassiotis, A. (2014). Drug treatments in people with intellectual disability and challenging behaviour: time to rethink? *British Medical Journal*, 348, G4323.

Wigham, S., Hatton, C., Taylor, J.L (2011). The effects of traumatizing life events on people with intellectual disabilities: a systematic review. *Journal of Mental Health Research in Intellectual Disabilities*, 4, 19–39.

Willner, P., Rose, J., Jahoda, A., et al. (2013). Group-based cognitive-behavioural anger management for people with mild to moderate intellectual disabilities: cluster randomised controlled trial. *British Journal of Psychiatry*, 203, 288–296.

World Health Organization. (1992).*The ICD-10 Classification of Mental and Behavioural Disorders: Clinical Descriptions and Diagnostic Guidelines*. Geneva: World Health Organization.

World Health Organization. (1996). *ICD-10 Guide for Mental Retardation*. At: http://www.who.int/iris/handle/10665/63000

Xenitidis, K., Thornicroft, G., Leese, M., et al. (2000). Reliability and validity of the CANDID – a needs assessment instrument for adults with learning disabilities and mental health problems. *British Journal of Psychiatry*, 176, 473–478.

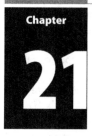

Chapter

21

The interface between medical and psychiatric disorders

Jessica A. Hellings and Seema Jain

Introduction

Individuals of all ages with intellectual disabilities (ID) require both acute and long-term high-level services to treat their complex medical and psychiatric needs, and to minimize impacts of neuropsychiatric and medical comorbidity on their cognitive, health, and mobility limitations. Increasingly, the scientific evidence base is expanded by studies linking brain disorders to somatic disease states such as obesity, autoimmune disorders, and gut–brain influences.

In general, access to clinical care of all types for patients with ID remains limited by several critical factors (Kwok and Cheung, 2007), notably: (1) inadequate training of healthcare professionals, including psychiatrists (Marrus et al., 2013); (2) limited availability of appropriate and accessible transportation; (3) physical barriers to healthcare and exercise facilities to accommodate individuals with mobility issues; (4) high turnover rates of support staff, who also lack sufficient training; (5) the phenomenon known as diagnostic overshadowing (Reiss et al., 1982), which describes incorrect attribution of a treatable psychiatric illness to the underlying disability; and (6) under-recognition of, and failure to address, past trauma, disrupted attachments, and loss of identity, all of which contribute to ongoing psychiatric illness and behavioral challenges (Harvey, 2012).

Individuals with ID may lack abilities needed to make informed choices, and also basic autonomy over healthcare decision-making and medication use. An example is limitation in the ability to request a trial of tapering-off of medications causing adverse side effects or those prescribed for concurrent problems such as seasonal allergies, depression, or indigestion. The average number of physical and psychiatric diagnoses combined in individuals with ID is 10; likewise, the average number of medications received on a daily basis is 10. Emergency department use by individuals with disabling conditions accounts for a relatively high amount of expenditures (Rasch et al., 2013).

Vision and oral-health needs

In a study by Owens et al. (2006), only 28% of children with ID had normal vision compared to 75% of typically developing children. The authors found that refractive errors were the commonest cause of decreased vision, notably hyperopia, myopia, and

Psychiatric and Behavioral Disorders in Intellectual and Developmental Disabilities, ed. Colin Hemmings and Nick Bouras. Published by Cambridge University Press. © Cambridge University Press 2016.

astigmatism, and that 27–52% of persons with ID had a refractive error compared to 4–25% of the US general population. In addition, other vision problems, including strabismus, cataracts, and keratoconus, were more prevalent in the population with ID in comparison with the general population. Poor vision may account for repeated falling and also compounds intellectual and physical disabilities.

A study by Hulland and Sigal (2000) found that oral-health needs are also greater in persons with ID. The study showed that 18–84% of people with ID had untreated dental caries compared to 16–55% in the general population. Periodontal disease is common, and can produce fever, discomfort, and challenging behaviors, and is often missed in those with communication deficits (Prater and Zylstra, 2006). Oral bacteria also play a role in cardiac disease, which in turn also impacts brain health and function.

Deficiencies in oral healthcare behavior resulting in poor oral hygiene are common in persons with ID. Limited ability to understand the prophylactic importance of tooth brushing may be accompanied by poor physical coordination in persons with ID, both contributing to suboptimal oral hygiene. For outpatient dental appointments in uncooperative patients, the administration of a low dose of benzodiazepine, such as 1–2 mg of alprazolam an hour before appointments, may improve cooperation. In some cases, hospitalization may be necessary to perform dental care under anesthesia.

Healthcare screenings

Basic healthcare screenings such as mammograms and Pap smears occur at lower rates in individuals with developmental disabilities. Women with ID have higher risks for leukemia, and for other tumors including breast, uterine, and colorectal cancers (Rajan, 2013). Comorbidities render colonoscopy preparation and examination difficult; discussion of each patient's individual issues prior to the event is needed. Only 19% of those with ID over age 50 years have had colorectal screenings (Fischer et al., 2012). Individuals with ID living with parents or independently are much less likely to have received preventive services than those in institutional community-based settings.

Cancer risks

Duff et al. (2001) found higher rates of gastrointestinal (GI) cancer in institutionalized persons with ID than in the general population, and also a significant number of deaths due to perforated stomach ulcers. They postulated that common *Helicobacter pylori* infections in institutionalized populations may account for this observation, and a different approach may be needed to eradicate this infection in persons with ID.

A population study conducted in Finland followed 2173 persons with ID from 1967 to 1997 for cancer incidence (Patja et al., 2001). The investigators found an increased risk of thyroid and gallbladder cancers, but a decreased risk of prostate, lung, and urinary tract cancers. The incidence of cancers overall was comparable to that in the general population. The reduced risk of lung cancer was likely explained by lower rates of smoking (9% versus 37% in the general population).

Although previous studies had reported up to a threefold increased rate of GI cancers in persons with ID, this study did not confirm an overall higher risk for GI cancers. However, there was increased risk identified for some cancer subtypes, notably of the gallbladder, esophagus, and undefined GI cancers. There is an increase in risk of esophageal cancers, correlated with an increased incidence of gastroesophageal reflux disease (GERD) and Barrett's esophagus. The increase in gallbladder cancer rates may relate to the increased use of medications that affect hepatic enzyme function and also the increased overweight and fatty liver risk in persons with ID, as well as a higher incidence of gallstones.

Medical conditions impacting behavior/psychiatric illness with aging

Emotional supports normally protect against health problems, including heart disease and depression. However, individuals with ID have been shown to have significantly fewer emotional supports, as well as loss of key parental and grandparental supports with aging.

Individuals with long-term disabilities and especially immobility are more likely to experience early onset of obesity, coronary heart disease, diabetes, stroke, osteoporosis, arthritis, renal disease, various forms of cancer, infections, and injuries.

A Canadian study comparing the prevalence of chronic health conditions in people with and without ID found reported higher rates of thyroid disorder and heart disease than was reported in the general population (Morin et al., 2012). Food allergies, migraines, arthritis, and back pain were less likely to be reported in individuals with ID, although this finding could be explained partly by communication difficulties. Individuals with Down syndrome are also more prone to autoimmune diseases, including hypothyroidism, juvenile rheumatoid arthritis, and celiac disease, as well as blood dyscrasias.

Pain syndromes

Persons with ID often lack adequate pain treatment, and their pain prevalence is higher than in the general population (Baldridge and Andrasik, 2010). In the setting of cognitive and communication impairments in patients, healthcare professionals must employ a high index of suspicion and explore all possible sources of pain as contributors to observed challenging behaviors.

Menstrual cramps and discomfort can produce or worsen self-injurious behavior, aggression, or agitation (Carr et al., 2003). Hormonal interventions, for example the levonorgestrel intrauterine system (Mirena®), may be employed to alleviate these problems (Pillal et al., 2010). Hormonal treatments may, however, also worsen moodiness and can cause deep vein thrombosis or strokes, especially if the dummy pills are skipped.

Approximately 70% of those with mobility problems associated with their disability are likely to have osteoporosis or osteopenia, which predisposes to hip, spine, and disk degeneration, and fractures. Individuals aging with cerebral palsy are more likely than the general population to suffer fractures (Murphy et al., 1995). Persons with ID and Down syndrome, hypogonadism, and those receiving antiepileptics or the ketogenic diet for seizure control are also at increased risk for osteoporosis.

Migraine or cluster headaches may be difficult to elicit in persons with ID owing to their impaired communication skills; sometimes they suffer rare but severe explosive outbursts accompanied by self-injury and aggression. Prophylactic treatments for headache may be helpful in such cases (Baldridge and Andrasik, 2010).

Neurological problems

Neurological conditions associated with ID and behavioral deterioration may include hyponatremia (related to medications or compulsive polydipsia), seizures, hydrocephalus, ventriculo-peritoneal shunt blockage, headaches, transient ischemic attacks, brain tumors, and encephalitis. These may present as acute, intermittent, or chronic mental status changes.

Antiseizure medications, including phenobarbital, phenytoin, mysoline, carbamazepine, and oxcarbazepine, may produce hyperactivity and behavioral worsening (Trimble and Cull, 1988). Topiramate may produce cognitive dulling, behavioral worsening, and renal calculi. Alzheimer's disease has early onset in the late 30s in many adults with Down syndrome (Lott and Head, 2001).

Gastrointestinal problems

Gastrointestinal problems are common in ID, especially if autism spectrum disorders (ASD) and also present. Reflux esophagitis, reverse peristalsis, *H. pylori* infections, irritable bowel syndrome, fecal impaction, bloating, abdominal discomfort, nausea, constipation, and bowel obstruction may all present with behavioral problems, including self-injury. Pica (ingestion of non-food objects) may result in cessation of eating and drinking, for example if an object obstructs the esophagus.

Persons with ID and physical disabilities may suffer from swallowing difficulties, with associated choking, impaired hydration, and malnutrition (Kennedy et al., 1997). Aspiration may be silent, and lead to bronchitis, pneumonia, or even death, and requires that clinicians use a high index of suspicion when treating persons with ID and accompanying neurological disorders, including cerebral palsy (Chaney and Eyman, 2000).

Constipation and accompanying fecal impaction may produce associated unexplained behavioral changes, and are common in this patient population (Bohmer et al., 2001). Avoidance of white flour products and the simple dietary addition of pears and plums to replace apples and bananas may be helpful. Medical causes and medication side effects should also be considered.

Gastroesophageal reflux disease (GERD) may produce unexplained changes in behavior, and the individual with poor communication skills may be unable to communicate their discomfort. Cough, choking, and sore throat may be other associated signs of GERD, which also is common in individuals with Down syndrome (Bohmer et al., 2000).

Food allergies, including gluten and lactose intolerance, should be investigated if suspected. Liver disease, including hepatitis B infection, may account for sudden appetite and food preference changes. Celiac disease, an autoimmune disease produced by gluten antibodies and malabsorption of nutrients due to intestinal damage, may produce malaise, fatigue, anemia, hepatitis, arthritis, GI symptoms such as irritable bowel syndrome, peripheral neuropathy, and skin rash (Green and Jones, 2010). Psychiatric symptoms may include refusals related to the associated pervasive tiredness, as well as anxiety, panic disorder, depression, and psychosis (Carta et al., 2002; Genuis and Lobo, 2014). More studies are needed to clarify the relationship between gluten sensitivity, gluten intolerance, and ASD etiology or worsening.

Eating disorders

As defined by The *International Classification of Diseases and Related Health Problems, Tenth Revision* (ICD-10) (World Health Organization, 1992), eating disorders are diagnosed in 1–4% of young women in the general population. However, eating disorders are identified in 3–42% of persons with ID in institutions and 1–19% of those with ID in the community. Of persons with ID, 2–35% are obese and 5–43% are underweight (Gravestock, 2000).

Substance abuse

In mental health settings, substance-abusing persons with ID make up between 1% and 34% of the client population (Slayter, 2010). Persons with mild to moderate ID are more likely to develop substance abuse than those with more severe ID who have less independence in the community. There are risks of drug interactions and substance abuse in individuals with ID if they are receiving psychotropic medications. Clients with substance abuse in general are more likely to receive treatment, and also to remain in treatment, than are clients with substance abuse and ID. Substance-abuse treatment in persons with ID should highlight family education, applied behavior analysis, safety management, and social and communication skills development.

Sexuality and sexually transmitted diseases

Sexually transmitted diseases can occur in persons with ID, although they are commonly overlooked (Prater and Zylstra, 2006). Issues such as sexuality are underexplored in patients with ID in general.

Medication side effects

See also Chapter 13.

Drug interactions should be borne in mind when prescribing drug treatments and reviewing medication regimens. Medication side effects not already discussed may include allergy, skin rashes, and akathisia (motor restlessness). Lithium treatment in individuals with ID is more likely to produce disabling tremor, thirst and wetting, and toxicity, which goes undiagnosed longer and may be life-threatening. Several antiseizure agents induce hepatic enzymes to metabolize medications of multiple types, not only psychotropic medications, significantly more rapidly. These include phenobarbital, phenytoin, carbamazepine, and oxcarbazepine. Thus, the effective doses of other medications metabolized by the liver will be unknown, albeit lower. Conversely, the selective serotonin reuptake inhibitors (SSRIs) paroxetine, fluoxetine, and sertraline inhibit the liver enzyme cytochrome P450 2D6, thus raising effective doses of medications metabolized by that enzyme. For example, concomitant benzodiazepines may cause more sedation than expected, and atypical antipsychotics then produce even more excessive weight gain and associated morbidity and mortality.

Clinical approach

On an individual level, it is vital for clinicians to get to know each patient, and to ask detailed questions pertaining to medical and psychiatric illnesses, but also to explore details of his or her life on all levels. Viewing the person as a whole should also include questions regarding sleep, diet, exercise, and activities enjoyed, as well as family supports and pets. Individuals with hearing impairment may favor conducting interviews in written format over use of sign language, for example, if they can write. Engaging the person directly at their ability level with respect and adequate time empowers them to communicate directly regarding their problems, and to make better health choices. Many important details are elicited simply by chatting to the patient and their caregivers.

Spiritual beliefs and their impact on well-being and health should also be explored (Gaventa and Coulter, 2002; Peach, 2003). This may also be vital in serving other cultures; for example, certain African cultures' beliefs that spirits of ancestors control one's life, as well as an individual's health and disease. As an example, a child with autism and ID was once tied outside to a tree so that evil spirits would not enter the family home.

The psychiatric professional using the biopsychosocial–spiritual approach (Lennox, 2007) needs to focus on details of all types of symptoms, and to sort them into categories of: (i) psychiatric disorder(s); (ii) medical/neurological illnesses, including possible seizures; (iii) medication-related side effects; (iv) environmental-related stressors. Thereafter, appropriate interventions, tests, or referrals can be made. Details to be clarified include any changes coincident with the time of onset or exacerbation of problems, and associated factors that improve or worsen the symptoms. Reliable caregivers' input is vital in elucidating these clues.

Importance of genetic evaluation and testing

See also Chapter 18.

Genetic evaluation and testing is indicated for every individual identified with a developmental disability. A genetic cause for ID can be identified in up to 40% of cases, which may then inform psychiatric and medical treatments as well as necessary ongoing health screenings, such as for carcinoma in certain cases. Every gene can now be studied, in a microarray, to identify nucleotide deletions, duplications, and copy number variants (Butler et al., 2012). As part of a genetic evaluation, a detailed extended family history is obtained, as well as a detailed developmental, medical, and psychiatric history, and a thorough physical examination and other appropriate tests such as blood tests or brain imaging. Specific DNA studies are ordered from one or more blood samples, including for the FMR1 mutation to exclude fragile X in all males with ID, and for the Rett syndrome, MECP2 gene-deletion screening in all females with ASD. A karyotype, or whole chromosome study, may identify congenital syndromes such as Down syndrome, Klinefelter syndrome (XXY), Turner syndrome (XO), or supermale (XYY).

Adults with Down syndrome are at risk of developing Alzheimer's dementia in their late 30s. Individuals of all ages with Down syndrome also often manifest obsessions about one or more other individuals, which may interfere with their functioning and requires further study. Individuals with fragile X syndrome are prone to attention-deficit/hyperactivity disorder (ADHD), bipolar disorder, obsessive-compulsive disorder (OCD), and mitral valve prolapse, as well as Parkinson-like brain disease in later life. The most severe type of Prader–Willi syndrome (PWS) results from deletion at 15p11–13, which is associated with severe OCD, accompanied by explosive outbursts, insatiable appetite, morbid obesity, type 2 diabetes, scoliosis, and skin picking. Fluoxetine may be useful for such problems (Hellings and Warnock, 1994). Maternal duplication in the same chromosomal region leads to a less severe form of PWS, which, however, is associated with development of psychosis in adulthood. Individuals with deletion of 16p13.3 may have Rubinstein–Taybi syndrome, with characteristic broadening of the thumbs and halluces, and facial features of a beaked nose and downward-slanting eyes, as well as proneness to develop bipolar disorder (Levitas and Reid, 1998; Hellings et al., 2002).

Many congenital syndromes are now associated with behavioral phenotypes. More than 20 congenital syndromes are associated with obesity. The prescription of psychotropic medications producing marked weight gain, such as atypical antipsychotic drugs (Hellings et al., 2001, 2010; Correll et al., 2009) in adolescents and adults, should be minimized in these cases; for example, by keeping doses low, and potentially augmenting with low-dose loxapine (Stahl, 2002; Hellings et al., 2015).

An interesting, recent development is the finding that an individual may have a gene defect, such as the *MECP2* gene-associated deletion of Rett syndrome, but not manifest the syndrome phenotypically. This is thought to be due to epigenetic influences on gene expression, including environmental factors, which are still to be elucidated.

Psychiatric illness in ID

Overall, psychiatric illness is more common in individuals with ID in comparison with the general population (Zaman et al., 2007). At the same time, the most common presentations of aggression, destructive behavior, and self-injury are symptoms that occur in association with several psychiatric disorders, physical illness, and seizure disorders in this population. It is up to the clinician to elicit and clarify symptom categories to make diagnoses that can inform selection of treatments; for example, inattention, distractibility, and impulsivity-type symptoms for ADHD, or bipolar disorder symptoms of irritable, expansive, or euphoric mood associated with sleep, appetite, motor, and sexual activity symptoms. Impulsivity associated with both disorders impacts poor choices, but treatment differs greatly depending on diagnosis.

Excessive dosing of bipolar disorder treatments, for example in what is often a mistaken diagnosis of bipolar disorder, leads to weight gain associated with atypical antipsychotic and mood-stabilizing drugs. Obesity in turn leads to worsened immobility, metabolic syndrome, type 2 diabetes, sleep apnea, arthritis, cardiovascular diseases and stroke, and various types of carcinoma. All of these conditions restrict the individual's lifestyle even more, and worsen psychiatric and behavioral challenges. Loxapine is a classical antipsychotic that has atypical antipsychotic properties in low doses of 5–15 mg/day (Stahl, 2002), and an open prospective pilot study showed weight neutrality and atypical antipsychotic-sparing properties, together with beneficial effects on irritability and aggression (Hellings et al., 2015). In addition, studies suggest beneficial effects of loxapine on brain health; notably in a pluripotent stem cell study, loxapine produced neural sprouting, in contrast to risperidone, clozapine, olanzapine, and thioridazine (Brennand et al., 2011), and significant increases in brain-derived neurotrophic factor (BDNF) were observed in a subset in the Hellings et al. (2015) study, warranting further studies.

Collateral information is vital for making accurate physical and psychiatric diagnoses, and leading questions should be avoided. In addition, idiosyncratic use of language may be confused with psychosis; for example, "my leg is dizzy," which may mean many things. All possible collateral information sources should be tapped in order to clarify predisposing, precipitating, and perpetuating factors related to changes in psychiatric and/or physical problems. It is vital to examine the patient thoroughly, and to order a collection of blood tests, an electrocardiogram (ECG), and sleep-deprived electro-encephalogram (EEG), magnetic resonance imaging (MRI) scan or other tests, as needed. Early referral to appropriate specialists is necessary for potentially serious cases, including to neurologists, gastroenterologists, geneticists, and endocrinologists.

Another problem is that in all but the mildest cases, combination treatments are needed utilizing psychotropic medications in low doses, for optimal results; however, combination studies are lacking. For bipolar disorder, a combination of low-dose antipsychotic drug, lithium, and divalproex may be needed (Hellings, 1999). Also, in many cases, gabapentin can be substituted for lithium together with the divalproex and low-dose antipsychotic, which produces fewer side effects than lithium in this population (Hellings, 2006). For ADHD, especially in treatment-resistant cases referred to tertiary referral centers, amitriptyline together with low-dose stimulant and low-dose risperidone or aripiprazole can be useful if used cautiously together with amitriptyline blood level and monitoring of QTc on ECG (Bhatti et al., 2013).

Conclusions

The complex interplay between psychiatric and medical problems in a patient with ID and medical and psychiatric comorbidities demands a holistic but also highly detailed approach. The clinician must target and treat psychiatric and physical problems, and arrange for nutritional and preventive health strategies for vision, hearing, dental, and other routine health screenings. If needed, a low dose of benzodiazepine, such as alprazolam 1–2 mg, may be given an hour before healthcare visits and medical or dental procedures in order to increase the likelihood of success.

Medical problems in persons with ID include epilepsy, hydrocephalus, cerebral palsy and mobility issues, thyroid disease, respiratory problems, obesity and diabetes mellitus, GI disorders, various types of cancer, and psychiatric illness. All of these conditions, which often co-occur in this population, may cause behavioral changes, aggression, agitation, and self-injury. Sexuality issues are underexplored, and sexually transmitted diseases can occur.

Key summary points

- Comorbidity of medical conditions is generally increased in people with ID overall.
- More evidence is now available regarding specific cancer relative risks in people with ID.
- Certain medical conditions are decreased in people with ID often associated with lifestyle habits, such as reduced smoking.
- Impaired communication means that medical conditions may often present atypically.
- Comorbidity increases the complexity of assessment and treatment of medical and psychiatric conditions.

References

Baldridge, K.H. and Andrasik, F. (2010). Pain assessment in people with intellectual or developmental disabilities. *American Journal of Nursing*, 110(12), 28–35.

Bhatti, I., Thome, A., Oxler-Smith, P., et al. (2013). A retrospective study of amitriptyline in youth with autism spectrum disorders. *Journal of Autism and Developmental Disorders*, 43(5), 1017–1027.

Bohmer, C.J., Klinkenberg-Knol, E.C., Niezende Boer, M.C., Meuwissen, S.G. (2000). Gastroesophageal reflux disease in intellectually disabled individuals: how often, how serious, how manageable? *American Journal of Gastroenterology*, 95, 1868–1872.

Bohmer, C.J., Taminiau, J.A., Klinkenberg-Knol, E.C., Meuwissen, S.G. (2001). The prevalence of constipation in institutionalized people with intellectual disability. *Journal of Intellectual Disability Research*, 45(3), 212–218.

Brennand, K.J., Simone, A., Jou, J., et al. (2011). Modeling schizophrenia using human induced pluripotent stem cells. *Nature*, 12(7346), 221–225.

Butler, M.G., Youngs, E., Roberts, J.L., Hellings, J.A. (2012). Assessment and treatment in autism spectrum disorders: a focus on genetics and psychiatry. *Autism Research and Treatment*, DOI: 10.1155/2012/242537.

Carr, E.G., Smith, C.E., Giacin, T.A., Whelan, B.M., Pancari, J. (2003). Menstrual discomfort as a biological setting event for severe problem behavior: assessment and intervention. *American Journal on Mental Retardation*, 108, 17–33.

Carta, M.G., Hardey, M.C., Boi, M.F., et al., (2002). Association between panic disorder, major depressive disorder and celiac disease. *Journal of Psychosomatic Research*, 53(3), 789–793.

Chaney, R.H. and Eyman, R.K. (2000). Patterns in mortality over 60 years among persons with mental retardation in a residential facility. *Mental Retardation*, 38, 289–293.

Correll, CU., Manu, P., Olshansky, V., et al. (2009). Cardiometabolic risk of second-generation antipsychotic medications during first-time use in children and adolescents. *Journal of the American Medical Association*, 302(16), 1765–1773.

Duff, M., Scheepers, M., Cooper, M., Hoghton, M., Baddeley, P. (2001). *Helicobacter pylori*: has the killer escaped from the institution? A possible cause of increased stomach cancer in a population with intellectual disability. *Journal of Intellectual Disability Research*, 45(3), 219–225.

Fischer, L.S., Becker, A., Paraguya, M., Chukwu, C. (2012). Colonoscopy and colorectal cancer screening in adults with intellectual and developmental disabilities: review of a series of cases and recommendations for examination. *Intellectual and Developmental Disabilities*, 50(5), 383–390.

Gaventa, W.C. and Coulter, D.L. (2002). *Spirituality and Intellectual Disability: International Perspectives on the Effect of Culture and Religion on Healing Body, Mind, and Soul*. New York, NY: Haworth Pastoral Press.

Genuis, S.J. and Lobo, R.A. (2014). Gluten sensitivity presenting as a neuropsychiatric disorder. *Gastroeneterology Research and Practice*, DOI: 10.1155/2014/293206.

Gravestock, S. (2000). Eating disorders in adults with intellectual disability. *Journal of Intellectual Disability Research*, 44(6), 625–637.

Green, P.H.R. and Jones, R. (2010). *Celiac Disease: A Hidden Epidemic*. New York, NY: Harper Collins Publishers.

Harvey, K. (2012). *Trauma-Informed Behavioral Interventions: What Works and What Doesn't*. Washington, DC: American Association on Intellectual and Developmental Disabilities.

Hellings, J.A. (1999). Psychopharmacology of mood disorders in persons with mental retardation and autism. *Mental Retardation and Developmental Disabilities Research Reviews*, 5, 270–278.

Hellings, J.A. (2006). Much improved outcome with gabapentin–divalproex combination in adults with bipolar disorders and developmental disabilities. *Journal of Clinical Psychopharmacology*, 26(3), 344–346.

Hellings, J.A. and Warnock, J.K. (1994). Self-injurious behavior and serotonin in Prader–Willi syndrome. *Psychopharmacology Bulletin*, 30(2), 245–250.

Hellings, J.A., Zarcone, J.R., Crandall, K., Wallace, D., Schroeder, S.R. (2001). Weight gain in a controlled study of risperidone in children, adolescents and adults with mental retardation and autism. *Journal of Child and Adolescent Psychopharmacology*, 1(3), 229–238.

Hellings, J.A., Hossain, S., Martin, J.K., Baratang, R.R. (2002). Psychopathology, GABA, and the Rubinstein–Taybi syndrome: a review and case study. *American Journal of Medical Genetics Part A*, 114(2), 190–195.

Hellings, J.A., Cardona, A., Schroeder, S.R. (2010). Long-term safety and adverse events of risperidone in children, adolescents and adults with pervasive developmental disorders. *Journal of Mental Health Research in Intellectual Disabiities*, 3, 132–144.

Hellings, J.A., Reed, G., Cain, S.E., et al. (2015). Loxapine add-on for adolescents and adults with autism spectrum disorders, aggression and irritability. *Journal of Child and Adolescent Psychopharmacology*, 25(2), 150–159.

Hulland, S. and Sigal, M.J. (2000). Hospital-based dental care for persons with disabilities: a study of patient selection criteria. *Special Care Dentist*, 20, 131–138.

Kennedy, M., McCombie, L., Dawes, P., McConnell, K.N., Dunnigan, M.G. (1997). Nutritional support for patients with intellectual disability and nutrition/dysphagia disorders in community care. *Journal of Intellectual Disabiity Research*, 41(5), 430–436.

Kwok, H. and Cheung, P.W. (2007). Co-morbidity of psychiatric disorder and medical illness in people with intellectual disabilities. *Current Opinion in Psychiatry*, 20(5), 443–449.

Lennox, N. (2007). The interface between medical and psychiatric disorders in people with intellectual disabilities. In N. Bouras and G. Holt (eds.), *Psychiatric and Behavioural Disorders in Intellectual and Developmental Disabilities*, second edition. Cambridge: Cambridge University Press.

Levitas, A.S. and Reid, C.S. (1998). Rubinstein–Taybi syndrome and psychiatric disorders. *Journal of Intellectual Disability Research*, 42, 284–292.

Lott, I.T. and Head, E. (2001). Down syndrome and Alzheimers disease: link between development and ageing. *Mental Retardation and Developmental Disability Research Reviews*, 7(3), 172–178.

Marrus, N., Veenstra-Vanderweele, J., Hellings, J.A., et al. (2013). Training of child and adolescent psychiatry fellows in autism and intellectual disabilities. *Autism*, 18(4), 471–475.

Morin, D., Merineau-Cote, J., Ouelhette-Kuntz, H., et al. (2012). A comparison of the prevalence of chronic diseases among people with and without intellectual disabilities. *American Journal on Intellectual and Developmental Disabilities*, 117(6), 455–463.

Murphy, K.P., Molnar, G.E., Lankasky, K. (1995). Medical and functional status of adults with cerebral palsy. *Developmental Medicine and Child Neurology*, 37, 1075–1084.

Owens, P.L, Kerker, B.D., Zigler, E., et al. (2006). Vision and oral health needs of individuals with intellectual disability. *Mental Retardation and Developmental Disabilities Research Reviews*, 12, 28–40.

Patja, K., Eero, P., Iivanainen, M. (2001). Cancer incidence among people with intellectual disability. *Journal of Intellectual Disability Research*, 45(4), 300–307.

Peach, H.G. (2003). Religion, spirituality, and health. *Medical Journal of Australia*, 178, 415–416.

Pillal, M., O'Brien, K., Hill, E. (2010). The levonorgestrel intrauterine system (Mirena) for the treatment of menstrual problems in adolescents with medical disorders, or physical or learning disabilities. *BJOG: An International Journal of Obstetrics and Gynecology*, 117(2), 216–221.

Prater, C.D. and Zylstra, R.G. (2006). Medical care of adults with mental retardation. *American Family Physician*, 73(12), 2175–2183.

Rajan, D. (2013). Women with disabilities less likely to be screened for cancer. *Health and Wellness*, Canadian Breast Cancer Network. At: http://www.thestar.com/life/health_wellness/2013/07/16/women_with_

disabilities_less_likely_to_be_screened_for_cancer.html

Rasch, E.K., Gulley, S.P., Chan, L. (2013). Use of emergency departments among working age adults with disabilities: a problem of access and services needs. *Health Services Research*, 48(4), 1334–1358.

Reiss, S., Levitan, G.W., Szyszko, J. (1982). Emotional disturbance and mental retardation: diagnostic overshadowing. *American Journal of Mental Deficiency*, 86(6), 567–574.

Slayter, E.M. (2010). Disparities in access to substance abuse treatment among people with intellectual disabilities and serious mental illness. *Health and Social Work*, 35(1), 49–59.

Stahl, S.M. (2002). *Essential Psychopharmacology of Antipsychotics and Mood Stabilizers*. New York, NY: Cambridge University Press.

Trimble, M.R. and Cull, C. (1988). Children of school age: the influence of antiepileptic drugs on behavior and intellect. *Epilepsia*, 29(Suppl.), 15–19.

World Health Organization. (1992).*The ICD-10 Classification of Mental and Behavioural Disorders: Clinical Descriptions and Diagnostic Guidelines*. Geneva: World Health Organization.

Zaman, S.H., Holt, G., Bouras, N. (2007). Managing mental health problems in people with intellectual disabilities. In A. Carr, G. O'Reilly, P.N. Walsh, J. McEvoy (eds.), *The Handbook of Intellectual Disability and Clinical Psychology Practice*. London: Routledge.

Special topics

Epilepsy

Frank M. C. Besag

Introduction

Epilepsy is common in people with intellectual disabilities (ID) and ID is common in people with epilepsy. The rate of psychiatric disorder is high in the general population of children with epilepsy but is much higher in those with ID. This implies that a great proportion of people who have both ID and epilepsy will require psychiatric services and will be demanding of resources. Because each of the three conditions, namely epilepsy, ID, and psychiatric disorder, covers a wide spectrum, there is a significant variation in the nature and severity of the difficulties encountered. Epilepsy becomes much more prevalent, and is also increasingly likely to be refractory to treatment, as the degree of ID increases. Epilepsy syndromes vary from the relatively benign to the very handicapping, and also vary greatly in the range of associated psychiatric disorders. Many behavioral phenotypes are associated with ID and epilepsy. There is an increasing recognition of the role of genetics in influencing outcome in terms of behavioral phenotype, range of ID, and type of epilepsy. Management of the individual with epilepsy, ID, and psychiatric disorder is influenced not only by the genetic and disease/disorder-related factors but also by situational/environmental factors.

Epidemiology

Sillanpää (1992) revealed ID in 31.4% in an unselected population of children in Finland. Murphy et al. (1995) reported similar results from Atlanta, USA. They estimated the prevalence of epilepsy in 10-year-old children and found that 35% had another developmental disability: ID, cerebral palsy, visual impairment, or hearing impairment. Berg (2008), using a broader criterion of IQ <80, carried out a prospective study of children with newly diagnosed epilepsy: 451 of the children (73.6%) were considered to have normal cognitive function. Russ et al. (2012) analyzed data on 91 605 children in the USA from birth to 17 years of age, including 977 children reported to have a seizure disorder; of the latter, 51% had developmental delay. Sillanpää also studied ID in adults who had childhood-onset epilepsy. He found that learning problems of one type or another were common, occurring in 76%, of whom half had ID (Sillanpää, 2004).

A different approach is to examine the prevalence of epilepsy in people with ID, rather than the prevalence of ID in people with epilepsy.

Psychiatric and Behavioral Disorders in Intellectual and Developmental Disabilities, ed. Colin Hemmings and Nick Bouras. Published by Cambridge University Press. © Cambridge University Press 2016.

A number of the classical older studies made it clear that the greater the degree of ID, the higher the prevalence of epilepsy. Some of these studies referred to the risk of having one or more epileptic seizures, rather than the risk of developing established epilepsy. For example, Richardson et al. (1980), in a population of children in the UK, found that one or more epileptic seizures occurred in 4% of those with normal intelligence, 11% in those with borderline intelligence, and 27% in those with ID. They also reported that more severe ID was associated with more frequent seizures at a younger age and over a longer time span. Goulden et al. (1991) in the USA, carried out a prospective cohort study of 221 children with ID in whom 33 (15%) developed epilepsy by the age of 22 years. The cumulative incidence of epilepsy was 9% at 5 years, 11% at 10 years, 13% at 15 years, and 15% at 22 years. In those with severe ID, two or more seizures occurred in 35% and one or more in 44%. Steffenburg et al. (1995) assessed all children with ID from 6 to 13 years in a defined geographical area in Sweden, using patient registers. They identified 378 children, of whom 98 had active epilepsy. Epilepsy had been diagnosed in 15% of those with mild ID and in 45% of those with severe ID. McGrother et al. (2006), in a UK population-based prevalence study, found an epilepsy prevalence of 26%. They also commented that, of these subjects, 68% continued to have seizures despite antiepileptic medication, suggesting that the epilepsy was more difficult to treat in the ID population.

The relationships between epilepsy and ID

Can epilepsy cause ID?

The most dramatic situation in which epilepsy can result in intellectual deterioration is when prolonged status epilepticus causes permanent brain damage. Experienced epileptologists will be aware of several personal cases of young people who have apparently been developing normally until they have a prolonged epileptic seizure, following which they have very significant or even profound ID. However, epidemiological studies have produced mixed results in relation to this. The implication is that some children may have prolonged epileptic seizures without sustaining obvious brain damage (Maytal et al., 1989). However, it is also clear that other children do sustain permanent brain damage and acquire ID after a single prolonged seizure. In the circumstances, the current practice of viewing every prolonged seizure as being a medical emergency appears to be entirely appropriate. Prolonged seizures can occur in a particular epilepsy syndrome, namely Panayiotopoulos syndrome, with an apparently benign outcome (Panayiotopoulos, 2000). However, this should be viewed as an exceptional syndrome.

Can repeated seizures that are not prolonged cause ID?

It appears that some children with severe epilepsy plateau in their development; the result of this is that the mental age remains relatively stationary while the chronological age continues to rise. Consequently, the IQ, because it a quotient, falls; Maria Fowler described such a group of children several years ago (Besag, 1988). The reasons for this "stagnation" of mental age remain unclear. Extensive study of the original group by the author of this chapter (unpublished studies) failed to reveal any unequivocal cause, although there was a suggestion that frequent nocturnal and/or diurnal epileptiform discharges might have been associated with this fall in IQ.

It is important to distinguish between permanent intellectual impairment and what has been termed "state-dependent" intellectual impairment. The latter can result from sedative medication, in which case a medication review is necessary, or it can be caused by the epilepsy itself. The important distinguishing factor of "state-dependent ID" is that it is potentially treatable and reversible. The epileptic phenomena that can result in state-dependent intellectual impairment include very frequent absence seizures, transitory cognitive impairment, frequent localized discharges, frequent hemispheric discharges, postictal state-dependent cognitive impairment and electrical status epilepticus of slow-wave sleep (ESES), or continuous spike-waves in slow-wave sleep (CSWS) (Besag, 2011).

Over recent years, the term "epileptic encephalopathy" has been used. This was defined by the International League Against Epilepsy taskforce (Engel and ILAE, 2001) as "a condition in which the epileptiform EEG abnormalities themselves are believed to contribute to a progressive disturbance in cerebral function." A number of epilepsy syndromes were listed as providing examples of epileptic encephalopathy, including early myoclonic encephalopathy, early infantile epileptic encephalopathy (Ohtahara syndrome), West syndrome, Dravet syndrome, migrating partial seizures in infancy, myoclonic status in non-progressive encephalopathies, Lennox–Gastaut syndrome, Landau–Kleffner syndrome, and epilepsy with CSWS. The author of this chapter has challenged the term "epileptic encephalopathy," because it might be taken to imply that there is necessarily some type of permanent brain pathology, which is irreversible. In some cases this may be true; however, in other cases the "encephalopathy" appears to be at least partially reversible. For example, in a report of a series of children with the Landau–Kleffner syndrome (acquired epileptic aphasia) some of the children appeared to recover completely, or almost completely, following the novel surgical procedure of multiple subpial transection (Morrell et al., 1989). What is important is that if the epilepsy itself is causing intellectual impairment in a reversible way, the epilepsy should be treated promptly and effectively, to avoid the possibility of permanent damage (Besag, 2011).

Can ID cause epilepsy?

Intellectual diabilities cannot cause epilepsy. The fact that ID are associated with brain dysfunction increases the probability of epilepsy developing.

Can an underlying disorder result in both ID and epilepsy?

There are several ways in which underlying factors can lead both to epilepsy and ID. Some of these will be discussed here.

Brain trauma

Annegers et al. (1998) surveyed 4541 children and adults with traumatic brain injury involving loss of consciousness, post-traumatic amnesia, or skull fracture. The standardized incident ratio of seizures was 1.5 after mild injuries, 2.9 after moderate injuries, and 17.0 after severe injuries. This study left no doubt about the conclusion that the severity of the brain injury determined the likelihood of subsequent seizures. Because the severity of the brain injury is also linked to the subsequent severity of ID, again, the severity of the ID is likely to be related to the probability of seizure occurrence. In the case of traumatic brain injury, there is a clear-cut cause for both the intellectual impairment and the seizures. In the majority of patients who have both epilepsy and ID, the cause will not be so obvious.

Genetics

Zuberi (2013) commented that epilepsy is now associated with several hundred chromosomal abnormalities. Most of these have not been categorized into a clear clinical phenotype. Many of these disorders are associated with ID and epilepsy together. It would not be unreasonable to describe the variety and number of genetic disorders being identified in people with epilepsy and ID as bewildering. There are, however, some very well-defined syndromes.

Does knowledge of the genetics affect treatment and prognosis? In most cases neither treatment nor prognosis is influenced in a major way by the genetic knowledge, although such information can sometimes be of considerable value in informing genetic counseling. For a small number of genetic syndromes, however, treatment and prognosis can be affected. Most cases of Dravet syndrome (severe myoclonic epilepsy of infancy) are caused by mutations in the *SCN1A* gene. This is a sodium-channel gene. Antiepileptic drugs that act on the sodium channel tend to make seizures worse in this syndrome. This consequently provides one of the few examples of how knowledge of the genetics might influence treatment. Another example is that of tuberous sclerosis complex, the majority of cases of which are the result of mutations in the hamartin gene on chromosome 9 or the tuberin gene on chromosome 16. The gene abnormality results in cell overgrowth, with tubers in the brain and abnormal cell growth in a number of other tissues, including skin (leading to the characteristic facial fibromas, previously termed "adenoma sebaceum"), kidney, lung, and elsewhere. Both the kidney and the lung disease can be life-threatening. In addition, giant cell astrocytomas may develop and can block the outflow of cerebrospinal fluid (CSF) from the ventricular system, which may lead to hydrocephalus and severe neurological problems. Rapamicin (sirolimus) and the closely related drug everolimus can cause regression in the cell growth with, for example, regression of giant cell astrocytomas (Franz et al., 2006). There is great interest in using these medications to treat the epilepsy itself (Wong, 2010).

Although recent advances in genetics are remarkable, their influence in terms of management remains limited at present. It is interesting to note that the current author made the following comment several years ago: "We have yet to reach the stage at which every epilepsy syndrome has a known gene, perhaps coding for a known channelopathy, allowing the doctor to select the specific, scientifically targeted antiepileptic drug to correct the ion channel defect. Is this what the future holds for the treatment of epilepsy? Time will tell" (Besag, 1999).

Malformations of cortical development

Several malformations of cortical development are associated with the combination of epilepsy and ID (Aronica and Crino, 2014). Localized areas of cortical dysplasia may be amenable to surgical resection, sometimes with improvement not only of the epilepsy but also of cognition and behavior. The extreme example of this is hemimegalencephaly, in which one side of the brain is abnormally large. This malformation sometimes results in a storm of epileptiform electrical discharges from the abnormal side of the brain. Hemispherectomy (removal or disconnection of one half of the brain) can result in seizure freedom, improvement in behavior, and, in at least some cases, improvement of cognition.

Neuronal antibodies

One of the most remarkable advances in the investigation and management of epilepsy has been the discovery of the role of neuronal antibodies, of which the most commonly described are N-methyl-D-aspartate (NMDA) receptor antibodies and voltage-gated potassium-channel complex antibodies. Such antibodies can result in acute deterioration, often with seizures and typically with loss of cognitive skills. Other phenomena, such as mood changes, memory loss, and psychosis can occur (Vincent et al., 2004; Dalmau et al., 2008). Left untreated, some patients will go into coma and die. However, this is a potentially treatable condition, generally responding well to immunotherapy. In general, when managing epilepsy, although it may be possible to control seizures with medication, it is not possible to cure the epilepsy by medical means alone. However, the patient with epilepsy resulting from neuronal antibodies provides an exceptional example of epilepsy that can be cured by medical treatment, namely immunotherapy. Many clinicians may be troubled to reflect on the patients they have seen in the past who almost certainly had an encephalitis caused by neuronal antibodies, which was not diagnosed at the time because the knowledge was not available. This raises the interesting question of whether any person who deteriorates cognitively, in association with seizures or not, deserves to be tested for neuronal antibodies. In the view of the current author, unless there is an obvious cause for the cognitive deterioration, the answer to this question is that they should, indeed, undergo such testing. There is an argument for performing such testing very promptly so that treatment can be instituted before permanent damage occurs.

Why is the combination of epilepsy and ID important?

Refractory epilepsy

Epilepsy in people with ID tends to be more difficult to treat effectively. The probability of achieving seizure control will be less, emphasizing the importance of striking a balance between achieving the best possible seizure control while avoiding adverse effects of medication, notably the cognitive and behavioral adverse effects. For example, the seizures in Lennox–Gastaut syndrome, which is associated with ID, autistic features, and behavioral problems, are generally very refractory to treatment. Because of this, clinicians are tempted to prescribe higher doses and greater numbers of antiepileptic drugs which, in combination with the frequent seizures, impair intellectual abilities to an even greater extent. The general rule when managing epilepsy is to try to avoid poly-pharmacy. However, it is not uncommon for people with ID and epilepsy to require several antiepileptic medications; when carefully planned attempts are made to tail off any of the antiepileptic medications, the seizures become unequivocally worse, with consequent impairment of the quality of life of the individual. In contrast, it is not unusual to find that when one or more of the antiepileptic drugs is tailed off and discontinued in an individual with epilepsy and ID who is taking polypharmacy, the seizures are no worse and no better. The cognitive and behavioral adverse effects, on the other hand, may be much reduced by this approach. For those antiepileptic drugs that tend to exacerbate psychiatric or behavioral problems, it is particularly important to question whether any antiepileptic drug is improving the situation or making matters worse (Besag, 2001). Some antiepileptic drugs need to be tailed off slowly to decrease the chance of withdrawal seizures; for example, the benzodiazepines and barbiturates.

There are several epilepsy syndromes in which ID is common or even characteristic (Besag, 2004a). Four examples of such syndromes follow.

West syndrome

West syndrome comprises infantile spasms, ID, and hypsarrhythmia (high-voltage, disorganized slow-wave activity) on the electroencephalogram (EEG). The spasms can be flexor, mixed flexor–extensor, or extensor. Onset is usually under 12 months, typically around 3–7 months. ID has been reported in the majority of cases, typically 70–80%. The earlier the onset of the spasms and the longer the delay to treatment, the worse the outcome in terms of adaptive behavior at four years of age (O'Callaghan et al., 2011). Autism has commonly been reported in West syndrome. In those who have West syndrome as a result of tuberous sclerosis, those who are subsequently diagnosed as having autism tend to have temporal lobe tubers (Bolton et al., 2002). In West syndrome, the cognitive deterioration appears to coincide with the onset of the disorganized EEG pattern of hypsarrhythmia, and there is a strong indication that successful antiepileptic treatment that abolishes the hypsarrhythmia can result in significant improvement in cognitive ability (Jambaque et al., 2000). This implies that the challenge is to treat not only the spasms but also the EEG abnormality early and effectively. In those babies whose infantile spasms are caused by tuberous sclerosis, the rate of seizure freedom with vigabatrin is strikingly high (Chiron et al., 1997). The reason for this remains uncertain but is probably related to the genetics of tuberous sclerosis. Vigabatrin can also be effective if the infantile spasms are not the result of tuberous sclerosis, but the consensus is that, in this case, treatment with adrenocorticotropic hormone (ACTH) or prednisolone is more effective than vigabatrin.

Dravet syndrome (severe myoclonic epilepsy of infancy)

Seizure onset is typically with febrile convulsions or generalized clonic seizures in the first year of life, followed by myoclonic and/or partial and/or absence seizures between two and three years. The initial seizures may be prolonged. Although early EEG recordings do not usually show paroxysmal epileptiform abnormalities, recordings in the second year of life show interictal generalized spike–wave complexes and/or generalized polyspike–waves. Delayed development is also typically seen in the second year and is usually accompanied by unsteadiness (Dravet et al., 1992). A variety of defects in the *SCN1A* gene have been identified as causing this syndrome. Most individuals with Dravet syndrome have a defect in this sodium-channel gene and the seizures in this syndrome tend to be exacerbated by drugs that have sodium-channel-blocking properties, such as lamotrigine or carbamazepine.

Lennox–Gastaut syndrome

Onset is usually between one and nine years of age, with a peak at three to five years. This syndrome is characterized by multiple seizure types, including brief tonic, atonic, myoclonic, and atypical absence seizures. Axial tonic seizures are considered by some to be an essential diagnostic feature. The EEG is grossly abnormal, with diffuse slow spike–wave discharges in the waking record and fast rhythms of about 10 cycles per second in sleep. ID is usual. There is underlying permanent ID but there may be an additional, potentially reversible component of ID as a result of the frequent seizures. Again, the implication is that if the seizures were treated more successfully, the degree of ID would be somewhat less. Although some degree of seizure control has been achieved with antiepileptic drugs such as lamotrigine (Motte et al., 1997) and topiramate (Sachdeo et al., 1999), the seizures usually remain resistant to treatment. The apparent lack of motivation of young people with this syndrome is almost certainly the result of the frequent seizures rather than any inherent lack of will on the part of the individual (Besag, 2004a). Autistic features are commonly reported.

Landau–Kleffner syndrome of acquired epileptic aphasia

This syndrome usually presents after language acquisition, but before six years of age, with verbal auditory agnosia. Expressive language is typically affected, probably because the child cannot understand his or her own speech either; as a result, the child may become mute. The daytime EEG abnormalities are not necessarily particularly marked, but typically include spikes and spike–wave discharges, tending to occur in the temporal regions. However, the night-time EEG is usually grossly abnormal with electrical status epilepticus of slow-wave sleep, defined as at least 85% of slow-wave sleep being occupied by spike–wave discharges. This syndrome is unusual, because it has been reported that around one-third of the subjects do not present with seizures. The diagnosis could be missed if overnight EEG monitoring were not performed. Because of the verbal agnosia, there is marked loss of cognitive skills. Treatment with medication or surgery can result in a dramatic increase in skills, provided the electrical status epilepticus of slow-wave sleep has not continued for a very long period. Robinson et al. (2001) found that no child who had electrical status epilepticus of slow-wave sleep for longer than three years subsequently had normal speech development. Again, the implication is that early, effective antiepileptic treatment, with either medicine or surgery, should be implemented. The remarkable surgical treatment of multiple subpial transection is described by Morrell et al. (1989). Again, autistic features are frequently described in this syndrome.

Psychiatric disorders

Psychiatric disorder is commonly associated with the combination of epilepsy and ID. From the earliest studies of psychiatric disorders in epilepsy (Rutter et al., 1970) it became evident that the rate of psychiatric disorder was much higher in children who also had ID. This was confirmed in a subsequent population study in the UK (Davies et al., 2003). Although there is no doubt that the rate of psychiatric disorder in children with epilepsy is higher in those who also have ID, there has been some debate about whether the rate of psychiatric disorder in those with both epilepsy and ID is any greater than those who have a similar degree of ID without epilepsy. Some population studies suggest that the epilepsy does not increase the rate of psychiatric disorder (Deb and Hunter, 1991). However, epilepsy can be a key causative factor in some of the psychiatric phenomenology in a number of epilepsy syndromes, and if the epilepsy is treated effectively then the psychiatric symptoms may ameliorate or resolve (Besag, 2002, 2004a, 2008).

Treatment

With a few notable exceptions, the management of the epilepsy in those with and without ID is much the same. The exceptional situations are those in which the individual has lost cognitive skills because of electrical status epilepticus of slow-wave sleep/continuous spike-waves of slow-wave sleep, non-convulsive status epilepticus, or neuronal antibodies. Apart from these exceptions, the mainstay of treatment is antiepileptic medication. Some individuals will be suitable for neurosurgery, which may either be resective surgery, for example temporal lobectomy or frontal lobe resection, or the disconnection procedures, such as callosotomy (disconnection or partial disconnection of the two hemispheres), hemispherotomy (disconnection of one hemisphere), or multiple subpial transection. In the past, ID was considered to be a contraindication to surgery, but this is no longer the case.

In those who have epilepsy, ID, and psychiatric disorder, the choice of antiepileptic medication may be influenced by the psychiatric disorder. Some antiepileptic drugs, notably lamotrigine and carbamazepine, can have positive psychotropic properties. On the other hand, antiepileptic drugs can cause psychiatric or behavioral disturbance, probably to a greater extent in those individuals who have ID (Besag, 2004b; Piedad et al., 2012). For example, the benzodiazepine drugs, barbiturates, and vigabatrin can precipitate an attention-deficit/hyperactivity disorder (ADHD)-like presentation in children with ID and should be avoided if other options are available. Vigabatrin and topiramate can be associated with both depression and psychosis; risk factors include a personal or family history of psychiatric disorder and rapid escalation of the antiepileptic medication (Mula et al., 2003).

Conclusions

The combination of epilepsy, ID, and psychiatric or behavioral disorders is common. Appropriate management depends on the meticulous assessment of each individual patient. Any individual who has lost cognitive skills must be investigated thoroughly; unless a clear cause has been found, serious consideration should be given to overnight EEG monitoring and/or neuronal antibody testing. Treatment of those epilepsy and psychiatric disorders in individuals who also have ID can be challenging, but the outcome can be very rewarding.

Key summary points

- The rate of ID in people with epilepsy is high, typically greater than 30% in epidemiological studies.
- The frequency of epilepsy increases with the degree of ID; epilepsy also tends to become more difficult to treat as the degree of ID increases.
- The rate of psychiatric disorder is high in the general population of people with epilepsy, but is even higher in people who also have ID.
- Because of the high rate of psychiatric disorder, people with epilepsy and ID are often very demanding of resources.
- Management of the individual with epilepsy, ID, and psychiatric disorders is influenced not only by genetic and disease/disorder-related factors but also by situational/environmental factors.
- When treating epilepsy in people with ID, antiepileptic drugs that are liable to affect cognition or behavior adversely should be avoided or at least monitored carefully; the prescription of polypharmacy for resistant epilepsy should also be avoided, if possible.

References

Annegers, J.F., Hauser, W.A., Coan, S.P., Rocca, W.A. (1998). A population-based study of seizures after traumatic brain injuries. *New England Journal of Medicine*, 338, 20–24.

Aronica, E. and Crino, P.B. (2014). Epilepsy related to developmental tumors and malformations of cortical development. *Neurotherapeutics*, 11, 251–268.

Berg, A.T. (2008). Risk of recurrence after a first unprovoked seizure. *Epilepsia*, 49(Suppl. 1), 13–18.

Besag, F.M. (1988). Cognitive deterioration in children with epilepsy. In M. Trimble and E. Reynolds (eds.), *Epilepsy, Behaviour and Cognitive Function*. Chichester, West Sussex, UK: Wiley.

Besag, F.M. (1999). Advances in epilepsy. *Current Opinion in Psychiatry*, 12, 549–553.

Besag, F.M. (2001). Behavioural effects of the new anticonvulsants. *Drug Safety*, 24, 513–536.

Besag, F.M. (2002). Childhood epilepsy in relation to mental handicap and behavioural disorders. *Journal of Child Psychology and Psychiatry and Allied Disciplines*, 43, 103–131.

Besag, F.M. (2004a). Behavioral aspects of pediatric epilepsy syndromes. *Epilepsy and Behavior*, 5(Suppl.), 13.

Besag, F.M. (2004b). Behavioural effects of the newer antiepileptic drugs: an update. *Expert Opinion on Drug Safety*, 3, 1–8.

Besag, F.M. (2008). Behavioral aspects of pediatric epilepsy syndromes. In S.C. Schachter, G.L. Homes, G.A.K. Trenite (eds.), *Behavioral Aspects of Epilepsy. Principles and Practice*. New York, NY: Demos.

Besag, F.M. (2011). Subtle cognitive and behavioral effects of epilepsy. In M. Trimble and B. Schmitz (eds.), *The Neuropsychiatry of Epilepsy*, second edition. Cambridge: Cambridge University Press.

Bolton, P.F., Park, R.J., Higgins, J.N., Griffiths, P.D., Pickles, A. (2002). Neuro-epileptic determinants of autism spectrum disorders in tuberous sclerosis complex. *Brain*, 125, 1247–1255.

Chiron, C., Dumas, C., Jambaque, I., Mumford, J., Dulac, O. (1997). Randomized trial comparing vigabatrin and hydrocortisone in infantile spasms due to tuberous sclerosis. *Epilepsy Research*, 26, 389–395.

Dalmau, J., Gleichman, A.J., Hughes, E.G., et al. (2008). Anti-NMDA-receptor encephalitis: case series and analysis of the effects of antibodies. *Lancet Neurology*, 7, 1091–1098.

Davies, S., Heyman, I., Goodman, R. (2003). A population survey of mental health problems in children with epilepsy. *Developmental Medicine and Child Neurology*, 45, 292–295.

Deb, S. and Hunter, D. (1991). Psychopathology of people with mental handicap and epilepsy. I: maladaptive behaviour. *British Journal of Psychiatry*, 159, 822–826.

Dravet, C., Bueau, M., Guerrini, R., Giraud, N., Roger, J. (1992). Severe myoclonic epilepsy in infants. In J. Roger, M. Bureau, C. Dravet, et al. (eds.), *Epileptic Syndromes in Infancy, Childhood and Adolescence*, second edition. London: John Libbey and Company.

Engel, J., Jr. and the International League Against Epilepsy. (2001). A proposed diagnostic scheme for people with epileptic seizures and with epilepsy: report of the ILAE Task Force on Classification and Terminology. *Epilepsia*, 42, 796–803.

Franz, D.N., Leonard, J., Tudor, C., et al. (2006). Rapamycin causes regression of astrocytomas in tuberous sclerosis complex. *Annals of Neurology*, 59, 490–498.

Goulden, K.J., Shinnar, S., Koller, H., Katz, M., Richardson, S.A. (1991). Epilepsy in children with mental retardation: a cohort study. *Epilepsia*, 32, 690–697.

Jambaque, I., Chiron, C., Dumas, C., Mumford, J., Dulac, O. (2000). Mental and behavioural outcome of infantile epilepsy treated by vigabatrin in tuberous sclerosis patients. *Epilepsy Research*, 38, 151–160.

Maytal, J., Shinnar, S., Moshe, S.L., Alvarez, L.A. (1989). Low morbidity and mortality of status epilepticus in children. *Pediatrics*, 83, 323–331.

McGrother, C.W., Bhaumik, S., Thorp, C.F., et al. (2006). Epilepsy in adults with intellectual disabilities: prevalence, associations and service implications. *Seizure*, 15, 376–386.

Morrell, F., Whisler, W.W., Bleck, T.P. (1989). Multiple subpial transection: a new approach to the surgical treatment of focal epilepsy. *Journal of Neurosurgery*, 70, 231–239.

Motte, J., Trevathan, E., Arvidsson, J.F., et al. (1997). Lamotrigine for generalized seizures associated with the Lennox–Gastaut syndrome. Lamictal Lennox-Gastaut Study Group. *New England Journal of Medicine*, 337, 1807–1812. [Published erratum appears in *New England Journal of Medicine*, 1998, 339(12), 851–852.]

Mula, M., Trimble, M.R., Lhatoo, S.D., Sander, J.W. (2003). Topiramate and psychiatric adverse events in patients with epilepsy. *Epilepsia*, 44, 659–663.

Murphy, C.C., Trevathan, E., Yeargin-Allsopp, M. (1995). Prevalence of epilepsy and epileptic seizures in 10-year-old children: results from the Metropolitan Atlanta Developmental Disabilities Study. *Epilepsia*, 36, 866–872.

O'Callaghan, F.J., Lux, A.L., Darke, K., et al. (2011). The effect of lead time to treatment and of age of onset on developmental outcome at four years in infantile spasms: evidence from the United Kingdom Infantile Spasms Study. *Epilepsia*, 52, 1359–1364.

Panayiotopoulos, C.P. (2000). Benign childhood epileptic syndromes with occipital spikes: new classification proposed by the International League Against Epilepsy. *Journal of Child Neurology*, 15, 548–552.

Piedad, J., Rickards, H., Besag, F.M., Cavanna, A.E. (2012). Beneficial and adverse psychotropic effects of antiepileptic drugs in patients with epilepsy: a summary of prevalence, underlying mechanisms and data limitations. *CNS Drugs*, 26, 319–335.

Richardson, S.A., Koller, H., Katz, M., McLaren, J. (1980). Seizures and epilepsy in a mentally retarded population over the first 22 years of life. *Applied Research in Mental Retardation*, 1, 123–138.

Robinson, R.O., Baird, G., Robinson, G., Simonoff, E. (2001). Landau–Kleffner syndrome: course and correlates with outcome. *Developmental Medicine and Child Neurology*, 43, 243–247.

Russ, S.A., Larson, K., Halfon, N. (2012). A national profile of childhood epilepsy and seizure disorder. *Pediatrics*, 129, 256–264.

Rutter, M., Graham, P., Yule, W. (1970). *A Neuropsychiatric Study in Childhood*. London: Heinemann Medical.

Sachdeo, R.C., Glauser, T.A., Ritter, F., et al. (1999). A double-blind, randomized trial of topiramate in Lennox–Gastaut syndrome. Topiramate YL Study Group. *Neurology*, 52, 1882–1887.

Sillanpää, M. (1992). Epilepsy in children: prevalence, disability, and handicap. *Epilepsia*, 33, 444–449.

Sillanpää, M. (2004). Learning disability: occurrence and long-term consequences in childhood-onset epilepsy. *Epilepsy and Behavior*, 5, 937–944.

Steffenburg, U., Hagberg, G., Viggedal, G., Kyllerman, M. (1995). Active epilepsy in mentally retarded children. I. Prevalence and additional neuro-impairments. *Acta Paediatrica*, 84, 1147–1152.

Vincent, A., Buckley, C., Schott, J.M., et al. (2004). Potassium channel antibody-associated encephalopathy: a potentially immunotherapy-responsive form of limbic encephalitis. *Brain*, 127, 701–712.

Wong, M. (2010). Mammalian target of rapamycin (mTOR) inhibition as a potential antiepileptogenic therapy: from tuberous sclerosis to common acquired epilepsies. *Epilepsia*, 51, 27–36.

Zuberi, S.M. (2013). Chromosome disorders associated with epilepsy. *Handbook of Clinical Neurology*, 111, 543–548.

Chapter

23

Specialized and mainstream mental health services

Johanna Lake, Carly McMorris, and Yona Lunsky

Introduction

This chapter outlines developments in mainstream and specialized inpatient and outpatient services for individuals with intellectual disabilities (ID). In the 21st century, any discussion of mental health services for individuals with ID should include consideration of where and how such services are provided. Historically, this was not a significant issue because all services for those with ID were provided in segregated, institutional settings. Around the world, the past 50 years have seen a gradual shift in healthcare provision for this population, recognizing that ID in itself is not a psychiatric disorder, and that services should be community-based whenever possible (Cumella, 2007). The closure of institutions has led to increased use of mainstream health services in many jurisdictions, particularly when specialized services have not been readily available.

Mainstream (sometimes referred to as "generic") mental health services refer to existing mental health services available to the general population, though models of care may vary by jurisdiction. These services may be quite broad in scope, such as psychiatric consultation or medication follow-up services offered through a local community mental health clinic, or a psychiatric inpatient unit in a general hospital, or elsewhere. Other mainstream services may focus on a particular diagnostic category (e.g., a first episode psychosis program, or an inpatient addiction service), a particular demographic (e.g., a women's mental health unit or an adolescent psychiatry service), or a particular type of intervention (e.g., cognitive-behavioral therapy for inpatients with depression, or dialectical behavior therapy for outpatients with borderline personality disorder). Depending on the service, there may or may not also be various disciplines involved in care. Such services can be focused or specialized, but are considered "mainstream," because they are not offered or designed specifically for those with ID. Specialized services, in contrast, refer to mental health services developed for and restricted to individuals with ID. Like mainstream services, they may focus on a particular disorder, demographic or therapeutic modality, or they may be more general. Practice guidelines suggest that these services take a biopsychosocial approach, that they be interdisciplinary in scope, and that they include, to some extent, caregivers as well as individuals with ID (Deb et al., 2001; Sullivan et al., 2011; National Institute for Health and Clinical Excellence, 2012). This chapter begins with a review of what is known about the clinical profiles of inpatients and outpatients with ID using mainstream and specialized services.

Psychiatric and Behavioral Disorders in Intellectual and Developmental Disabilities, ed. Colin Hemmings and Nick Bouras. Published by Cambridge University Press. © Cambridge University Press 2016.

The next section summarizes research on clinical outcomes in the two program models, while the final two sections discuss which services are best for which people, and areas which require further exploration.

Patient profiles

Inpatient mainstream and specialized services

Many individuals with ID present with comorbid mental health issues, putting them at greater risk for inpatient admission. Given the heterogeneous and complex nature of this population, many individuals with ID are admitted to specialized inpatient units to receive treatment tailored to their needs; however, a large number of these individuals are still admitted to mainstream services. Although there are many demographic similarities between individuals admitted to the two service models (Xenitidis et al., 2004; Hemmings et al., 2009; White et al., 2010), there remain some key clinical differences. In general, male patients account for the majority of admissions to both types of services (Alexander et al., 2001; Hemmings et al., 2009). Individuals with ID in both inpatient units tend to be under the age of 50, with the majority in their 20s to mid 30s (Lunsky and Balogh, 2010; Bakken and Martinsen, 2013); however, those admitted to specialized units tend to be younger than those in mainstream units (Lunsky et al., 2010). Individuals with ID admitted to specialized inpatient units are typically living with family (Hemmings, et al., 2009), single, and have an unstable employment history (Lunsky et al., 2008). The majority of studies report that level of ID does not differ between inpatients with ID in mainstream and specialized units, with most inpatients having mild to moderate ID in both programs (Hemmings et al., 2009; Charlot et al., 2011; Bakken and Martinsen, 2013). However, Alexander et al. (2001) found that individuals admitted to specialized inpatient units were more likely to have severe ID. Aggression is the primary reason for referral for those admitted into both programs (Lunsky et al., 2008; Charlot et al., 2011), but other problem behaviors, such as self-injury, risk to self and others, and property destruction, are also frequent reasons for admission (White et al., 2010; Charlot et al., 2011). In terms of psychiatric diagnoses, individuals with ID who also have a diagnosis of autism spectrum disorders (ASD) or a comorbid mood disorder are more likely to be admitted to specialized inpatient programs (Alexander et al., 2001; Lunsky et al., 2008; Charlot et al., 2011), while those with a psychotic disorder or addiction issues are more likely to be admitted to mainstream programs (Lunsky et al., 2008; White et al., 2010). The one large-scale study comparing patient profiles in the two types of services reported that inpatients in specialized programs were rated as requiring more intensive mental health supports than those in mainstream programs (Lunsky et al., 2008).

Outpatient mainstream and specialized services

Less is known about the demographic and clinical profiles of individuals with ID in outpatient mainstream and specialized services, as few studies have specifically examined and compared the patient profiles of these two services. Findings from this limited literature demonstrate that similar to inpatient services, differences exist between mainstream and specialized outpatient programs. Specifically, outpatients in specialized programs tend to be younger, male, single (Lunsky et al., 2011), living at home with family at time of referral (Russell et al., 2011), and present with disruptive or aggressive behavior as the primary reason for referral (Russell et al., 2011). In terms of psychiatric diagnoses, one study found that individuals in specialized programs were more likely to have a mood or anxiety disorder, whereas those in mainstream programs were more likely to have a psychotic disorder or comorbid medical issues (Lunsky et al., 2011). In this study, outpatients in specialized programs also had more intensive mental health care needs than those in mainstream programs.

Clinical outcomes

Inpatient mainstream and specialized services

Across countries and studies, individuals with ID in specialized inpatient settings consistently document greater clinical improvement (i.e., psychopathology, severity of mental health symptoms, behavior impairment, or level of functioning) compared to individuals in mainstream settings (Xenitidis et al., 2004; Hall et al., 2006; White et al., 2010; Gabriels et al., 2012). Positive outcomes have also been described by caregivers, hospital staff, and patients receiving specialized services (Longo and Scior, 2004; Parkes et al., 2007; Samuels et al., 2007; Siegel et al., 2014). For mean length of stay (LOS), studies comparing specialized and mainstream inpatient services remain varied. Some studies report a shorter mean LOS for inpatients with ID in specialized inpatient units (Gabriels et al., 2012), others a longer mean LOS (Alexander et al., 2001; Xenitidis et al., 2004; Hemmings et al., 2009; White et al., 2010), and some no differences (Addington et al., 1993; Burge et al., 2002). These differences may be explained, in part, by variation in the clinical characteristics of the populations studied. Related to readmission rates, a US study of children with ASD and ID reported lower one-year readmission rates in a specialized versus mainstream psychiatry unit (Gabriels et al., 2012). At discharge, inpatients in mainstream settings were more likely to return to the family home (Hemmings et al., 2009), while inpatients in specialized settings were more likely to be discharged to out-of-area placements (Xenitidis et al., 2004). In Ontario, inpatients with ID receiving care in specialized units were also more likely to have medications reduced at discharge compared to inpatients receiving mainstream services (White et al., 2010).

In terms of quality of care and satisfaction with services, results for specialized and mainstream inpatient services have been mixed. Findings of a UK study examining three specialized ID units and seven mainstream psychiatry wards identified a number of positives and negatives for each service (Longo and Scior, 2004). While specialized units were described as positive, caring, and practical, these units left some patients feeling isolated. Mainstream wards, by contrast, were described as supportive of peer relationships, but left some patients feeling disempowered and vulnerable. Caregivers rated specialized units more positively because of good discharge planning and clear/open communication, while mainstream units were rated more negatively because of poor discharge planning and concerns for safety.

Outpatient mainstream and specialized services

We know less about outpatient care, despite the fact that most individuals receive care in outpatient rather than inpatient settings. Part of the reason for this is because of significant variation in outpatient programs, both mainstream and specialized, making comparisons difficult. In some jurisdictions, "mainstream psychiatric care" simply means that an individual with ID receives a consultation from a psychiatrist, but receives most of their mental health care otherwise, from their family doctor. One type of outpatient psychiatric service could be psychotropic medication prescribing and monitoring, which is quite common for the ID population (Cobigo et al., 2013). Mainstream psychiatric outpatient care may also refer to more enhanced outpatient services, such as assertive community treatment (ACT), or a combination of medication monitoring and psychotherapy. Some research has shown that enhanced clinical services, for example intensive case management, have greater benefits for individuals with ID than individuals without ID. In the UK700 trial, adults with mild ID or borderline IQ who received intensive case management had reduced hospital admissions, fewer days spent in hospital, lower costs, and greater satisfaction than adults who received standard case management only (Hassiotis et al., 2001). This difference was not evident for individuals without ID in the same trial.

Outcomes for patients with ID in specialized outpatient settings are generally positive, with a number of studies reporting improvements in adaptive and maladaptive functioning (Coelho et al., 1993), increased patient satisfaction, and decreased use of inpatient services (Holden and Neff, 2000). For example, results of a randomized controlled trial of a specialist behavior therapy team for adults with ID and challenging behavior resulted in significant reductions in challenging behavior and hyperactivity (Hassiotis et al., 2009). Findings also demonstrated that specialist behavior therapy in addition to psychiatric treatment was more effective in reducing aggressive behavior than psychiatric treatment alone. Two studies of individuals with ID receiving either ACT or standard community treatment (Martin et al., 2005; Oliver et al., 2005), failed to find differences in patient functioning, carer burden, and unmet need across services; however, eligibility constraints and similarities between ACT and community services, may have impacted the studies' ability to detect differences. There is emerging evidence that providing specialized psychotherapy interventions can benefit individuals with ID (Vereenooghe and Langdon, 2013), but very few studies have compared whether manualized interventions for those with ID are more effective than mainstream outpatient care.

Models of patient services for individuals with ID: who is best served where?

Mainstream inpatient and outpatient services: strengths and limitations

There is considerable debate over the adequacy and suitability of mainstream inpatient and outpatient services for individuals with ID. While mainstream services have certain advantages, they also come with considerable limitations. The most obvious and arguably significant strength of mainstream services is their capacity to serve and support a large number of individuals with ID. It has also been argued that mainstream services may be less stigmatizing for patients with ID (Chaplin, 2004; Hemmings et al., 2009). Limitations of mainstream services include lack of training and expertise in ID, inadequate resources to modify or support patients with cognitive limitations, and unsupportive or unhelpful staff attitudes (Lunsky et al., 2006; Jess et al., 2008; Chaplin, 2009, 2011; Hemmings et al., 2009). Mainstream services have also been criticized for their inability to serve patients with ID who have complex needs (e.g., behavior challenges, comorbid medical or psychiatric issues, communication impairments, severe or profound ID) and who, as a result, may require more intensive or individualized treatment.

Specialized inpatient and outpatient services: strengths and limitations

One of the major advantages of specialized services is their size and staff-to-patient ratio. Specialized services tend to be smaller and have a higher staff-to-patient ratio than mainstream services, which better facilitates client-centered care, patient safety, and allows services to be individually tailored to patient needs and level of cognitive or adaptive functioning (Xenditidis et al., 2004). Specialized services also employ interdisciplinary teams with knowledge, experience, and expertise working with individuals with ID and comorbid mental health issues (Chaplin, 2009, 2011).

Although there is substantial literature supporting the effectiveness of specialized services, certain disadvantages must also be considered. Specifically, specialized services do not typically have the capacity to service everyone who is referred. Similarly, given that individuals in specialized programs sometimes have longer length of stays, this can translate into longer wait times for patients awaiting services (Mackenzie-Davies and Mansell, 2007). While specialized services typically involve professionals who have more experience in ID, some specialized programs have encountered difficulty with staff retention (Mackenzie-Davies and Mansell, 2007). Specialized units exclusive to patients with ID can be very stressful, particularly when aggression, the most common reason for referral, is high (Hensel et al., 2014). Lastly, specialized services do not build capacity in mainstream services, and may in fact reduce the skills of healthcare providers outside these programs over time (Mackenzie-Davies and Mansell, 2007).

Integrated/hybrid service models of care

As in the general population, only a small proportion of individuals with ID will require inpatient services, leaving most individuals receiving care on an outpatient basis. As noted in the discussion on mainstream and specialized inpatient and outpatient services above, the question is not *which service* is better, but which *service* is better for *whom*. The literature largely supports the idea that specialized services are best suited to individuals with more severe disabilities (profound or severe ID), those who have limited or no verbal communication, and individuals with complex medical or psychiatric needs that present challenges to diagnosis and treatment. Individuals with mild or moderate ID, and those who have a clear psychiatric diagnosis, may be adequately served by mainstream services. It could be further argued that specialized services within mainstream mental health services which are diagnosis-specific (e.g., schizophrenia or anxiety disorders) or treatment-specific (e.g., cognitive-behavioral therapy for mood, dialectical behavior therapy for bipolar disorder) may also represent a good option, since they have the expertise and resources to support these specific populations. Because it may be difficult for specialized services to accommodate individuals with ID in their programs, some mainstream programs have also opted to include specialized ID consultation services as part of their programming.

In the UK, a number of integrated service models of care have started to emerge (Alexander et al., 2002; Hall et al., 2006; Davidson and O'Hara, 2007; Chaplin, 2009). These "hybrid" services enable mental health services to work collaboratively with ID services to deliver care that is effective for *all* individuals with ID. Although the individual programs themselves may vary, all models maintain a range of both mainstream and specialized services. For example, Hall et al. (2006) developed and evaluated an integrated model of care where adult mental health services worked collaboratively with ID services. The foundation of the model was the provision of specific beds for adults with mild ID and mental health issues within a general psychiatric ward and an associated community "virtual team" comprised of professionals in ID and other mental health professionals. In a review of this integrated service compared to patients in a mainstream psychiatry ward without specialist beds, patients in the integrated service experienced greater social contact, felt more comfortable, and settled more easily into the hospital environment (Parkes et al., 2007). Staff and caregivers also rated the integrated service more positively, reporting that the unit felt safe and that most patients were able to connect with individuals without ID (Samuels et al., 2007). In another UK study, a survey of consultants in the psychiatry of learning disability revealed that integrated mental health services were the most preferred management option, followed by specialist learning disability trusts (Alexander et al., 2002). Similarly, outcomes of a recent integrated care pathway-based inpatient service for individuals with ID resulted in more timely assessments, increased capacity for admission, reduced LOS, and better patient outcomes (Devapriam et al., 2014).

Key elements of successful integrated programs include those that incorporate staff training in ID, interdisciplinary teams, clear care pathways, and close links with community services for people with ID (e.g., residential, vocational, respite) (Alexander et al., 2002; Hall et al., 2006; Davidson and O'Hara, 2007; Jess et al., 2008). Studying what has worked in other successful mental health services, such as intensive case management and early intervention programs for individuals with psychosis (Bouras and Holt, 2004; Jess et al., 2008; Devapriam et al., 2014), will also be important in developing effective integrated programs. Additionally, what works best may be jurisdiction-specific. For example, national and provincial/state policies and funding for mental health or disability services will impact how services are provided. It would be easier to support mainstream programs if all clinicians received some training in ID and became comfortable working with the population. That, combined with access to specialized consultation as needed, would greatly improve the willingness and capacity of all healthcare providers. Finally, bridging the gap between mainstream and specialized services will require knowledge, resources, and mentorship from professionals with specialist knowledge and experience in ID, in both inpatient and outpatient settings.

Conclusions

Variation in the delivery of services, the client groups studied, and the measures used to evaluate these programs, has made direct comparison of mainstream and specialized services for individuals with ID difficult. While there is general agreement that mainstream services should have the capacity and willingness to provide care for at least some individuals with ID, there remain circumstances where these services alone are not adequate. Studies to date suggest that individuals with severe disabilities and those with more complex needs may be better served in specialized settings, leaving mainstream services to provide care to those with fewer needs or less severe disabilities. One way to bridge the gap between the two models is through the development of integrated or hybrid models of care where mental health and ID services work together to provide a continuum of services. Evidence for these programs is beginning to emerge where integrated programs have demonstrated reductions in LOS, improved patient outcomes, and greater staff and caregiver satisfaction (Davidson and O'Hara, 2007; Parkes et al., 2007; Samuels et al., 2007; Devapriam et al., 2014). Going forward, it will be important to study what has worked well in successful integrated programs and how to adapt those elements to different jurisdictions.

Key summary points

- Most individuals with ID in mainstream and in specialized inpatient units are male, young adults, have mild to moderate ID, and present with challenging behavior.
- Inpatients and outpatients with ID receiving specialized services tend to be younger, single, living with family, and have a diagnosis of ASD or a mood disorder. Inpatients and outpatients with ID in mainstream settings are more likely to have a psychotic disorder or substance abuse issues.
- Most studies comparing outcomes of inpatients with ID in specialized services to mainstream services document greater clinical improvement in specialized settings.
- Findings for length of inpatient stay are varied, and studies describing satisfaction with services suggest that there are positive and negative aspects to both programs.
- Mainstream outpatient services have greater capacity to serve individuals with ID and may be less stigmatizing, but lack training, resources, and expertise in ID. Specialized services, by contrast, have greater expertise in ID, access to interdisciplinary teams, and more tailored programing, but may stigmatize individuals with ID and lead to longer wait times.
- Mainstream services appear best suited to provide care for individuals with mild or moderate ID, while specialized services may be better equipped for individuals with ID who have more severe disabilities and/or complex medical or psychiatric needs.
- An emerging literature supports the development of integrated models of care that enable mental health and ID services to work together to provide a range of mainstream and specialized services.

References

Addington, D., Addington, J.M., Ens, I. (1993). Mentally retarded patients on general hospital psychiatric units. *Canadian Journal of Psychiatry*, 38, 134–136.

Alexander, R.T., Piachaud, J., Singh, I. (2001). Two districts, two models: in-patient care in the psychiatry of learning disability. *British Journal of Developmental Disabilities*, 47, 105–110.

Alexander, R.T., Regan, A., Gangadharan, S., Bhaumik, S. (2002). Psychiatry of learning disability – a future with mental health? *Psychiatric Bulletin*, 26, 299–301.

Bakken, T.L. and Martinsen, H. (2013). Adults with intellectual disabilities and mental illness in psychiatric inpatient units: empirical studies of patient characteristics and psychiatric diagnoses from 1996 to 2011. *International Journal of Developmental Disabilities*, 59, 179–190.

Bouras, N. and Holt, G. (2004). Mental health services for adults with learning disabilities. *British Journal of Psychiatry*, 184, 291–292.

Burge, P., Ouellette-Kuntz, H., Saeed, H., et al. (2002). Acute psychiatric inpatient care for people with a dual diagnosis: patient profiles and lengths of stay. *Canadian Journal of Psychiatry*, 47, 243–249.

Charlot, L., Abend, S., Ravin, P., et al. (2011). Non-psychiatric health problems among psychiatric inpatients with intellectual disabilities. *Journal of Intellectual Disability Research*, 55, 199–209.

Chaplin, R. (2004). General psychiatric services for adults with intellectual disability and mental illness. *Journal of Intellectual Disability Research*, 48, 1–10.

Chaplin, R. (2009). New research into general psychiatry services for adults with intellectual disability and mental illness. *Journal of Intellectual Disability Research*, 53, 189–199.

Chaplin, R. (2011). Mental health services for people with intellectual disabilities. *Current Opinion in Psychiatry*, 24, 372–376.

Cobigo, V., Ouellette-Kuntz, H.M.J., Lake, J.K., Wilton, A.S., Lunsky, Y. (2013). Medication use. In Y. Lunsky, J.E. Klein-Geltink, E.A. Yates (eds.), *Atlas on the Primary Care of Adults with Developmental Disabilities in Ontario*. Toronto, ON: Institute for Clinical Evaluative Sciences.

Coelho, R.J., Kelley, P.S., Deatsman-Kelley, C. (1993). An experimental investigation of an innovative community treatment model for persons with a dual diagnosis (DD/I). *Journal of Rehabilitation*, 54, 37–42.

Cumella, S. (2007). Mental health and intellectual disabilities: the development of services. In N. Bouras and G. Holt (eds.), *Psychiatric and Behavioural Disorders in Intellectual and Developmental Disabilities*, second edition. Cambridge: Cambridge University Press.

Davidson, P.W. and O'Hara, J. (2007). Clinical services for people with intellectual disabilities and psychiatric or severe behaviour disorders. In N. Bouras and G. Holt (eds.), *Psychiatric and Behavioural Disorders in Intellectual and Developmental Disabilities*, second edition. Cambridge: Cambridge University Press.

Deb, S., Matthews, T., Holt, G., Bouras, N. (2001). *Practice Guidelines for the Assessment and Diagnosis of Mental Health Problems in Adults with Intellectual Disability*. Brighton, UK: Pavilion.

Devapriam, J., Alexander, R., Gumber, R., Pither, J., Gangadharan, S. (2014). Impact of care pathway-based approach on outcomes in a specialist intellectual disability inpatient unit. *Journal of Intellectual Disabilities*, 18(3), 211–220.

Gabriels, R.L., Agnew, J.A., Beresford, C., et al. (2012). Improving psychiatric hospital care for pediatric patients with autism spectrum disorders and intellectual disabilities. *Autism Research and Treatment*, ID: 685053, 1–7.

Hall, I., Parkes, C., Samuels, S., Hassiotis, A. (2006). Working across boundaries: clinical outcomes for an integrated mental health source for people with intellectual disabilities. *Journal of Intellectual Disability Research*, 50, 598–607.

Hassiotis, A., Ukoumunne, O.C., Byford, S., et al. (2001). Intellectual functioning and outcome of patients with severe psychotic illness randomized to intensive case management: report from the UK700 trial. *British Journal of Psychiatry*, 178, 166–171.

Hassiotis, A., Robotham, D., Ganagasbey, A., et al. (2009). Randomized single-blind, controlled trial of a specialist behavior therapy team for challenging behaviour in adults with intellectual disabilities. *American Journal of Psychiatry*, 166, 1278–1285.

Hemmings, C.P., O'Hara, J., McCarthy, J., et al. (2009). Comparison of adults with intellectual disabilities and mental health problems admitted to specialist and generic inpatient units. *British Journal of Learning Disabilities*, 37, 123–128.

Hensel, J.M., Lunsky, Y., Dewa, C.S. (2014). The mediating effect of severity of client aggression on burnout between hospital inpatient and community residential staff who support adults with intellectual disabilities. *Journal of Clinical Nursing*, 23, 1332–1341.

Holden, P. and Neff, J.A. (2000). Intensive outpatient treatment of persons with mental retardation and psychiatric disorder: a preliminary study. *Mental Retardation*, 38, 27–32.

Jess, G., Torr, J., Cooper, S.A., et al. (2008). Specialist versus generic models of psychiatry training and service provision for people with intellectual disabilities. *Journal of Applied Research in Intellectual Disabilities*, 21, 183–193.

Longo, S. and Scior, K. (2004). In-patient psychiatric care for individuals with intellectual disabilities: the service users' and carers' perspectives. *Journal of Mental Health*, 13, 211–221.

Lunsky, Y. and Balogh, R. (2010). Dual diagnosis: a national study of psychiatric hospitalization patterns of people with developmental disabilities. *Canadian Journal of Psychiatry*, 55, 721–728.

Lunsky, Y., Bradley, E., Durbin, J., et al. (2006). The clinical profile and service needs of hospitalized adults with mental retardation and a psychiatric diagnosis. *Psychiatric Services*, 57, 77–83.

Lunsky, Y., Bradley, E., Durbin, J., Koegl, C. (2008). A comparison of patients with intellectual disability receiving specialized and general services in Ontario's psychiatric hospitals. *Journal of Intellectual Disability Research*, 52, 1003–1012.

Lunsky, Y. White, S.E., Palucka, A.M. Weiss, J. Bockus, S., Gofine, T. (2010). Clinical outcomes of a specialized inpatient unit for adults with mild to severe intellectual disability and mental illness. *Journal of Intellectual Disability Research*, 54, 60–69.

Lunsky, Y., Gracey, C., Bradley, E., Koegl, C., Durbin, J. (2011). A comparison of outpatients with intellectual disability receiving specialised and general services in Ontario's psychiatric hospitals. *Journal of Intellectual Disability Research*, 55, 242–247.

Mackenzie-Davies, N. and Mansell, J. (2007). Assessment and treatment units for people with intellectual disabilities and challenging behaviour in England: an exploratory survey. *Journal of Intellectual Disability Research*, 51, 802–811.

Martin, G., Costello, H., Leese, M., et al. (2005). An exploratory study of assertive community treatment for people with intellectual disability and psychiatric disorders: conceptual, clinical, and service issues. *Journal of Intellectual Disability Research*, 49, 516–524.

National Institute for Health and Clinical Excellence (NICE). (2012). *Autism: Recognition, Referral, Diagnosis and Management of Adults on the Autism Spectrum. NICE Guideline [CG142].* At http://guidance.nice.org.uk/cg142

Oliver, P., Piachaud, J., Tyrer, P., et al. (2005). Randomized controlled trials of assertive community treatment in intellectual disability: the TACTILD study. *Journal of Intellectual Disability Research*, 49, 507–515.

Parkes, C., Samuels, S., Hassiotis, A. (2007). Incorporating the views of service users in the development of an integrated psychiatric service for people with learning disabilities. *British Journal of Learning Disabilities*, 35, 23–29.

Russell, A.T., Hahn, J.E., Hayward, K. (2011). Psychiatric services for individuals with intellectual and developmental disabilities: medication management. *Journal of Mental Health Research in Intellectual Disabilities*, 4, 265–289.

Samuels, S., Hall, I., Parkes, C., Hassiotis, A. (2007). Professional staff and carers' views of an integrated mental health service for adults with learning disabilities. *The Psychiatrist*, 31, 13–16.

Siegel, M., Milligan, B., Chemelski, B., et al. (2014). Specialized inpatient psychiatry for serious behavioral disturbance in autism and intellectual disability. *Journal of Autism and Developmental Disorders*, 44(12), 3026–3032.

Sullivan, W.F., Berg, J.M., Bradley, E., et al. (2011). Primary care of adults with developmental disabilities: Canadian consensus guidelines. *Canadian Family Physician*, 57, 541–553.

Vereenooghe, L. and Langdon, P.E. (2013). Psychological therapies for people with intellectual disabilities: a systematic review and meta-analysis. *Research in Developmental Disabilities*, 34, 4085–4102.

White, S.E., Lunsky, Y., Grieve, C. (2010). Profiles of patients with intellectual disability and mental illness in specialized and generic units in an Ontario psychiatric hospital. *Journal of Mental Health Research*, 3, 117–131.

Xenitidis, K., Gratsa, A., Bouras, N., et al. (2004). Psychiatric inpatient care for adults with intellectual disabilities: generic or specialized units. *Journal of Intellectual Disability Research*, 48, 11–18.

Service users' and carers' experiences of mental health services

Katrina Scior

Introduction

A decade ago dissatisfaction among people with intellectual disabilities (ID), and their family and paid carers, with mental health service provision was first noted (Cole, 2002; Foundation for People with Learning Disabilities, 2003; Chaplin, 2004; Longo and Scior, 2004; Scior and Longo, 2005). However, it is only relatively recently that the experiences of service users with ID have received greater attention in service development and improvement. In parallel, over the past five years there has been an increased attempt to obtain first-hand accounts of mental health service use from service users and carers (Donner et al., 2010; Chinn et al., 2011; Stenfert Kroese and Rose, 2011; Bonell et al., 2012; Stenfert Kroese et al., 2013). The present chapter summarizes what we know about the experiences of people with ID who require support to meet their mental health needs. It will also account for the experiences of family and paid carers who provide support to people with ID affected by comorbid mental health problems. As there is no unitary service model for treatment and support, evidence on provision by mainstream mental health services and specialist ID services will be considered, where available, as will inpatient and community-based services. Two subgroups who have been identified as finding it particularly difficult to access mental health assessment and treatment are young people with ID in the transition from child to adult services, and people with ID from Black and minority ethnic communities. Hence, their experiences and needs will find particular mention in this chapter. As this chapter's focus is on the experiences of service users and carers, where possible these are represented in their own words.

Why pay attention to the experiences of service users and carers?

This may seem an odd question to pose, given that policy documents these days emphasize the need to listen to service users and their family and paid carers in evaluating service provision and identifying areas for development. However, the fact that a chapter on service user and carer experiences appears for the first time only in this, the third edition of a highly regarded textbook on ID and mental health, leads one to question why such a chapter seems necessary, or rather why it seems necessary only now. One explanation for this somewhat belated shift away from viewing service user experiences as an optional "add on," is recognition that it is not only morally and ethically right

Psychiatric and Behavioral Disorders in Intellectual and Developmental Disabilities, ed. Colin Hemmings and Nick Bouras. Published by Cambridge University Press. © Cambridge University Press 2016.

to ask those who use services about their experiences, but that, not surprisingly, basing improvement to the quality of services on feedback provided by service users may well contribute to improved outcomes (National Institute for Health and Clinical Excellence, 2011). Recent commissioning guidance goes as far as stating that the quality of mental health services should be measured from the perspective of the individual with ID and their family (Joint Commissioning Panel for Mental Health, 2013).

In the UK, guidance by the National Institute for Health and Clinical Excellence (NICE) has detailed the level of service that people using mental health services through the National Health Service (NHS) should expect to receive (National Institute for Health and Clinical Excellence, 2011). This guidance includes the following qualities that services should impart to adults experiencing mental health problems across all care pathways, that is, across community, crisis, and inpatient services: empathy, dignity, and respect; shared decision-making and self-management; and combating stigma. The guidance notes that "improving service user experience is unlikely to incur significant cost, and is more often related to challenging and improving the *values* or *culture* of an organisation" (National Institute for Health and Clinical Excellence, 2011). Given that people with ID are increasingly expected to access mainstream mental health services wherever possible (Joint Commissioning Panel for Mental Health, 2013), arguably they should be equally entitled to expect the core service qualities set out above. The limited evidence available on the experiences of people with ID who use mental health services suggests, though, that empathy, dignity, and respect is something individual staff impart, but it is by no means a common experience. Furthermore, shared decision-making and supporting self-management is something many services for people with ID struggle with at the best of times, and find even harder to practice when service users present with additional mental health problems. As core values are helpful but often difficult to translate into everyday practice, this chapter will aim to set out what specific aspects of service provision make for good practice, as perceived by service users and carers.

How do service users with ID and carers experience mental health services?

In trying to understand the experiences of people with ID who require mental health services, it is important to emphasize how bewildering and frightening the onset of mental health problems can be for individuals who, due to their pre-existing cognitive and communication impairments, may find the world around them and their own emotional and mental state hard to understand at the best of times. Similarly, for their families and carers, this is often a time of intense confusion and distress. Some parents vividly expressed this in Faust and Scior (2008):

> "I remember it was so confusing, like my little boy had just changed into a monster . . . I felt lost . . . it felt like we were struggling on in the dark, blind if you like." and "At the time I continually thought he was acting. And that sounds ludicrous now I say it. How could I have thought that? But we really didn't know what to do. We had no idea what was happening, what help we could get. I just thought he was bad, I didn't know what to think."

Against this background, the frustration experienced in response to often very extended but unanswered calls for help made by people with ID, and their family and paid carers, can be fully appreciated. Faust and Scior (2008) reported accounts from numerous parents who felt that, even when they were very explicit about their sense of desperation, their pleas for help often fell on deaf ears. They concluded that *"often parents felt that services simply 'paid lip service' to their pleas, pretending to take their concerns seriously to placate them ... There was general agreement that a crisis had to be reached before services would intervene and offer the appropriate help."* Other studies similarly noted service users' and carers' perception that huge barriers had to be overcome to access mental health support (Longo and Scior, 2004; Donner et al., 2010).

Focusing specifically on inpatient mental health services, feeling disempowered, lacking in control, and with little to do for much of the time, are experiences shared by most psychiatric inpatients, regardless of their intellectual functioning (Quirk and Lelliott, 2001; Gilburt et al., 2008). However, admissions to mainstream psychiatric wards appear to present additional challenges for people with ID, including a common tendency to attribute presenting problems to the person's ID, rather than recognizing their mental health needs, and a misplaced "assumption of competence," which can lead to a failure to meet even basic needs.

As Chaplin (2009) notes, even in countries where specialized ID services are highly developed, people with ID still not infrequently use general psychiatric inpatient services. A study by Longo and Scior (2004) compared the experiences of 30 adults with mental health problems and their carers of seven general psychiatric wards and three specialist assessment and treatment units in the UK. They found that staff in specialist units were more likely to be described as caring and willing to provide practical help. Those admitted to general psychiatric wards were more likely to find staff unfriendly or neglectful, and to feel disempowered and lacking in freedom. Of note, a sense of isolation was a more common feature of specialist provision, while supportive relationships with other inpatients were more common on general wards.

Opportunities for social contact were similarly rated a positive feature of general psychiatric wards by service users in Parkes et al. (2007) and Vos et al. (2007). However, some service users may be painfully aware of being viewed as different and "deficient" by fellow inpatients, as noted by these participants in a study by Donner et al. (2010): *"They judged me. I'm different to them."* and *"I had a few friends but most people tormented me and called me names."*

Recognition of the additional and unique support needs of individuals with ID who require mental health care is the fundamental basis for services making reasonable adjustments, now a legal requirement (in the UK). Where this does not happen, people with ID can often be faced with inappropriate expectations. A participant in Donner et al.'s (2010) study observed that *"the nurses (on a mainstream psychiatric ward) took the line 'you've got to be independent, you've got to do it, I'm not going to do it for you.' It wasn't even a case of 'you do what you can do and I'll help with the rest'."* A family carer had this to say: *"all the others could do things for themselves, he couldn't and he was just left to it you know. He just didn't know how to do anything. I went in one day and there was sick all over the floor of his room, he was sitting on the chair with just a pair of pants on and I couldn't find any clothes for him and he was freezing."*

In contrast, in Parkes et al.'s (2007) study, users of an inpatient service with four dedicated beds for people with ID within a mainstream psychiatric ward described a less frightening experience and greater involvement in their treatment and the decision-making process than in the pre-existing general adult inpatient service. Of note, they were supported by nurses who had received additional training in ID, and access to specialized ID services was high. They also felt able to make friends with fellow inpatients without ID.

Suggestions that specialist inpatient services necessarily offer a positive experience should be viewed with great caution though. A study by Chinn et al. (2011) examined the experiences of 17 individuals with ID placed in out-of-area inpatient settings, often far from home. Of the participants, 80% had a mild ID and 75% had been compulsorily detained. The authors (Chinn et al., 2011) noted that they *"were particularly struck by the very negative reports from participants of their treatment by staff. They reported staff using very derogatory language and responding to service users with a lack of respect, fairness and consistency. Descriptions of warm and supportive relationships with staff were missing from most of the accounts"* (p. 57). Given that for many participants the admission was triggered by aggressive behavior and physical assaults on others, this complaint by one participant seems very concerning: *"Asked for anger management groups once, but nothing happened. I feel I could use something like that to deal with my aggression ... nothing seemed to be done about it"* (p. 55). Instead, the most widespread intervention in the inpatient units was medication, with all 17 participants taking some form of psychotropic medication.

Perhaps surprisingly, few studies have examined the experiences of individuals with ID who use community-based mental health services. A study of community services for adults with psychosis and ID found that service users, carers, and professionals largely agreed as to what makes for good services but expressed different priorities. The six service users who participated in a focus group prioritized advice, practical help, and having more of a say. The five carers who participated in a separate focus group emphasized the need for good communication between all involved, and for service personnel to know the service user well as a person (Hemmings et al., 2009).

While concerns have repeatedly been expressed about negative attitudes within mainstream services towards providing psychological therapies for this service user group since Bender (1983) first talked of *"therapeutic disdain,"* little comparative first-hand evidence is available to elucidate how people with ID view the accessibility and quality of therapies received. At a time when people with ID are increasingly expected to access mainstream services, for example to receive psychological therapy as part of large-scale programs such as England's *Improving Access to Psychological Therapies* (IAPTs), it seems incumbent to examine to what extent their experiences match the vision set out in good practice guidance (Department of Health, 2009).

Experiences of specific subgroups

One specific group that merits attention are young people with ID who are in the transition period from childhood to adulthood. They have consistently been shown to be at much increased risk for mental health problems compared to their typically developing peers (Emerson and Hatton, 2007). Numerous authors have noted concern about a failure to provide mental health services for these young people and their families (Allington-Smith, 2006), with as many as two-thirds of young people affected receiving no specialist mental health input during the transition from child to adult services (McCarthy and Boyd, 2002).

It has been observed elsewhere that people with ID from Black and ethnic minority communities often experience double discrimination (Azmi et al., 1997; Mir et al., 2001). A study by Bonell et al. (2012) studied the experiences of users of specialist community-based mental health services for adults with ID. While White participants were generally positive about the services and care they received, Black service users reported more varied, and generally less positive, experiences of services. All of the 11 White service users felt involved in their assessment and all except one felt involved in decisions about their treatment, but only three-quarters of the 13 Black participants did. Furthermore, 9 of the 11 White service users disagreed strongly with the suggestion that when they showed signs of feeling worried staff would rather offer them medication than talk to them, yet less than half of Black service users disagreed with this statement.

What makes for good experiences?

In a project funded by the Judith Trust, Stenfert Kroese and colleagues (Stenfert Kroese and Rose, 2011; Stenfert Kroese et al., 2013) conducted 23 focus groups with service users with ID and a variety of staff, as well as individual interviews with 16 service users and 38 paid carers. Their central aim was to invite service users and paid carers to describe what they view as good services and how services should be improved. Their key conclusions were that for mental health services to be good, staff need to have a real interest in the people they support; they need to have the ability to be open and honest, yet gentle and sensitive; they need to be able to spend time with service users and listen to what they have to say. The value of experiencing staff as genuinely interested was expressed by this participant in their study: *"Some staff I wouldn't go to because they have a bad attitude. I go to staff who listen to you and not judge you"* (Stenfert Kroese and Rose, 2011, p. 13). The impact of positive interactions with staff was also evident in the accounts of service users in Parkes et al.'s (2007) study: *"You could talk to the nurses, if you had problems you used to talk to them you know"* (p. 27), and *"They'd done their best to help me get well. They were caring nurses, they were very kind"* (p. 27). A further important staff quality noted by Stenfert Kroese and colleagues (Stenfert Kroese and Rose, 2011; Stenfert Kroese et al., 2013) concerns the provision of support in a way that is "competence promoting" rather than "competence inhibiting." In the words of a participant in their study: *"... are helpful, helping their client to do their job"* and *"... show you what to do instead of just telling you"* (Stenfert Kroese and Rose, 2011, p. 14).

It cannot be stressed enough that in order to impart qualities such as empathy, dignity, and respect, and to practice shared decision-making, mental health staff need to be treated well themselves, and need to be provided with good supervision and ongoing training (Stenfert Kroese and Rose, 2011; Stenfert Kroese et al., 2013). In order to make reasonable adjustments and provide person-centered support, without doubt, they will need to be able to dedicate time to service users with ID, and to be empowered to prioritize direct interactions over procedural and administrative duties.

Conclusions

This chapter has summarized first-hand accounts of the experiences of service users with ID, and family and paid carers, of mental health services. To date, such evidence is limited and mostly derived from small, local samples. Some of the studies cited are 10 or more years old, and it is possible that negative experiences of mental health services are less common, although recent evidence indicates that they are by no means a thing of the past. As is now formally recognized, good experiences are likely to make for better outcomes. Hence, exploring the experiences of service users and carers should be central to the evaluation of services, rather than viewed as an optional extra.

Several studies have explored service users' and carers' experiences of inpatient services. They suggest that specialist services tailored to the needs of this population can make for better experiences, but some offer alarmingly poor care. Disappointingly, very little is known regarding what people with ID make of community services and psychological therapies delivered via mainstream or specialist services. At a time when huge resources are devoted to improving access to psychological therapies for all, a failure to examine whether "all" includes people with ID is a major omission that should be addressed.

Key summary points

- Timely access to mental health services is viewed as a major challenge by many service users and carers.
- First-hand evidence on their experiences is limited and mostly derived from small, local studies.
- While studies have compared inpatient services provided in mainstream mental health and specialist ID settings, comparative evidence on community services is lacking.
- Staff attitudes and behavior are central to a good experience, and making time, listening actively, and providing support that recognizes the additional needs of service users with ID yet promotes their competence should be central to reasonable adjustments made in mainstream mental health services.
- Further research is needed into the experiences of people with ID of community services, including psychological therapy services.

References

Allington-Smith, P. (2006). Mental health of children with learning disabilities. *Advances in Psychiatric Treatment*, 12, 130–140.

Azmi, S., Hatton, C., Emerson, E., Caine, A. (1997). Listening to adolescents and adults with intellectual disability in South Asian communities. *Journal of Applied Research in Intellectual Disability*, 10, 250–263.

Bender, M. (1983). The unoffered chair: the history of therapeutic disdain towards people with a learning difficulty. *Clinical Psychology Forum*, 54, 7–12.

Bonell, S., Underwood, L., Radhakrishnan, V., McCarthy, J. (2012). Experiences of mental health services by people with intellectual disabilities from different ethnic groups: a Delphi consultation. *Journal of Intellectual Disability Research*, 56, 902–909.

Chaplin, R. (2004). General psychiatric services for adults with intellectual disability and mental illness. *Journal of Intellectual Disability Research*, 48, 1–10.

Chaplin, R. (2009). New research into general psychiatric services for adults with intellectual disability and mental illness. *Journal of Intellectual Disability Research*, 53, 189–199.

Chinn, D,. Hall, I., Ali, A., Hassell, H., Patkas, I. (2011). Psychiatric in-patients away from home: accounts by people with intellectual disabilities in specialist hospitals outside their home localities. *Journal of Applied Research in Intellectual Disabilities*, 24, 50–60.

Cole, A. (2002). *Include Us Too: Developing and Improving Services to Meet the Mental Health Needs of People with Learning Disabilities*. London: Foundation for People with Learning Disabilities.

Department of Health. (2009). *Improving Access to Psychological Therapies: Learning Disabilities Positive Practice Guide*. London: Department of Health.

Donner, B., Mutter, R., Scior, K. (2010). Mainstream in-patient mental health admissions for people with learning disabilities: service user, carer and provider experiences. *Journal of Applied Research in Intellectual Disabilities*, 23, 214–225.

Emerson, E. and Hatton, C. (2007). Mental health of children and adolescents with intellectual disabilities in Britain. *British Journal of Psychiatry*, 191, 493–499.

Faust, H. and Scior, K. (2008). Mental health problems in young people with learning disabilities: the impact on parents. *Journal of Applied Research in Intellectual Disabilities*, 21, 414–424.

Foundation for People with Learning Disabilities (2003). *Working Together: Developing and Providing Services for People with Learning Disabilities and Mental Health Problems*. London: Mental Health Foundation.

Gilburt, H., Rose, D., Slade, M. (2008). The importance of relationships in mental health care: a qualitative study of service users' experiences of psychiatric hospital admission in the UK. *BMC Health Services Research*, 8, 92.

Hemmings, C., Underwood, L., Bouras, N. (2009). What should community services provide for adults with psychosis and learning disabilities? A comparison of the views of service users, carers and professionals. *Advances in Mental Health and Learning Disabilities*, 3, 22–27.

Joint Commissioning Panel for Mental Health. (2013). *Guidance for Commissioners of Mental Health Services for People with Learning Disabilities*. At: http://www.jcpmh.info/good-services/learning-disabilities-services/

Longo, S. and Scior, K. (2004). In-patient psychiatric care for individuals with intellectual disabilities: the service users' and carers' perspectives. *Journal of Mental Health*, 13, 211–221.

McCarthy, J. and Boyd, J. (2002). Mental health services and young people with intellectual disability: is it time to do better?

Journal of Intellectual Disability Research, 46, 250–256.

Mir, G., Nocon, A., Ahmad, W., Jones, L. (2001) *Learning Difficulties and Ethnicity: Report to the Department of Health*. London: Department of Health.

National Institute for Health and Clinical Excellence (2011). *Service User Experience in Adult Mental Health: Improving the Experience of Care for People Using Adult NHS Mental Health Services. NICE Guideline [CG 136]*. Manchester, UK: National Institute for Health and Clinical Excellence.

Parkes, C., Samuels, S., Hassiotis, A., Lynggaard, H., Hall, I. (2007). Incorporating the views of service users in the development of an integrated psychiatric service for people with learning disabilities. *British Journal of Learning Disabilities*, 35, 23–29.

Quirk, A. and Lelliott, P. (2001). What do we know about life on acute psychiatric wards in the UK? A review of the research evidence. *Social Science and Medicine*, 53, 1565–1574.

Scior, K. and Longo, S. (2005). In-patient psychiatric care: what we can learn from people with learning disabilities and their carers. *Tizard Learning Disability Review*, 10, 22–33.

Stenfert Kroese, B. and Rose, J. (2011). *Mental Health Services for People with Adults with Learning Disabilities*. London: The Judith Trust.

Stenfert Kroese, B., Rose, J., Heer, K., O'Brien, A. (2013). Mental health services for adults with intellectual disabilities – what do service users and staff think of them? *Journal of Applied Research in Intellectual Disabilities*, 26, 3–13.

Vos, A., Markar, N., Bartlett, L. (2007). A survey on the learning disability service user's view of admission to an acute psychiatric ward. *British Journal of Developmental Disabilities*, 53, 71–76.

Chapter

25

Carer and family perspectives

Gemma L. Unwin, Shoumitro Deb, and John Rose

Introduction

Psychiatric and behavioral disorders can be a major concern for families and carers of people with intellectual disabilities (ID). Such difficulties are a common source of stress and negative emotions in carers. Challenging behaviors, which can often be the outward manifestation of mental health problems, present major difficulties for families and carers. People with ID may receive a "diagnosis" of behavioral disorder rather than a psychiatric diagnosis. The present chapter will focus upon the impact of challenging behaviors on carers. Studies have shown that behavioral or psychiatric problems are important sources of stress experienced by caregivers and that stress intensifies with the increasing severity of a carer's experience (Hayden and Goldman, 1996; Heller et al., 1997a; Lecavalier et al., 2006; Cudré-Maroux, 2011). Psychiatric and behavioral disorders are related to carer burden, coping, and are perceived to have a negative impact on families (McIntyre et al., 2002; Maes et al., 2003; Unwin and Deb, 2011; Hartley et al., 2012). In residential care settings the presence of challenging behavior and interpersonal difficulties are related to lower job satisfaction, increased anxiety, emotional exhaustion, depersonalization/cynicism, and staff burnout (Jenkins et al., 1997; Mitchell and Hastings, 2001; Rose et al., 2004; Mills and Rose, 2011; Vassos and Nankervis, 2012).

Personal and situational variables, stress, and burnout

Whilst studies report a relationship between psychiatric or behavioral disorders and negative outcomes for carers, other studies suggest that a range of factors, such as carer cognitive variables, human and social capital, socioeconomic position, and carer satisfaction, mediate this relationship (e.g., Ben-Zur et al., 2005; Devereux et al., 2009; Hill and Rose, 2009; Hatton et al., 2010). Studies investigating the attribution model (Weiner, 2006; Dagnan et al., 2013) have suggested that internal judgments about the control individuals have over challenging behaviors can predict staff response and subsequent placement breakdown, with carers more likely to help where the behavior is perceived as out of the control of the person (Phillips and Rose, 2010; Cudré-Maroux, 2011). However, the results obtained using this model have been inconsistent with some researchers failing to find a clear relationship between attributions and helping behavior (e.g., Rose and Rose 2005).

Psychiatric and Behavioral Disorders in Intellectual and Developmental Disabilities, ed. Colin Hemmings and Nick Bouras. Published by Cambridge University Press. © Cambridge University Press 2016.

Other models are starting to be used to investigate the complex relationship between challenging behavior, psychiatric disorder, and stress in carers (e.g., Hill and Rose, 2010; Rose 2011). This includes a model of stress in parent–child interactions developed by Mash and Johnston (1990). This model has been used to demonstrate the mediation of the relationship between challenging behavior and carer stress and burnout by carer cognitive variables. It consists of four elements, including a client's characteristics such as challenging behavior, environmental characteristics, and parent characteristics that might include a variety of psychological variables, such as attributions or locus of control, with interactive stressor burnout as an outcome. These links are considered reciprocal, and while they recognize that other factors may be influential, they consider that these variables are likely to be the most important influence on the development of carer–child interactive stress. This model has been used to demonstrate predictive utility in mothers of younger children with ID (Hassall et al., 2005), in adult children living at home with parents (Hill and Rose, 2010), and for care staff (Mills and Rose, 2011; Rose et al., 2013). A review of this model suggests that a number of cognitive variables such as locus of control, fear of assault, and self efficacy mediate the relationship between challenging behavior and stress, and they can also mediate the relationship between environmental variables such as family support and organizational climate and stress.

Another promising area for the exploration of the relationship between challenging behavior/psychiatric disorder and stress is the adaptation of the self-regulation theory of illness behavior (Leventhal et al., 1984, 1992), which has been used to develop a measure, the Challenging Behaviour Perception Questionnaire (Williams and Rose, 2007) that explores the impact of challenging behavior on a range of staff–carer cognitions. This questionnaire has recently been adapted for use with parents (Nelson, 2013) and makes available a number of concepts to explore in the relationship between challenging behavior and stress. These include consequences for the carer and client, changes in the behavior over the course of time, control, and carer emotional reactions. Nelson, (2013) has also shown that parental beliefs about the consequences of the observed challenging behavior on the child itself was a significant mediator of the relationship between challenging behavior and parental stress.

Current research would therefore suggest that there is a relationship between psychiatric disorders, challenging behavior, and stress and burnout in both parents and carers; however, this relationship is complex. There are a range of variables that will influence the relationship, particularly a range of cognitive variables. That is, it is often possible to ameliorate the impact of caring for someone with psychiatric difficulties and corresponding challenging behavior if the carer is supported to see the behavior in a different way. This provides clinicians with an additional means of supporting carers, especially when underlying psychiatric and behavioral problems prove resistant to treatment.

Positive aspects of caring

Positive aspects of caring have received less recognition than stress and burnout. Hastings and Taunt (2002) suggested a model based on the idea that positive perceptions can be used by families as strategies to help them cope with the experience of raising children with disabilities. Specific research has been slowly developing. High levels of satisfaction and uplift as a result of caring and quality of life have been reported by family carers (Jokinen and Brown, 2005; Unwin and Deb, 2011). Furthermore, relationships may not always be unidirectional, with the person with ID perceived to be a source of support to the family (Heller et al., 1997b; Jokinen and Brown, 2005). Hastings et al. (2005) have developed the Positive Contributions Scale (PCS) in an attempt to quantify the contributions of children with ID to their families. They suggest that the measure has reasonable reliability and construct validity. Mothers generally reported more positive contributions to the family than fathers; however, there was clear evidence that their children were making a positive contribution to their families. Todd and Jones (2003) suggest that whilst parent caregivers may be potent advocates for their offspring, they may be more reserved and hesitant about expressing their own needs. Therefore, research needs to focus on further elucidating the experience of caring in this context, to ensure that caregivers are appropriately supported by services.

There has been less research on the positive aspects of caring for employed staff; however, Hastings and Horne (2004) have developed a measure, the Staff Positive Contributions Questionnaire (SPCQ), which could be used to further measure the positive contributions that people with ID make to staff. Indeed, other research has asked staff to evaluate their relationships with their clients, other staff, and the organization they worked for. Thomas and Rose (2010) based their research on equity theory, which asks staff to compare how much they put into their work compared to what they get back. Staff perceived that they contributed more to all of their relationships than they received, but it was the imbalance in their relationships with their colleagues and the organization that had a greater impact on their levels of burnout.

Direct carer's perceptions of the causes for aggressive challenging behavior

A recent study investigated the motivations and antecedents that trigger aggressive challenging behavior amongst adults with ID by interviewing their carers, including both paid and family carers (Unwin, 2013). The aim was to explore the knowledge and understandings of paid and family carers, to contrast these with existing models of challenging behavior, and to identify potential gaps in knowledge that could be targets for intervention with carers. Few studies have explored the perspectives of carers in this way and have instead concentrated on the psychological consequences of providing care. Unwin (2013) conducted structured interviews with 100 carers (56 paid care workers and 44 family carers) of adults with ID who were in contact with specialist health services for the management of aggressive behavior. Carers were asked to generate a list of what they perceived as contextual factors or motivations for aggressive behavior. The term "triggers" was used for carers as it was felt to be more understandable, less technical, and broader than other terms used in the literature such as "contextual variable" or "setting event." Similarly, the term "motivates" was used instead of "functions" for the same reasons. Triggers were described as referring to predisposing events as well as situations or circumstances which precipitate and sometimes perpetuate aggressive behavior.

Six main themes were extracted from the thematic analysis, namely, external environment, internal environment, expression of volition, specific activities/events, characteristics of ID, and predictability of behavior (Unwin, 2013). The carers interviewed identified a wide range of triggers, demonstrating some knowledge of the determinants of behavior. However, knowledge varied, with 41% of carers describing the aggressive behavior as unpredictable. The carers in the study cared for individuals who were in contact with specialist services; therefore, they may have received some psychosocial education from health professionals and may not be representative of the wider population of carers. The study also included both family and paid carers; it is not known whether family carers were less likely to identify triggers and more likely to perceive the behavior as unpredictable.

The results demonstrate convergence with existing literature on contextual variables (McAtee et al., 2004; McGill et al., 2005; Embregts et al., 2009b); however, some differences were evident when compared to the functional analysis literature. Unwin (2013) describes an external environment theme, related to features of the person's immediate physical environment and the social environment. Carers perceived the social environment to be the most common trigger, which included interactions with others, how others interact with individuals, and interactions observed by individuals. The carers interviewed often cited attention as a motivator and suggested that much behavior was "attention seeking": to initiate interaction or "get a reaction," whether this was negative or positive. Other carers did not identify attention as a function but rather identified a lack of attention or others getting attention as a trigger. Carers also identified features of the social context, such as the presence of certain staff members, other service users, or conflicts with others.

Attention has been reported to be a common function for challenging behavior (e.g., Embregts et al., 2009a; Matson et al., 2011; McClean and Grey, 2012); however, carers in the study by Unwin (2013) did not always describe attention-controlled motivation. Studies have also suggested that aggressive behavior is most commonly maintained by the need to escape external stimuli (e.g., Matson et al., 2011; Rojahn et al., 2012). The presence of certain individuals or witnessing conflict may relate to escape functions, but carers did not perceive behaviors in these terms and instead focused on observable features of the social environment. The physical environment also encompassed observable visual, auditory, and spatial triggers, such as loud, unexpected noises, busy environments, the proximity of others, and specific stimuli such as ambulances (Unwin, 2013). Such ecological variables have often been cited but rarely studied. It could be asserted that the escape function was also activated in response to many of these triggers; however, this understanding was not evident from the carers' accounts.

In the same study, carers identified triggers relating to the expression of volition, which included both goal-directed behavior and limits to volition imposed by others, often in response to the person being encouraged to do something, or the person wanting to do something. Much of the "expression of volition" described by Unwin (2013) could relate to a tangible function, as people exhibited aggressive behavior when they were not able to fulfill their desires; their behavior may have the aim of achieving that desire; however, few carers described this process. Few carers identified goal-directed behavior in relation to trying to achieve something (tangible) or avoid something (escape); rather, they identified "demands not being met" or "requests being denied." Unwin (2013) also describes a "specific activities and events" theme, which includes various activities of daily living, medical appointments, vacations, and special events. The author highlights that such triggers may provoke an escape function; however, carers did not provide any qualification as to how such activities and events trigger behavior. The emergence of these themes highlights the reduced autonomy of people with ID and the reliance on carers for access to activities and items. Carers understood this to be a source of tension, and further research should explore different approaches to managing these issues that would be acceptable to people with ID and avoid reinforcing the behavior.

Carers can most reliably identify physical functions for behavior such as pain, discomfort, and hunger (Matson and Wilkins, 2009), but physical functions are rarely considered in the literature (Matson et al., 2011). Unwin (2013) describes an "internal environment" theme from carers' accounts, which includes similar aversive physical states and medical conditions as well as emotional states that were identified by 58% of carers. McGill et al. (2005) reported on the tendency for functional analysis to neglect personal-setting events, especially emotional states. Carers in the study by Unwin (2013) often implicated underlying anxiety, agitation, and stress as triggering aggressive behavior, which indicates empathy amongst carers. However, without understanding the function of the behavior, carers may inadvertently reinforce behavior by providing or withdrawing attention/activities when aggressive behavior is expressed contingent on an underlying emotional state.

Carers are often relied upon to inform functional analysis (Rojahn et al., 2012). The study by Unwin (2013) indicates that carers can identify a range of contextual variables; however, some may struggle to identify triggers without prompting, and carers may not consider functional determinants of behavior, other than in relation to seeking attention. Authors have commented on the complexities of locating functions for behavior and suggested that a contextual approach may be useful in practice (McGill et al., 2005; Unwin, 2013). Commonly, carers are responsible for implementing behavioral plans on a day-to-day basis, but the lack of behavioral knowledge may present barriers to their successful implementation (McClean and Grey, 2012; Hutchinson et al., 2014; Willems et al., 2014). The acceptability of support plans to carers has been found to be the most salient factor relating to effectiveness (McClean and Grey, 2012).

Training and support for carers

Current evidence suggests low levels of behavioral and mental health knowledge and training amongst paid carers (Quigley et al., 2001; Allen et al., 2005; Stenfert Kroese et al., 2013); it can be asserted that informal carers have less knowledge and training. Training could help carers start to link contextual variables with functions for behavior; however, this is a complex task and may require psychological input. Carers may also benefit from training and information about potential contextual triggers to help them think more about personal and environmental conditions and their own role in the environment. Training could work on two levels: an educative/knowledge level and an attitudinal/attributional level.

Behavioral training packages for paid carers have been developed and have been shown to improve knowledge, attitudes, attributions, and understanding (Costello et al., 2007; Kalsy et al., 2007; Lowe et al., 2007b; Rose, 2014), improve the sense of empowerment, self-efficacy, and empathy (Hutchinson et al., 2014), and have resulted in improved behavioral support plans and reduced levels of challenging behavior (Lowe et al., 2007b; McClean and Grey, 2012). However, access to such training remains limited, can be resource-intensive, can be costly to services, and it is unlikely that family carers have access to such training. Little research has evaluated training for family carers, but research suggests that training can be effective in changing parental attitudes

(Rose, 1990). Training is also likely to support carers so that they are more confident in their approach and are able to cope more effectively in conceptualizing challenging behavior. As a result, carers are much less likely to experience higher levels of stress and burnout.

Supporting carers to identify and understand the role of contextual variables in precipitating behavior may represent a sustainable, widely implementable approach. Improving such knowledge may help to bridge the gap between highly trained health professionals and direct caregivers by developing a common language and shared understanding. Improving understanding of behavior may also improve carer's sense of self-efficacy, and shift their locus of control. Carers may become more involved in the development of behavioral support plans, which may improve investment and subsequent fidelity to the behavioral plan (Hieneman and Dunlap, 2000; Holt et al., 2005). Such plans, developed by direct carers rather than other professionals, may have a better "contextual fit," being developed in the environments in which they are to be implemented (McClean et al., 2005).

Conclusions

Behavioral and psychiatric disorders are key factors affecting carer experience and are associated with negative psychological consequences. While family carers appear to be rather resilient and, despite challenges, experience positive effects from their caring role, it is important to note that significant burden and stress are still present. Carer attributes, such as locus of control and self-efficacy, may mediate relationships between behavioral disorders and stress. Such psychological variables are subject to change with training in behavioral techniques. Carers can identify contextual triggers for aggressive behavior; supporting carers to develop contextually informed support may provide an accessible approach to facilitate mutual understanding and reduce stress and burnout in carers (see also Chapter 20).

Key summary points

- Psychiatric and behavioral disorders among people with ID are related to negative outcomes for carers such as stress, burden, and burnout. However, the relationships are complex.
- The caring role can also produce positive effects, with high levels of satisfaction with caring, uplift, and quality of life reported amongst family carers. However, there is currently little research into the positive aspects of caring.
- Carer cognitive variables, such as locus of control, fear of assault, self-efficacy, and beliefs about the consequences of challenging behaviors, mediate the relationship between challenging behavior and stress.
- Carer cognitive variables may be a target for intervention, especially where psychiatric or behavioral disorders are resistant to treatment.
- Behavioral and mental health training has been shown to improve knowledge, attitudes, attributions, self-efficacy, and empathy.
- One area for intervention may be to improve carers' identification and understanding of contextual variables to develop behavioral support plans to deliver contextually informed care.

References

Allen, D., James, W., Evans, J., Hawkins, S., Jenkins, R. (2005). Positive behavioural support: definition, current status and future directions. *Learning Disability Review*, 10(2), 4–11.

Ben-Zur, H., Duvdevany, I., Lury, L. (2005). Associations of social support and hardiness with mental health among mothers of adult children with intellectual disability. *Journal of Intellectual Disability Research*, 49, 54–62.

Costello, H., Bouras, N., Davis, H. (2007). The role of training in improving community staff awareness of mental health problems in people with intellectual disabilities. *Journal of Applied Research in Intellectual Disabilities*, 20, 228–235.

Cudré-Maroux, A. (2011). Staff and challenging behaviours of people with developmental disabilities: influence of individual and contextual factors on the transactional stress process. *British Journal of Developmental Disabilities*, 57(1), 21–40.

Dagnan, D., Hull, A., McDonnell, A. (2013). The Controllability Beliefs Scale used with carers of people with intellectual disabilities: psychometric properties. *Journal of Intellectual Disability Research*, 57(5), 422–428.

Devereux, J.M., Hastings, R.P., Noone, S.J., Firth, A., Totskia, V. (2009). Social support and coping as mediators or moderators of the impact of work stressors on burnout in intellectual disability support staff. *Research in Developmental Disabilities*, 30, 367–377.

Embregts, P.J.C.M., Didden, R., Huitink, C., Nieuwenhuijzen, M.V. (2009a). Aggressive behaviour in individuals with moderate to borderline intellectual disabilities who live in a residential facility: an evaluation of functional variables. *Research in Developmental Disabilities*, 30(4), 682–688.

Embregts, P.J.C.M., Didden, R., Huitink, C., Schreuder, N. (2009b). Contextual variables affecting aggressive behaviour in individuals with mild to borderline intellectual disabilities who live in a residential facility. *Journal of Intellectual Disability Research*, 53(3), 255–264.

Hartley, S.L., Barker, E.T., Baker, J.K., Seltzer, M.M., Greenberg, J.S. (2012). Marital satisfaction and life circumstances of grown children with autism across 7 years. *Journal of Family Psychology*, 26(5), 688–697.

Hassall, R., Rose, J., McDonald, J. (2005). Parenting stress in mothers of children with an intellectual disability: the effects of parental cognitions in relation to child characteristics and family support. *Journal of Intellectual Disability Research*, 48(6), 405–418.

Hastings, R. and Horne, S. (2004) Positive perceptions held by support staff in community mental retardation services. *American Journal on Mental Retardation*, 109, 53–62.

Hastings, R. and Taunt, H.M. (2002). Positive perceptions in families of children with developmental disabilities. *American Journal on Mental Retardation*, 107(2), 116–127.

Hastings, R.P., Beck, A., Hill, C. (2005). Positive contributions made by children with an intellectual disability in the family: mothers' and fathers' perceptions. *Journal of Intellectual Disabilities*, 9(2), 155–165.

Hatton, C., Emerson, E., Kirby, S., et al. (2010). Majority and minority ethnic family carers of adults with intellectual disabilities: perceptions of challenging behaviour and family impact. *Journal of Applied Research in Intellectual Disabilities*, 23, 63–74.

Hayden, M. and Goldman, J. (1996). Families of adults with mental retardation: stress levels and needs for services. *Social Work*, 41, 657–667.

Heller, T., Hsieh, K., Rowitz, L. (1997a). Maternal and paternal caregiving of persons with mental retardation across the lifespan. *Family Relations*, 46, 407–415.

Heller, T., Miller, A.B., Factor, A. (1997b). Adults with mental retardation as supports to their parents: effects on parental caregiving appraisal. *Mental Retardation*, 35, 338–346.

Hieneman, M. and Dunlap, G. (2000). Factors affecting the outcomes of community-based behavioral support. II. Factor category importance. *Journal of Positive Behavior Interventions*, 3(2), 67–74.

Hill, C. and Rose, J. (2009). Parenting stress in mothers of adults with an intellectual disability: parental cognitions in relation to child characteristics and family support. *Journal of Intellectual Disability Research*, 53(12), 969–980.

Hill, C. and Rose, J. (2010). Parenting stress models and their application to parents of adults with intellectual disabilities. *British Journal of Developmental Disabilities*, 56(110), 19–37.

Holt, G., Hardy, S., Bouras, N. (2005). *Mental Health in Learning Disabilities: A Reader.* Brighton, East Sussex, UK: Pavilion Publishing.

Hutchinson, L.M., Hastings, R.P., Hunt, P.H., et al. (2014). Who's challenging who? Changing attitudes towards those whose behaviour challenges. *Journal of Intellectual Disability Research*, 58(2), 99–109.

Jenkins, R., Rose, J., Lovell, C. (1997). Psychological well-being of staff working with people who have challenging behaviour. *Journal of Intellectual Disability Research*, 41, 502–511.

Jokinen, N.S. and Brown, R.I. (2005). Family quality of life from the perspective of older parents. *Journal of Intellectual Disability Research*, 49(10), 789–793.

Kalsy, S., Heath, R., Adams, D., Oliver, C. (2007). Effects of training on controllability attributions of behavioural excesses and deficits shown by adults with Down syndrome and dementia. *Journal of Applied Research in Intellectual Disabilities*, 20, 64–68.

Lecavalier, L., Leone, S., Wiltz, J. (2006). The impact of behaviour problems on caregiver stress in young people with autism spectrum disorders. *Journal of Intellectual Disability Research*, 50(3), 172–183.

Leventhal, H., Nerenz, D.R., Steel, D.J. (1984). Illness representations and coping with health threats. In A. Baum, S.E., Taylor, J.E. Singer (eds.), *Handbook of Psychology and Health*, Vol. 4. Hillsdale, NJ: Erlbaum.

Leventhal, H., Diefenbach, M., Leventhal, E. (1992). Illness cognition: using common

sense to understand treatment adherence and affect cognition interactions. *Cognitive Therapy and Research*, 16, 143–163.

Lowe, K., Jones, E., Allen, D., et al. (2007b). Staff training in positive behaviour support: impact on attitudes and knowledge. *Journal of Applied Research in Intellectual Disabilities*, 20, 30–40.

Maes, B., Broekman, T.G., Dösen, A., Nauts, J. (2003). Caregiving burden of families looking after persons with intellectual disability and behavioural or psychiatric problems. *Journal of Intellectual Disability Research*, 47(6), 447–455.

Mash, E.J. and Johnston, C. (1990). Determinants of parenting stress: illustrations from families of hyperactive children and physically abused children. *Journal of Clinical Child Psychology*, 19, 313–328.

Matson, J.L. and Wilkins, J. (2009). Factors associated with Questions About Behaviour Function for functional assessment of low and high rate challenging behaviours in adults with intellectual disability. *Behaviour Modification*, 33, 207–218.

Matson, J.L., Kozlowski, A.M., Worley, J.A., et al. (2011). What is the evidence for environmental causes of challenging behaviours in person with intellectual disabilities and autism spectrum disorders? *Research in Developmental Disabilities*, 32, 693–698.

McAtee, M., Carr, E.G., Schulte, C., Dunlap, G. (2004). A Contextual Assessment Inventory for problem behaviour: initial development. *Journal of Positive Behaviour Interventions*, 6, 148–165.

McClean, B. and Grey, I. (2012). A component analysis of positive behaviour support plans. *Journal of Intellectual and Developmental Disability*, 37(3), 221–231.

McClean, B., Dench, C., Grey, I., et al. (2005). Person focused training: a model for delivering positive behavioural supports to people with challenging behaviours. *Journal of Intellectual Disability Research*, 49(5), 340–352.

McGill, P., Teer, K., Rye, L., Hughes, D. (2005). Staff reports of setting events associated with challenging behaviour. *Behaviour Modification*, 29, 599–615.

McIntyre, L.L., Blacher, J., Baker, B.L. (2002). Behaviour/mental health problems in young adults with intellectual disability: the impact on families. *Journal of Intellectual Disability Research*, 46(3), 239–249.

Mills, S. and Rose, J. (2011). The relationship between challenging behaviour, burnout and cognitive variables in staff working with people who have intellectual disabilities. *Journal of Intellectual Disability Research*, 55(9), 844–857.

Mitchell, G. and Hastings, R.P. (2001). Coping, burnout, and emotion in staff working in community services for people with challenging behaviours. *American Journal on Mental Retardation*, 106(5), 448–459.

Nelson, L. (2013). The relationship between challenging behaviour, cognitions and stress in mothers of individuals with intellectual disabilities. D.Clin.Psy. thesis. Birmingham, UK: University of Birmingham.

Phillips, N. and Rose, J. (2010). Predicting placement breakdown: individual and environmental factors associated with the success or failure of community residential placements for adults with intellectual disabilities. *Journal of Applied Research in Intellectual Disabilities*, 23, 201–213.

Quigley, A., Murray, G.C., MacKenzie, K., Elloit, G. (2001). Staff knowledge about symptoms of mental health problems in people with learning disabilities. *Journal of Learning Disabilities*, 5, 235–244.

Rojahn, J., Zaja, R.H., Turygin, N., Moore, L., van Ingen, D.J. (2012). Functions of maladaptive behaviour in intellectual and developmental disabilities: behaviour categories and topographies. *Research in Developmental Disabilities*, 33, 2020–2027.

Rose, D. and Rose, J. (2005). Staff in services for people with intellectual disabilities: the impact of stress on attributions and challenging behaviour. *Journal of Intellectual Disability Research*, 49(11), 827–838.

Rose, D., Home, S., Rose, J.L., Hastings, R.P. (2004). Negative emotional reactions to challenging behaviour and staff burnout: two replication studies. *Journal of Applied Research in Intellectual Disabilities*, 17, 219–223.

Rose, J. (1990). Accepting and developing the sexuality of people with mental handicaps: working with parents. *Mental Handicap*, 18(1), 4–6.

Rose, J. (2011). How do staff psychological factors influence outcomes for people with developmental and intellectual disabilities in residential services? *Current Opinion in Psychiatry*, 24(5), 403–407.

Rose, J., Mills, S., Silva, D., Thompson, L. (2013). Testing a model to understand the link between client characteristics, organisational variables, staff cognitions and burnout in care staff. *Research in Developmental Disabilities*, 34(3), 940–947.

Rose, J., Gallivan, A., Wright, D., Blake, J. (2014). An evaluation of short training course in positive behavioural support. *International Journal of Developmental Disabilities*, 60(1), 35–42.

Stenfert Kroese, B., Rose, J., Heer, K., O'Brien, A. (2013). Mental health services for adults with intellectual disabilities – what do service users and staff think of them? *Journal of Applied Research in Intellectual Disabilities*, 26(1), 3–13.

Thomas, K. and Rose, J.L. (2010). The relationship between reciprocity and the emotional and behavioural responses of staff. *Journal of Applied Research in Intellectual Disabilities*, 23(2), 167–179.

Todd, S. and Jones, S. (2003). "Mum's the word!": maternal accounts of dealing with the professional world. *Journal of Applied Research in Intellectual Disabilities*, 16, 229–244.

Unwin, G.L. (2013). A longitudinal observational study of aggressive behaviour in adults with intellectual disabilities. PhD thesis. Birmingham, UK: University of Birthmingham. At etheses.bham.ac.uk

Unwin, G.L. and Deb, S. (2011). Family caregiver uplift and burden: associations with aggressive behaviour in adults with intellectual disability. *Journal of Mental Health Research in Intellectual Disability*, 4(3), 186–205.

Vassos, M.V. and Nankervis, K.L. (2012). Investigating the importance of various individual, interpersonal, organisational and demographic variables when predicting job burnout in disability support workers. *Research in Developmental Disabilities*, 33, 1780–1791.

Weiner, B. (2006). *Social Motivation, Justice and the Moral Emotions: An Attributional Approach*. Mahwah, NJ: Lawrence Erlbaum.

Willems, A.P.A.M., Embregts, P.J.C.M., Bosman, A.M.T., Hendriks, A.H.C. (2014). The analysis of challenging relations: influences on interactive behaviour of staff towards clients with intellectual disabilities. *Journal of Intellectual Disability Research*, 58(11), 1072–1082.

Williams, R.J. and Rose, J.L. (2007). The development of a questionnaire to assess the perceptions of care staff towards people with intellectual disabilities who display challenging behaviour. *Journal of Intellectual Disabilities*, 11, 197–211.

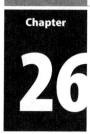

Chapter

Reflections

Colin Hemmings

Introduction

Definitions and terminology matter. The study and practice of the mental health of intellectual disabilities (ID) probably suffers to some extent from the complication of terminology arising from dual (or multiple) diagnosis. The title of this book itself reflects that complexity. It is not possible to easily capture the complexity of the field in terms that will be to the point and universally accepted. Accordingly, there is no worldwide consensus as to whether a recognizable "mental health of ID" field exists or whether, for example, it is now more of a "neurodevelopmental" field. People are not suddenly remarkably different because of a change of one point on an IQ scale. Such "fields" of research and practice are always artificially drawn to some extent; they consist in reality of multiple overlapping areas. Where the boundaries should be drawn and which terminology should be used is inevitably controversial (see Chapter 2 by Marco Bertelli et al.). A prime example is the uncertain place in services of people with autism spectrum disorders but without ID.

If we accept though that there is, or should be, a "mental health of ID" field of practice and research, with reasonably definable boundaries, then this would be distinct from the general medical health care of people with ID and from their education and social care. It is the author's view, as of many others but no means all, that the "mental health" (problems) term should encompass behavioral problems carrying significant risk or distress. This then is the "field" to which will be referred to in this chapter. The preceding chapters in this new edition have shown how knowledge about this field of the mental health of ID continues to advance. Clinicians and researchers working with people with ID are gradually more able to draw on evidence derived direct from the care of people with ID. There is less need for extrapolation from the evidence base of generic mental health care.

This final chapter is an opportunity for the author to reflect on where this field is now. The chapter will include the author's views on the ongoing central debate about the relationships between mental health problems and behavioral problems, on how services might further develop, and on what some of the ongoing research should be.

Basic tenets

It is important to understand how this field has evolved to date (see Chapter 1 by Nick Bouras). This is surely more difficult than for many others, as services for people with

Psychiatric and Behavioral Disorders in Intellectual and Developmental Disabilities, ed. Colin Hemmings and Nick Bouras. Published by Cambridge University Press. © Cambridge University Press 2016.

ID vary so much, especially between a few high-income countries and the rest of the world. A major trend witnessed in most high-income countries has been the process of deinstutionalization of ID services, occurring mainly in the latter part of the 20th century. Driven by multiple influences, it was made possible by clinicians who were committed to the development of improved care for this ultra-marginalized group of patients. Considering there had been virtually no community care previously, a huge amount was achieved in a relatively short period. In this era there was also simultaneously a great deal of research interest into the epidemiology of mental disorders and challenging behaviors in people with ID. Previous suggestions of institutionalization being the major precipitant and perpetuator of mental health problems in people with ID did not stand the test of time.

What became abundantly clear over this period was that: (i) people with ID could (and did) have coexisting mental health problems; and (ii) people with ID actually have an increased prevalence of many mental disorders. These two facts have been well documented previously and, indeed, have arguably become two of the basic tenets of the modern field of the "mental health of ID" (MHID). It can be argued though that it is still the case, even well into the 21st century, that these tenets are still not universally understood, especially by those not trained in the mental health aspects of ID.

Even from within the field some have continued to challenge the evidence that mental health problems are more common in ID. Jason Buckles (see Chapter 3) has reviewed the most recent epidemiological research and highlighted the problems of both over- and underestimating the prevalence of mental disorders in people with ID. The evidence available has been boosted substantially by recent large-scale population-based studies. What has emerged now is a more nuanced understanding that some mental disorders appear increased in people with ID, whilst the prevalence of other mental disorders is more or less the same as in people with more typical IQ. What is clearly increased is the prevalence of behavioral problems. It is evident that when problem or challenging behaviors are not included, the increased prevalence in mental disorders overall in people with ID is less marked. Thus, the key is always how challenging behaviors are conceptualized and classified (see also Chapter 20 by Sally-Ann Cooper).

"Mental health" and "challenging behaviors"

One of the most enduring clinical and research questions has been, "*To what extent should mental illness and behavioral problems be considered separately in people with ID?*" The term, "behavioral equivalents," was used for some years until there was a backlash against it. Evidence was not forthcoming to substantiate challenging behaviors as equivalents of psychiatric symptoms. The author would agree that we have now witnessed the "end of behavioral equivalents." Nonetheless, challenging behaviors are associated with mental illness overall, so a preferred (but less emphatic) term instead might be behavioral "correlates." These still retain some utility for assessment and treatment. Like the increased prevalence of mental disorders overall, the overlap between mental health problems and challenging behaviors in people with ID should neither be overplayed nor underplayed; mental illness is but one cause or consequence of challenging behaviors from very many. The relationships between them though are arguably still underinvestigated.

The distinction that should be made between behavioral problems and mental illness remains then one of the key issues (and tensions) for the field. It has huge clinical and service implications. It sometimes, unfortunately, becomes the basis of professional rivalries. Some of this is probably driven by lingering antimedical attitudes and the stigma of mental illness by association. Perhaps motivated by the harm caused by lazy labeling and poor quality mental health care, some still try to deny the extent of dual diagnosis. Unfortunately this only lets down people with ID. There has been research that appears at least partly motivated by an intention to prove that medication is mostly harmful and ineffective for people with ID. It is difficult to accept this, not least because of the low-powered and methodological gaps of existing studies.

The truth is that it will always be impossible to neatly separate out mental health and behavioral problems in people with ID. The need for a holistic (biopsychosocial) approach, including coordinated multidisciplinary input, is arguably no greater in the whole of health care than for people with ID and mental health problems. But very often concurrent trends are contradictory; for example, the desirability of holistic practice or care exists widely in staff or carers' minds whilst there is a concurrent process in services towards more and more super-specialization. Various ways of understanding, such as the "medical" or "behavioral" or other "models," are different aids that should be applied simultaneously to provide insights at different levels of mental health problems. Problems can be approached from the "biological" level (e.g., genetics, neuroimaging, receptors) up to the "psychosocial" level (e.g., cognitive processes, beliefs), and even the "political" level (e.g., law, policy). A unimodal practice or narrow understanding will cause incomplete and, thus, poor practice.

Service provision

Levi-Strauss (1966) famously suggested that humans tended towards binary (and oppositional) thinking. Service provision for those dually disadvantaged by ID and coexisting mental health problems is still heavily determined by widespread binary thinking. Unfortunately it continues to prove remarkably difficult for many to remember that people can have both ID and mental health problems. In many low-income countries there can be very little provided for the care of the dually diagnosed. In high-income countries mental health and ID (or developmental) services mostly continue to operate separately with quite different cultures. Where there are stand-alone, dedicated services for the dually diagnosed, the mental health and challenging behavior components are often split, leading to a fragmentation of already scant resources (see also Chapter 23 by Johanna Lake et al.).

One can easily understand how services have varied so much between countries given the enormous differences in income, funding, and infrastructure, as well as in philosophies and culture. But service provision has also widely varied within countries and even between areas with similar demographics. This reflects the many different (and often competing) ideologies in the field. It is often fashionable to say that we should not have a "one size fits all" approach to service provision. It does stretch belief, however, to think that these widely varying services are likely to be equally effective or to provide equal value for money.

There have not been the same sorts of service developments for people with ID that have been seen in recent years, such as the formation of crisis resolution and home treatment services. Certainly this is at least partly due to resources. If mental health services are often on the margins of healthcare funding, then mental health of ID services can be said to be on the margins of those margins. But it has also partly been due to ID services having only relatively recently embraced service research. It still remains unclear how best to deliver mental health care for people with ID. The problem for dedicated mental health of ID services (where they exist) is that they are inevitably too small-scale to operate alone effectively. They will always tend to be squeezed between generic mental health and ID services, even if their clinicians work assiduously at both interfaces.

A major difficulty in overcoming the struggle of balancing between mental health and ID services is the differing opinions about who should provide mental health care and where mental health of ID service provision should lie primarily, whether alone or aligned more closely with one of these two larger "empires." With the stigma of mental illness and the long and sad history of abuse of people with ID, there can be overcompensation from ID staff and frequent subtle or even overt criticisms of generic mental health services. There can often be a stigmatizing attitude towards mental health staff from ID staff (Hassiotis et al., 2003). Given the marginalization of people with ID, this is an ironic kind of reverse stigmatization. Barr (2011) noted the perjorative connotations and use of the term, "mainstream." There are frequently assumptions made that the ongoing problems for people with ID accessing generic mental health services lie only with the mental health staff.

The best intentions to protect people with ID from abuse can cause some paradoxical effects. Increased scrutiny of inpatient units and the rise of the "safeguarding vulnerable people from abuse" agenda (e.g., Department of Health, 2012) are long overdue. But such efforts should only be motivated by the aim of better care, which includes necessary treatment of mental illness and challenging behaviors. They should not be influenced by antimedical or antihospital bias. Otherwise they may lead to commissioners becoming risk-averse to the opening and maintenance of local, quality inpatient services and may lead in turn to inadvertent outcomes, such as people being placed far from their homes when they need admissions. Staff in ID services should not just complain as outsiders about people with ID being misunderstood or neglected or stigmatized (or themselves by proxy) by mental health services, but instead take an active role in assisting these services.

There is widespread agreement of the need for better crisis services for people with ID, although simple data of this need is often lacking. But there is not universal support for developing new stand-alone "super-specialist" services, such as crisis services for people with ID (e.g., Hemmings and Al-Sheikh, 2013). The replication of super-specialization of services that is occurring in the generic mental health services of many high-income countries is unlikely in any case to occur for people with ID, owing to lack of critical mass and resources. It is the author's view, like many others, that the best way forward is in developing new and closer ways of joint working with staff in generic mental health services (Hemmings et al., 2014). Sometimes the mental health of ID staff might often be best situated directly within the wider mental health services. Depending on local factors, there could sometimes instead be new "hybrid" services (see also Chapter 23 by Johanna Lake et al.). The mental health of ID staff would then be more highly visible to their mental health colleagues (Flynn, 2010). They would concentrate on a core group with ID who need continuing mental health care, high support, and more intensive input at times. Their other main function would be to enhance the assessments of people with low IQ and a range of complex needs such as mental illness, autism spectrum disorders (ASD), attention-deficit/hyperactivity disorder (ADHD), personality disorders, and/or epilepsy. This may mean more assessment and management of people with borderline low IQ and/or ASD who would benefit from mental health of ID expertise (Flynn, 2010).

The author believes that it does not really make sense to artificially separate behavioral problems from mental health problems, nor indeed the care of the more severely intellectually disabled from those with milder ID. Any service dedicated to managing challenging behaviors in people with ID will always need access to medical input, including physical health assessment and medication, and sometimes inpatient care, no matter how well the behavioral management and environment can be improved. However, given the widespread enduring binary thinking discussed previously, those staff primarily concerned with challenging behavior without diagnosable mental illness might sometimes and in some areas be best placed separately from those dually trained staff working more embedded within mental health services. Although this is perhaps not ideal as a somewhat "forced" choice, it is not really possible in practice to be "all things to all people" when attitudes to dual diagnosis continue to be so resistant to change. In the end there are pros and cons to most service models, but what matters ultimately is that services, however they are configured, have clarity of purpose and clear care pathways that are understandable to everyone, including service users and carers, and clinicians who are not dually trained.

Perhaps mental health of ID staff can benefit paradoxically from the dedicated ID services in this era being as yet so undeveloped and, thus, perhaps less likely to be "entrenched." For example, ID services can hopefully show the way for generic mental health services in promoting meaningful service user and carer engagement and inclusion. Staff that work with people with ID are confronted with communication issues daily. It is, therefore, regularly and explicitly acknowledged in ID services that a major part of successful practice is thinking how to engage and to work with these communication difficulties. Being on a smaller scale and invariably containing committed individuals inspired to make positive changes, ID services can often be the forerunners of innovative practices. In this vein, mental health of ID clinicians and services should be in the vanguard of making smoother the care pathway transitions between inpatient and community mental health care, to make the reality of seamless "in-reach" and outreach between community and hospitals as the standard for health care in the 21st century.

Research

Following behind research in generic mental health care, research into the mental health aspects of ID was in the latter part of the 20th century largely concerned with classification, diagnosis, and epidemiology, and also the use of various rating instruments (see Chapter 4 by Heidi Hermans). One major difference in the ID field has been the major debate as to whether to use standardized or modified diagnostic criteria. The research emphasis shifted to some degree towards the end of the 20th century with advances in technology allowing attempts to understand more of the genetic basis of mental disorders. For example, there has been a large increase of research into behavioral phenotypes (see Chapter 18 by Robert Hodapp et al.) and the dementias in people with ID (see Chapter 5 by Jennifer Torr).

We still have yet to see, though, a large body of research into interventions and services in this specific patient group, including many evaluations of clinical outcomes and cost effectiveness (Hemmings, 2010). The mental health of ID field has tended to have a time lag for the evaluation and the adoption of interventions that have long become standard in generic mental health services. Well-documented examples have included the use of clozapine and antidementia medications, and cognitive-behavioral and other therapies. Often this delay is entirely understandable, as it occurs for multiple reasons. These include the relative lack of resources proportionate to clinical need and the very often unclear commissioning of services. Sometimes the time lag has not been so justified. Some staff in ID services have operated idiosyncratically without close scrutiny on the margins of "mainstream" health care, arguing that their practice was "a special case"; only belatedly has it been more widely considered obligatory for ID services to be evidence-based like everyone else.

Thus, the evidence base as it currently stands is even less substantial than perhaps many clinicians realize. For example, we still do not have published evidence to confirm beyond doubt widespread and longstanding clinician beliefs, such as tardive dyskinesia and neuromalignant syndrome (and even arguably all side effects in general due to antipsychotic medications) being more common in people with ID than in the general population. It is difficult also to assume, yet, that psychological treatments are all evidence-based alternatives or adjuncts to medication in people with ID. Relatively little about them has yet been studied in this specific patient group, although this is gradually changing (see Chapter 14 by Nigel Beail and Chapter 15 by Dave Dagnan).

There have been of course many well-documented difficulties in conducting research in people with ID, including funding and recruitment, and the difficulties of conducting randomized controlled trials (RCTs) (Robotham and Hassiotis, 2009). It is difficult to see how research in the mental health aspects of ID will provide the numbers required for sufficient RCTs and multicenter studies unless databases can be linked, and this type of large-scale research often needs government funding. Mental health research, including health services' research, has frequently excluded adults with ID (Lennox et al. 2005). Another research "problem" is the increasingly stringent ethical research safeguarding rightly intended to protect people with ID from abuse. Unfortunately, this may lead to the paradox of less research in people with ID being conducted and this unintended outcome is not in their best wider interests.

Given ongoing problems of research in people with ID, it is the author's view that we need to run "against the grain" to some extent and not discourage the smaller-scale research that has become increasingly unfashionable. There is a range of levels of evidence, not just RCTs. We should not forget, for example, that carefully written case studies and case series rich in observation and transparent for any biases or preconceived opinions, as well as expert opinions gathered systematically and small sample naturalistic studies, can all be important sources of evidence. Quantitative research often needs a grounding prepared by qualitative research to promote validity. Otherwise a risk in being research "purists" is that we might continue to have little or no evidence on which to base practice.

The research at the biological (and molecular) level of mental health problems is often now showing exciting new leads. Biologically orientated research (and similarly research in cognitive psychology) is also often the most likely to be funded. But it would be a mistake to not continue research in other areas, including those now perhaps considered slightly more old-fashioned for research. We should continue to research, for example, areas such as phenomenology, psychosocial determinants, psychoeducation, staff attitudes and training, diagnostic practices, treatment outcomes, and service-component effectiveness.

As an example, the recent research helping to improve detection of mental health problems in people with autism is invaluable (see Chapter 11 by Trine L. Bakken et al.). We have arrived at a time when ASD is finally being more recognized as an entity by clinicians who have not trained in developmental or ID services. But it is also essential that psychosis is not missed in people with ID and autism owing to a reverse type of diagnostic overshadowing by some staff trained in ID perhaps inclined to see only ASD where there is schizophrenia. Specific education and training in dual diagnosis is necessary, and further research is needed into the effectiveness of this training of staff in generic mental health and ID services (Werner and Stawski, 2012). We also need more research such as that by Crowley et al. (2008) into psychoeducation for service users, carers, and families (Jess et al. 2008; see also Chapter 24 by Katrina Scior and Chapter 25 by Gemma L. Unwin et al.). Carers' perspectives have been neglected, yet their opinions are often crucial in the care of people with ID (e.g., Inwang et al., 2013). It is important also to investigate the views and actions of staff in mental health and primary care services, and others often involved such as social workers, police, and paramedics, about their encounters with people with ID and mental health problems when they are in crisis. This might in turn clarify what particular training might be helpful for these staff at the crucial junctions in the pathways of care. In health services' research, a wider range of outcomes than hospital admissions needs to be investigated (Chaplin, 2011). Researchers in ID have historically found it difficult to compete for the huge grants needed for whole-service evaluations. A more realistic way forward in this sphere of research is to look at the modeling, piloting, and the evaluation of specific service components (Burns et al. 2006).

It has often been said, for example by Arthur Kleinman and other leading medical writers, that the greatest medical advances would take place simply if existing treatments were just used more effectively (Hemmings, 2005). We have not researched adequately such fundamental clinical issues such as adherence to interventions or factors promoting engagement in people with ID. We have not very often tried to understand how marked placebo responses might be being mediated. For example, it is the author's opinion that the NACHBID study (Neuroleptics in the Treatment of Aggressive Challenging Behaviour for People with Intellectual Disabilities; Tyrer et al. 2008) of the "ineffectiveness" of risperidone and haloperidol for aggression in people with ID, from the data, was overstated; partly because it was based on a very small sample drawn from multiple heterogeneous sites, but, more importantly, because there was an alternative conclusion that could be drawn from the data. The antipsychotic medication was in fact extraordinarily "effective" in reducing aggression as measured, although no more so than the placebo tablets. What was lost then was discussion of this enormous apparent positive placebo effect, seemingly caused through changes in the carers' attitudes and/or behaviors. This type of finding can and should be further investigated, rigorously and scientifically. It is the author's view that we also need more research into clinicians' diagnosing practices. For example, it is likely that diagnosing mental illness in the presence of epilepsy (e.g., Arshad et al., 2011) and ASD (e.g., Tsakanikos et al., 2006) is affected greatly by diagnostic overshadowing, which can of course occur in both ways; that is, to reduce or increase the detection of mental illness in a person with ID.

Research in the "mental health of ID" needs to become more interdisciplinary and multimodal. Some of the most interesting research into challenging behaviors (e.g., Lowry and Sovner, 1992) measured clinical progress using both behavioral assessments and symptomatic assessments simultaneously. Unfortunately, more than two decades later, this type of interdisciplinary research has remained rare. However, in an encouraging observation in Chapter 18, Robert M. Hodapp et al. note that "the previous more rigid cultural distinctions between the biomedical perspective and the psychosocial has shown encouraging signs of lessening" in research into behavioral phenotypes and genetic syndromes.

One principle that is helpful to bear in mind for research is what can this relatively small field of the mental health of ID teach the very large generic mental health field? Some research trends in wider mental services are already well advanced in staff working with people with ID. For example, some of the most active research into service users' and carers' perspectives and experiences is already taking place with people with ID (see Chapter 24 by Katrina Scior and Chapter 25 by Gemma L. Unwin et al.). Clinicians and researchers working with people with ID tend to be already keenly aware of the impact of life experiences on people with ID from events that others might just sometimes dismiss as trivial (see Chapter 9 by Philip Dodd and Fionnuala Kelly). ID staff have also arguably long considered the concepts and implementation of recovery, person-centered care, and empowerment. Very often research in people with ID and their carers can actually be among the first research studies of their types in any patient group (e.g., Chaplin et al., 2013; see also Chapter 8 by Jane McCarthy and Eddie Chaplin). This can be one way to boost funding and support, to show how insights gained from the care of people with ID might be helpful also to the wider population, and, therefore, another way of staff working with people with ID showing what they can "bring to the table" (Flynn, 2010).

Conclusions

This final chapter has been a reflection on the content of this book and has included a personal view about the possible evolution of services and what should guide future research. It would be very interesting and useful to ask a range of authors also with extensive knowledge of the literature to provide their own reflections, perhaps for a future edition of this book. Reading a well-known book like this gives an opportunity for all clinicians and researchers to take an overview and take stock. There are many grounds for realism about the rate of progress and even some grounds for disappointment. But there are also many grounds for optimism. The field will continue to develop, and in some areas this growth will likely be exponential. Time will tell if this means the field as covered in this book will become too large to be summarized in such an equivalent-sized and richly detailed textbook. Meanwhile, before a future edition hopefully, we will see improving access to assessments and treatments for people with ID and mental health problems, including in lower-income countries. We hope also that we will see the stigma and ignorance about people with ID gradually decreasing, and the expectation that people with ID deserve quality mental health care becoming more widespread.

Key summary points
- Service provision for those dually disadvantaged by ID and coexisting mental health problems is still heavily determined by widespread binary thinking.
- If mental health services are often on the margins of healthcare funding, then mental health of ID services can be said to be on the margins of those margins.

- It does not make sense to artificially separate behavioral problems from mental health problems, nor indeed the care of the more severely intellectually disabled from those with milder ID.
- Any service dedicated to managing challenging behaviors in people with ID will always need access to medical input, including physical health assessment and medication, and sometimes inpatient care, no matter how well the behavioral management and environment can be improved.
- We hope that we will see stigma and ignorance about people with ID gradually decreasing and the expectation that people with ID deserve quality mental health care becoming more widespread.

References

Arshad, S., Winterhalder, R., Underwood, L., et al. (2011). Epilepsy and intellectual disability: does epilepsy increase the likelihood of co-morbid psychopathology? *Research in Developmental Disabilities*, 3, 353–357.

Barr, O. (2011). What is "mainstream"? *Journal of Intellectual Disabilities*, 15, 155–156.

Burns, T., Catty, J., Wright, C. (2006). Deconstructing home-based care for mental illness: can one identify the effective ingredients? *Acta Psychiatrica Scandinavica*, 113(429, Suppl.), 33–35.

Chaplin, E., Chester, R., Tsakanikos, E., et al. (2013). Reliability and validity of the SAINT: a guided self-help tool for people with intellectual disabilities. *Journal of Mental Health Research in Intellectual Disabilities*, 6, 245–253.

Chaplin, R. (2011). Mental health services for people with intellectual disabilities. *Current Opinion in Psychiatry*, 24, 372–376.

Crowley, V., Rose, J., Smith, J., Hobster, K., Ansell, E. (2008). Psycho-educational groups for people with a dual diagnosis of psychosis and mild intellectual disability. *Journal of Intellectual Disabilities*, 12, 25–39.

Department of Health. (2012). *Transforming Care: A National Response to Winterbourne View Hospital*. London: Department of Health.

Flynn, A. (2010). This far, yet how much further? Reflections on the allure of the mainstream for people with intellectual disabilities and mental health needs. *Advances in Mental Health and Learning Disabilities*, 4, 9–14.

Hassiotis, A., Tyrer, P., Oliver, P. (2003). Psychiatric assertive outreach and learning disability services. *Advances in Psychiatric Treatment*, 9, 368–373.

Hemmings, C.P. (2005). Rethinking medical anthropology: how anthropology is failing medicine. *Anthropology and Medicine*, 2, 91–103.

Hemmings, C.P. (2010). Service use and outcomes. In N. Bouras and G. Holt (eds.), *Mental Health Services for Adults with Intellectual Disability: Strategies and Solutions (Maudsley Series)*. London: Psychology Press.

Hemmings, C.P. and Al-Sheikh, A. (2013). Expert opinions on community services for people with intellectual disabilities and mental health problems. *Advances in Mental Health and Intellectual Disabilities*, 7, 169–174.

Hemmings, C.P., Bouras, N., Craig, T. (2014). How should community mental health of intellectual disability services evolve? *International Journal of Environmental Research and Public Health*, 11, 8624–8631.

Inwang, F., Hemmings, C., Hvid, C. (2013). Using explanatory models in the care of a person with learning disabilities. *Advances in Mental Health and Learning Disabilities*, 7, 152–160.

Jess, G., Torr, J., Cooper, S.-A., et al. (2008). Specialist versus generic models of psychiatry training and service provision for people with intellectual disabilities.

Journal of Applied Research in Intellectual Disabilities, 21, 183–193.

Lennox, N., Taylor, M., Rey-Conde, T., et al. (2005). Beating the barriers: recruitment of people with intellectual disability to participate in research. *Journal of Intellectual Disability Research*, 49, 296–305.

Levi-Strauss, C. (1966). *The Savage Mind*. London: Weidenfeld and Nicolson.

Lowry, M.A. and Sovner, R. (1992). Severe behavior problems associated with rapid cycling bipolar diorders in two adults with profound mental retardation. *Journal Intellectual Disability Research*, 36, 269–281.

Robotham, D. and Hassiotis, A. (2009). Randomised controlled trials in learning disabilities: a review of participant experiences. *Advances in Mental Health and Learning Disabilities*, 3, 342–346.

Tsakanikos, E., Costello, H., Holt, G., et al. (2006). Psychopathology in adults with autism and intellectual disability. *Journal of Autism and Developmental Disorders*, 36, 1123–1129.

Tyrer, P., Oliver-Africano, P.C., Ahmed, Z., et al. (2008). Risperidone and haloperidol in the treatment of aggressive challenging behaviour in patients with intellectual disability: a randomised controlled trial. *Lancet*, 371, 57–63.

Werner, S. and Stawski, M. (2012) Mental health: knowledge, attitudes and training of professionals on dual diagnosis of intellectual disability and psychiatric disorder. *Journal of Intellectual Disability Research*, 56, 291–304.

Index

A–B–C charts, 172
A–B–C model of behavior, 171
Aberrant Behavior Checklist
    (ABC), 49
acetylcholinesterase inhibitors,
    59, 142
acute stress disorder, 100–1
adaptive functioning deficits,
    22, 24–6
ADHD. *See* attention-deficit/
    hyperactivity disorder
adjustment disorders, 101–2
Adult Behavior Checklist
    (ABCL), 50
affective disorders. *See* mood
    disorders
age of onset, as diagnostic
    criterion, 26
aging-related health problems,
    233
aggressive behavior, 209
    assessment in children, 185
    behavioral interventions,
        175
    carers' perceptions of
        causes, 271–3
    cognitive-behavioral
        interventions, 211–12
    course over time, 226
    inpatient admission, 253
    pharmacotherapy, 142, 187,
        285
    prevalence, 224
agoraphobia, 91
agreeableness (A), 112
alcohol misuse, 216
Alzheimer's disease, 57
    Down syndrome and, 57–60
    pharmacotherapy, 59, 142
American Association for
    Intellectual and
    Developmental Disorders
    (AAIDD), 16, 24, 27
American Psychiatric
    Association (APA), 5, 16,
    18
amphetamines, 134, 187
amyloid deposition, Down
    syndrome, 58

anger, interventions, 157,
    211–12
animal models, 202
anticonvulsants. *See*
    antiepileptic drugs
antidepressants, 141
    anxiety disorders, 93
    autism spectrum disorders,
        143
    children, 187
    depression, 83, 142
antiepileptic drugs
    behavioral problems, 140
    epilepsy, 249
    refractory epilepsy, 246
    side effects, 144, 234–5,
        249
    West syndrome, 247
antipsychotic agents
    anxiety disorders, 93
    children, 187
    extra-pyramidal side effects,
        70, 144
    first-generation (FGA), 140
    problem behaviors, 142,
        228, 285
    schizophrenia spectrum
        disorders, 70–1, 141
    second-generation. *See*
        atypical antipsychotics
antisocial behavior, 209, *See
    also* offending behavior
    assessment in children, 185
antisocial personality disorder,
    110–11
anxiety, 89, 99
    in autism spectrum
        disorders, 120–2
Anxiety, Depression and
    Mood Scale (ADAMS),
    47, 83
anxiety disorders, 89–96
    clinical presentation, 90–1
    diagnostic tools, 48, 91–7
    in autism spectrum
        disorders, 93, 121–5
    in children, 183
    in Williams syndrome,
        198–9

management and treatment,
    92–5
    pharmacotherapy, 93, 141
    prevalence, 90
    risk factors, 91
    stepped-care model, 93
Anxiety Disorders Interview
    Schedule, 184
apolipoprotein E4 (Apo E4)
    allele, 59
APP gene, increased
    expression, 58
Arc (National Association of
    Parents and Friends of
    Mentally Retarded
    Children), 2
aripiprazole, 140, 143
arson. *See* firesetting
Asian countries, service
    provision, 9
assertive community
    treatment (ACT), 71, 255
assessment
    behavioral, 171–9
    children with ID, 183–4
    epidemiological studies,
        37–9
assessment instruments and
    rating scales, 45–51
    choosing, 50
    new developments, 51
    screening, 46
    screening vs. diagnostic, 46
    self-report vs. informant-
        report, 45
    standardized diagnostic
        interviews, 50
Assessment of Dual Diagnosis
    (ADD), 47, 82–3
Assimilation of Problematic
    Experiences model, 153
asylums, 2
atomoxetine, 141
attention-deficit/
    hyperactivity disorder
    (ADHD), 129–35
    areas for future research,
        134
    assessment, 131–2

attention-deficit/
hyperactivity disorder (ADHD)
(cont.)
  diagnostic criteria, 129–30,
    185
  diagnostic validity in ID, 131
  epidemiology, 130
  impact, 131
  longitudinal course, 182
  management, 132–4
  pharmacotherapy, 133–4,
    141, 238
attention function, aggressive
  behavior, 272
attribution model, carer stress
  and, 269
atypical antipsychotics. See
  also risperidone
  bipolar disorder, 84
  problem behaviors, 140
  schizophrenia spectrum
    disorders, 70–1
  side effects, 70, 144
auditory hallucinations, 69
Australia, service provision, 9
Autism Diagnostic Instrument
  (ADI)/Autism Diagnostic
  Observation Schedule
  (ADOS), 184
autism spectrum disorders
  (ASD), 28–9, 119–26
  anxiety symptoms and
    disorders, 93, 120–5
  assessment tools, 29, 184
  clinical implications of
    mental illness, 123
  diagnosis of mental illness,
    121, 124
  differential diagnosis,
    28–9, 68, 120–1
  management and treatment,
    124–5
  pharmacotherapy, 125, 140–
    1, 144
  Prader–Willi syndrome, 201
  prevalence of mental illness,
    122–3
  risk of mental illness, 119–20
  service provision, 8, 253
aversive interventions,
  problem behaviors, 174
avoidant behavior, 102, 176

barbiturates, 140, 249
Beck Depression Inventory
  (BDI), 48, 92

Behavior Problems Inventory
  (BPI), 50
behavioral and psychological
  symptoms of dementia
  (BPSD), Down
  syndrome, 59
behavioral approach, 171–8
behavioral assessment, 171–2,
  177
behavioral equivalents, 79, 280
behavioral interventions,
  171, 172–8
  challenging behavior,
    174–6
  focusing on consequences,
    173–4
  for children, 187
  implementation in practice,
    176–7
  modifying antecedent
    stimuli, 173
  symptoms of psychiatric
    disorders, 176
behavioral phenotypes,
  196–202
  age-related changes, 198
  complex interactions,
    198
  examples, 198–201
  future areas for research,
    201–2
  multiple domains, 197
  social and family context,
    198
  total vs. partial specificity,
    197
  within-syndrome variability,
    197
behavioral problems. See
  problem behaviors
benzodiazepines, 93, 140, 249
bereavement, 103–5
beta-adrenergic blockers, 141,
  187
bipolar disorder
  assessment instruments, 83
  diagnostic features, 79–80
  epidemiology, 81
  etiology, 81
  pharmacotherapy, 84, 142,
    237–8
  psychosocial interventions,
    84
Bipolar Mood Chart, 83
birth complications,
  schizophrenia risk, 66

BOLD (Becoming Older with
  Learning Disability)
  study, 56–7
borderline intellectual
  functioning (BIF), 27
brain damage
  causing ID, 29
  prolonged seizures causing,
    243
  traumatic, epilepsy and ID,
    244
Brief Symptom Inventory
  (BSI), 46
burnout, carer, 270

CAMDEX-DS, 49
cancer
  risks, 233
  screening, 232
cannabis use, 66
carbamazepine, 140, 187
carers. See also family(ies);
  parents
  burden of psychosis and ID,
    71
  employed. See staff
  experiences of services,
    262–7
  impact of problem
    behaviors, 269–74
  perceptions of causes of
    aggression, 271–3
  positive aspects of caring,
    270–1
  stress, and cognitive
    variables, 269–70
  training and support, 133,
    186, 273–4
Cattell–Horn–Carroll model
  of intelligence, 23
celiac disease, 234
cerebral palsy, 29
challenging behavior. See
  problem behaviors
Challenging Behaviour
  Perception
  Questionnaire, 270
children, psychopathology of,
  181–92
  ADHD, 131, 133–4, 182
  case examples, 187–92
  clinical assessment, 183–4
  depression, 81, 183
  developmental level and
    cognitive ability, 184–5
  epilepsy, 242–3

management principles, 186–7
multiple disabilities and medical illness, 185
pharmacotherapy, 141, 143, 187
phenomenology, 182–3
prevalence, 181
psychosocial and family factors, 185–6
transitional services, 124, 265
cholinesterase inhibitors, 59, 142
citalopram, 83, 141
classification of ID, 15–21, 30
future perspectives, 17–19
neurodevelopmental perspective, 21
terminology, 19–21
classification of problem behaviors, 226–7
classification systems. See DSM-5; ICD-10; ICD-11
clomipramine, 142
clonidine, 141, 187
clozapine, 71, 83
cognitive assessment
children with ID, 184
diagnosis of ID, 24
longitudinal, in dementia, 56
cognitive-behavioral therapy (CBT), 161–7
adaptations for ID, 165
anger and aggression, 211–12
anxiety disorders, 94–5
autism spectrum disorders, 125
challenges of using, 162–5
depression, 84
development of trials, 165
firesetting behavior, 215
for children, 186
future directions, 166
impact of ID, 164–5
sexually aggressive behavior, 212–13
theoretical basis, 161–2
cognitive deficit models, 162
cognitive distortion models, 162
cognitive skills training, offenders, 216–17

communication impairments, autism, 119
community-based services. See also outpatient services
historical context, 2–4
implementing behavioral interventions, 176–7
normalization concept, 3–4
offender populations, 209
psychosis and ID, 71
service users' experiences, 265
community intellectual disability teams, 7
conduct disorder
assessment, 185
classification, 226
conscientiousness (C), 112
constipation, 234
Core and Cluster program, 4
cortical development, malformations of, 245
countertransference, 155–6
course of IDD, 27–8
criminal offending. See offending behavior
crisis services, 282

DASH-II, 47
anxiety disorders, 92
mood disorders, 83
schizophrenia spectrum disorders, 69
DBC. See Developmental Behavior Checklist
DC-LD (Diagnostic Criteria - Learning Disability)
ADHD, 130
anxiety disorders, 89
epidemiological studies, 36, 39–40
mood disorders, 78
schizophrenia spectrum disorders, 65, 69
deafness, 185
death, understanding of concept, 103
defense mechanisms, 154–6
defiant behavior, assessment, 185
deinstitutionalization, 3–13, 252, 280
impact on mental health problems, 4
normalization concept and, 4–13

offending behavior and, 209
delirium, 56
delusions, 69, 176
dementia, 55–60
diagnosis, 55–6
Down syndrome and, 57–60
epidemiological studies, 56–7
pharmacotherapy, 59, 142
prevalence and incidence, 56–7
risk factors, 57
screening instruments, 48–9
subtypes, 57
Dementia Questionnaire for Learning Disabilities (DMR), 48–9
Dementia Scale for Down Syndrome (DSDS), 48–9
dental care needs, 232
dependent personality disorder, 110
depression
assessment instruments, 47–8, 82–3
behavioral interventions, 176
diagnostic features, 78–9
etiology, 81–2
in autism spectrum disorders, 121–2, 124
in childhood, 81, 183
pharmacotherapy, 83, 142
prevalence, 80–1
psychosocial interventions, 84
risk factors, 163
depressive factor/dimension, 227–8
development of IDD, 27–8
Developmental Behavior Checklist (DBC), 50
adult version (DBC-A), 92
children, 182–3
Hyperactivity Index, 132–6
diagnosis, psychiatric
assessment instruments and rating scales, 45–51
autism spectrum disorders, 121, 124
children with ID, 182
epidemiological studies, 37–8

diagnosis, psychiatric (cont.)
ID/IDD, 21–9
Diagnostic and Statistical Manual of Mental Disorders, Fifth Edition. See DSM-5
Diagnostic Assessment for the Severely Handicapped–II. See DASH-II
diagnostic criteria for ID/IDD, 21–6
adaptive functioning, 24–6
age of onset, 26
intelligence, 22–4
Diagnostic Criteria for Psychiatric Disorders for Use with Adults with Learning Disabilities/ Mental Retardation. See DC-LD
Diagnostic Interview for Social and Communication Disorders (DISCO), 29
diagnostic interviews, structured, 46, 50
Diagnostic Manual – Intellectual Disability. See DM-ID
diagnostic overshadowing, 99, 124, 231
dialectical behavior therapy (DBT), personality disorders, 111
differential diagnosis of IDD, 28–9
differential reinforcement (DR), 173
difficulties, 20
DiGeorge syndrome (velocardiofacial syndrome), 67, 143
disability
concept of ID as a, 16–17
defined, 25
Disorders of Intellectual Development, 19, 30
divalproex, 84, 238
DM-ID (*Diagnostic Manual – Intellectual Disability*)
ADHD, 130
anxiety disorders, 89
epidemiological studies, 39
mood disorders, 78–9
PTSD, 102
schizophrenia spectrum disorders, 65

donepezil, 59, 142
Down syndrome, 236
age-related changes, 198
Alzheimer's disease, 57–60
animal model, 202
family and social context, 198
medical illness, 233
pharmacotherapy of dementia, 59, 142
schizophrenia spectrum disorders, 68
severe, adverse behavioral changes, 199–200
Dravet syndrome, 245, 247
drug therapy. See psychopharmacology
DSM-5
anxiety disorders, 89
applicability to children with ID, 182
classification of ID, 16, 30
diagnostic criteria for ID, 21–6
neurocognitive disorder, 55
neurodevelopmental disorders, 21
personality disorders, 111, 114
problem behaviors, 226
terminology for ID, 15, 18–20, 30
dual diagnosis, 5
Dual Disability Services, Australia, 9
DYRK1A gene, 58

Eastern Nebraska Community Office of Retardation (ENCOR), 4
eating disorders, 235
ego, 151–2
emotion dysregulation, 119, 228
emotion dysregulation– problem behavior, 227–8
emotional intelligence, Goleman's, 23
Emotional Problems Scale, 210
emotional states, triggering aggression, 273
epidemiology of psychiatric comorbidity in adults, 34–40

changes in diagnostic manuals and, 39
definition, measurement, and assessment methods, 37–8
geographical, cultural and linguistic spread, 39–40
inclusion of physiological assessment, 38–9
prevalence data, 35–6
sampling methodology, 37
studies reviewed, 34–5
epilepsy, 185, 242–9
as cause of ID, 243–4
disorders causing ID plus epilepsy, 244–6
epidemiology, 242–3
genetics, 245
ID as cause of, 244
psychiatric comorbidity, 225, 248
refractory, 246
syndromes, associated with ID, 246–8
treatment, 248–9
epileptic encephalopathy, 244
escape function, aggressive behavior, 272
ethnic minority status
schizophrenia risk, 66
service users' experiences, 266
eugenics, 2, 4
Europe, service provision, 7–8
everolimus, 245
extra-pyramidal side effects (EPSEs), 70, 144
extraversion/introversion (E), 112, 114

family therapy, 71, 186
family(ies). See also parents
behavioral phenotypes and, 198
childhood psychopathology and, 185–6
cognitive variables and stress, 269–70
experiences of services, 262–7
impact of problem behaviors, 269–74
perceptions of causes of aggression, 271–3
positive aspects of caring, 270–1

training and support, 133,
  186, 274
fear, 89
Fear Survey for Adults with
  Mental Retardation
  (FSAMR), 48, 92
fetal alcohol spectrum
  disorder, 143
firesetting, 209
  therapeutic interventions,
    214–15
Five Factor Model (FFM) of
  personality, 111–12, 114
5p-syndrome, 197
fluoxetine, 83
Flynn effect, 22–4
forensic populations, 207–18,
  See also offending
  behavior
  personality disorders,
    110–11
  prevalence of ID, 207
  psychotic illness and ID, 66
  recidivism rates, 207–8
forensic risk assessment,
  209–11
foster care, 185
fragile X syndrome (FXS), 236
  behavioral phenotype,
    197, 198
  pharmacotherapy, 142–3
free-association, 154
Freud, Sigmund, 151–2, 156
frontal type dementia, 57
functional analysis (FA) of
  behavior, 172
functional assessment
  questionnaires, 172
functional communication
  training (FCT), 173

Gardner model of intelligence,
  23
gastroesophageal reflux disease
  (GERD), 234
gastrointestinal (GI) cancer,
  233
gastrointestinal problems, 234
generalized anxiety disorder
  presentation, 90
  prevalence, 90
  Williams syndrome, 199
generic mental health services.
  See mainstream mental
  health services
genetic syndromes, 203–4

ADHD, 130
anxiety disorders, 91
as models for psychiatric
  disorders, 201–2
behavioral phenotypes,
  196–201
development and course, 28
epilepsy and ID, 245
evaluation and diagnosis,
  236–7
mood disorders, 82
schizophrenia spectrum
  disorders, 67–8
Glasgow Anxiety Scale for
  people with an
  Intellectual Disability
  (GAS-ID), 48, 92
Glasgow Depression Scale for
  people with a Learning
  Disability (GDS-LD), 48,
  82
global developmental delay
  (GDD), 29
goal-directed behavior, 273
Goleman's emotional
  intelligence, 23
grief
  complicated (pathological),
    103–5
  normal reactions to, 103
group-based interventions
  anger and aggression, 212
  firesetting behavior, 215
  sexually aggressive behavior,
    212–13
guanfacine, 141
guided self-help (GSH),
  anxiety disorders, 94–5

hallucinations, 69
haloperidol, 187, 285
Hamilton Depression Rating
  Scale, 48
HCR-20, 210
head trauma/head banging,
  repeated, 57
headache, 233
health condition, 16
  categorization of ID as,
    17–28
hearing impairment, 185
Helicobacter pylori infections,
  232
hemi-megalencephaly, 245
hemispherectomy, cranial, 29,
  245

historical perspective of
  services, 1–7
holistic approach, need for,
  281
Hospital Anxiety and
  Depression Scale
  (HADS), 92
hospital services. See inpatient
  services
human rights, 2
hybrid service models of care,
  256–7, 283
hyperkinetic disorder, 129
hyperphagia, 197, 200–1

ICD-10
  anxiety disorders, 89
  applicability to children
    with ID, 182
  classification of ID, 16,
    18–19
  diagnostic criteria for ID,
    21
  disability concept of ID and,
    17
  hyperkinetic disorder,
    129
  problem behaviors, 226–7
  revision working group.
    See under World Health
    Organization
ICD-11
  classification of ID, 17–19,
    30
  neurodevelopmental
    approach to ID, 21
  problem behaviors, 226
  proposed terminology for
    ID, 19–21, 30
  subtyping of IDD, 27
ID. See intellectual disabilities
IDD. See Intellectual
  Developmental Disorder
impairment, 20
Improving Access to
  Psychological Therapies
  (IAPTs) teams, 94
informant-report assessment
  instruments, 45
inpatient services
  clinical outcomes, 254
  patient profiles, 253
  schizophrenia spectrum
    disorders, 72
  service users' experiences,
    264–5

inpatient services (cont.)
  strengths and limitations,
    255–6
institutional care, 1–2, 252
  children living in, 186
  shift away from. See
    deinstitutionalization
integrated service models of
  care, 256–7, 283
Intellectual Developmental
  Disorder (IDD)
  as neurodevelopmental
    disorder, 21
  development and course,
    27–8
  diagnostic criteria, 21–6
  differential diagnosis, 28–9
  introduction by DSM-5, 15,
    18–20
  proposed use in ICD-11,
    20–1, 30
  subtyping, 26–7
intellectual disabilities (ID)
  as a health condition, 17–28
  classification, 15–21, 30
  diagnosis, 21–9
  differential diagnosis, 28–9
  disability concept, 16–17
  meta-syndrome concept, 18
  subtyping, 26–7
  terminology. See
    terminology for ID
Intellectual Disability
  (Intellectual
  Developmental Disorder)
  (ID (IDD))
  adoption by DSM-5, 16,
    19–20, 30
  diagnostic criteria, 21–6
intelligence, 22–4
intensive case management,
  255
internal objects, 156
International Classification of
  Diseases. See ICD
International Classification of
  Functioning, Disability
  and Health (ICF), 16, 20,
  24
international trends, service
  provision, 7–10
introversion. See extraversion/
  introversion
IQ score
  as diagnostic criterion for
    ID, 21–3

borderline intellectual
  functioning, 27
  limitations, 23–4
  offending behavior and, 208
  subtyping based on, 27
Ireland, service provision, 10
Itard, Jean, 2

Lancaster and Northgate
  Trauma Scales (LANTS),
  102–8
Landau–Kleffner syndrome,
  244, 248
Lennox–Gastaut syndrome,
  246, 248
Lesch–Nyhan syndrome, 197
Lewy body dementia, 57
life events, adverse, 99–100
  acute stress reaction,
    100–1
  adjustment disorders,
    101–2
  increased frequency, 100
  mood disorders, 82
  problem behaviors and,
    226
  schizophrenia risk, 66
life experiences, psychological
  impact, 163–4
lithium, 140, 187, 235
loxapine, 237

mainstream mental health
  services, 252
  attitudes of ID staff to, 282
  client groups suited to, 256
  clinical outcomes, 254–5
  historical context, 4–6
  patient profiles, 253–4
  service users' experiences,
    264–5
  strengths and limitations, 256
Malan's triangles, 156–7
malformations of cortical
  development, 245
mania. See also bipolar
  disorder
  assessment instruments, 83
  symptoms, 80
matrix model, for services, 6
Matson Evaluation of Drug
  Side Effects (MEDS), 70
MECP2 gene deletion,
  236, 237
medical conditions, comorbid,
  231–8

aging-related, 233
children, 185
clinical approach, 235–6
screening for, 232
medication. See
  psychopharmacology
memantine, 59, 142
menstrual cramps/discomfort,
  233
mental health of ID (MHID)
  field, 279–86
  basic tenets, 279–80
  definitions and terminology,
    279
  mental health vs.
    challenging behaviors,
    280–1
  research, 283–6
  service provision, 281–3
mental health of ID services.
  See services
mental health problems,
  comorbid. See psychiatric
  disorders, comorbid
mental retardation
  terminology, 15
  use in ICD-10, 16
metabolic syndrome, 70
meta-syndrome concept of ID,
  18
methylphenidate
  ADHD, 134, 141, 187
  velocardiofacial syndrome,
    143
migraine, 233
mild cognitive impairment,
  18
Mini Psychiatric Assessment
  Schedule for Adults with
  Developmental
  Disabilities (Mini PAS-
  ADD), 46
minocycline, 143
Monthly Sleep Chart, 83
Mood and Anxiety Semi-
  Structured (MASS)
  interview, 50, 83
mood disorders, 78–85
  assessment instruments,
    47–8, 82–3
  diagnostic features,
    78–80
  epidemiology, 80–1
  etiology, 81–2
  in autism spectrum
    disorders, 124

intervention and treatment, 83–4
pharmacotherapy, 83–4, 142
service provision, 254
Mood, Interest, and Pleasure Questionnaire (MIPQ), 48
mood stabilizers
behavioral problems, 140
bipolar disorder, 84, 142
side effects, 144
motivation
intrinsic vs. extrinsic, 113
values providing, 113
Motivation Assessment Scale (MAS), 172

naltrexone, 141–2
National Association for the Dually Diagnosed (NADD), 8
National Association of Parents and Friends of Mentally Retarded Children (Arc), 2
National Institute for Health and Care Excellence (NICE)
anxiety disorders, 93–4
depression, 83
quality of services, 263
negative symptoms, 69
NEO Personality Inventory (NEO-PI; NEO-PI-R), 110, 112
neurocognitive disorder, 55
neurodegenerative disorders, 29
neurodevelopmental disorders (NDD), 21
neurofibrillary tangles, 58
neurological problems, 234
neuronal antibodies, 246
neurosurgery, for epilepsy, 29, 245, 249
neuroticism (N), 112, 114
NICE. See National Institute for Health and Care Excellence
NMDA-receptor antibodies, 246
non-contingent reinforcement (NCR), 173–4
normalization, 3–4

Northgate, Cambridge, and Abertay Pathways (NCAP) project, 209

obesity, 237
object relations theory, 156
obsessive-compulsive disorder (OCD), 120, 122
offending behavior, 207–18
See also forensic populations
alcohol misuse, 216
cognitive skills training, 216–17
intellectual functioning and, 208
interventions, 209–17
nature, 209
psychodynamic psychotherapy, 153
recidivism rates, 207–8
risk assessment, 209–11
openness (O), 112
operant conditioning, 187
opiate antagonists, 141, 187
oppositional defiant disorder (ODD), 131, 226
oral health needs, 232
osteoporosis/osteopenia, 233
outpatient services. See also community-based services
clinical outcomes, 254–5
patient profiles, 253–4
strengths and limitations, 255–6
oxcarbazepine, 140

PAC (Psychopathology in Autism Checklist), 47–52, 121, 122–3
pain syndromes, 233
panic disorder, 90
parents. See also carers; family(ies)
experiences of services, 264
grief responses to death of, 104–5
mental health problems in, 186
positive aspects of caring, 270–1
stress and burnout, 270
training and support, 133, 186
paroxetine, 83

PAS-ADD, 38, 40, 50
anxiety disorders, 92
Checklist, 46
Clinical Interview, 50
Mini, 46
mood disorders, 83
schizophrenia spectrum disorders, 69
PCL-R, 111
periodontal disease, 232
personality
assessment, 111–14
Five Factor Model (FFM), 111–12, 114
psychiatric disorders and, 114
personality disorders, 109–11
difficulties in diagnosing, 109–10
factor analysis, 110
prevalence, 109–10
psychiatric disorders and, 114
treatment studies, 111
pharmacotherapy. See psychopharmacology
phobic anxiety disorders, 91
behavioral interventions, 176
Williams syndrome, 199
physical discomfort, triggering aggression, 273
pica, 226, 234
behavioral interventions, 175
PIMRA (Psychopathology Inventory for Mentally Retarded Adults), 47–52, 92
Pinel, Phillipe, 1
Planning, Attention, Simultaneous and Successive (PASS) model of intelligence, 23
Positive Contributions Scale (PCS), 271
post-traumatic stress disorder (PTSD), 102–3
acute stress disorder and, 101
autism spectrum disorders, 125
presentation and diagnosis, 102–3

Prader–Willi syndrome
(PWS), 200–1, 236
age-related changes, 198
autism spectrum disorders,
201
cognitive processing style,
197
hyperphagia, 197, 200–1
pharmacotherapy, 143
psychotic illness, 68, 201
severe psychiatric illness,
200–1
preference assessment, 172
pregabalin, 93
pregnancy complications,
schizophrenia risk, 66
prisoners. *See* forensic
populations
problem (challenging)
behaviors, 224–8
assessment tools, 49
behavioral interventions,
174–6
carer and family
perspectives, 269–74
carers' perceptions of
causes, 271–3
classification, 226–7
course over time, 226
Down syndrome, 199–200
interdisciplinary research,
286
management issues, 228
mental illness and, 224–8,
280–1
pharmacotherapy, 140–2,
228
prevalence in ID, 224
psychodynamic
psychotherapy, 153
services, 253, 255, 283
prolonged grief disorder,
103, 104
Psychiatric Assessment
Schedule for Adults with
Developmental
Disabilities.
See PAS-ADD
psychiatric disorders,
comorbid
ADHD, 131
autism spectrum disorders,
119–26
behavioral interventions, 176
carer and family
perspectives, 269–74

clinical approach, 237–40
diagnosis. *See* diagnosis,
psychiatric
epidemiology in adults,
34–40
epilepsy, 225, 248
historical perspective, 7–11
impact of
deinstitutionalization, 4
in children, 181–92
international trends in
services, 7–10
medical illness and,
231–8
personality, personality
disorders and, 114
pharmacotherapy, 141–2
prevalence, 35–6, 181,
280
problem behaviors and,
224–8, 280–1
psychoanalysis, 151
psychodynamic
psychotherapy, 151–8
evidence base, 152–4
information gathering,
154–5
recontextualization,
155–6
suitability criteria, 152
therapeutic frame, 154
therapists' activities,
154–7
Psychopathology checklists for
Adults with Intellectual
Disability (P-AID), 50
Psychopathology in Autism
Checklist (PAC), 47–52,
121–3
Psychopathology Inventory for
Mentally Retarded Adults
(PIMRA), 47, 92
psychopharmacology,
139–45
children with ID, 141, 143,
187
guidelines, 144–5
past, 140–1
side effects, 144, 235
specific ID-related
disorders, 142–4
specific psychiatric
disorders, 141–2
psychosocial factors,
psychopathology of
children, 185–6

psychosocial interventions
alcohol misuse, 216
anxiety disorders, 93–5
mood disorders, 84
schizophrenia spectrum
disorders, 71
psychotic illness. *See*
schizophrenia spectrum
disorders
psychotropic medication.
See psychopharmacology
PTSD. *See* post-traumatic
stress disorder

Questions About Behavioural
Function (QABF) scale,
172

rapamycin (sirolimus), 245
rating scales. *See* assessment
instruments and
recidivism rates, 207–8
recontextualization, 155–6
Reiss Screen for Maladaptive
Behaviour (RSMB),
47, 82
research, mental health of ID
field, 283–6
residential care. *See*
institutional care
response cost, 174
restraint, physical and
mechanical, 174
Rett syndrome, 197, 236–7
risk assessment, forensic,
209–11
risperidone
ADHD, 134
aggressive behavior, 142, 285
autism spectrum disorders,
140, 143
problem behaviors, 140,
142, 187
rivastigmine, 59
Royal College of Psychiatrists,
5, 10
*Diagnostic Criteria –
Learning Disability.*
See DC-LD
Rubinstein–Taybi syndrome,
237

SAINT self-help tool, 51, 95
scatterplots, behavioral, 171
schizophrenia spectrum
disorders (SSDs), 65–73

associated genetic
  conditions, 67–8
autism spectrum disorders
  and, 123–4
differential diagnosis, 68, 120
management, 70–1
neurodevelopmental model,
  66–7
outcome/prognosis, 72
pharmacotherapy, 70–1,
  141
Prader–Willi syndrome, 68,
  201
prevalence, 65–6
recognition and diagnosis,
  68–9
risk factors, 66
service provision, 71–2, 254
screening instruments, 45–9
anxiety disorders, 48
behavioral problems, 49
dementia, 48–9
mood disorders, 47–8
psychopathology, 46–7
vs. diagnostic instruments,
  46
screenings, basic healthcare,
  232
second-generation
  antipsychotics. See
  atypical antipsychotics
seizures. See also epilepsy
as cause of ID, 243–4
in Down syndrome
  dementia, 60
intellectual function and,
  243
selective serotonin reuptake
  inhibitors (SSRIs), 141,
  187
anxiety disorders, 93, 141
autism spectrum disorders,
  143
depression, 83
side effects, 235
self-injurious behavior (SIB)
behavioral interventions,
  175
course over time, 226
pharmacotherapy, 142, 187
prevalence in ID, 224
PTSD, 103
self-regulation theory of illness
  behavior, 270
self-report assessment
  instruments, 45

Self-Report Depression
  Questionnaire (SRDQ),
  48, 82
sensory stimulation,
  hypersensitivity to, 120
separation distress,
  bereavement-related, 103,
  105
service users, experiences of
  services, 262–7
services, 252–8, 281–3
barriers to access, 231
clinical outcomes, 254–5
community-based. See
  community-based
  services
deinstitutionalization. See
  deinstitutionalization
historical context, 1–7
integrated/hybrid models,
  256–7, 283
international trends, 7–10
mainstream. See
  mainstream mental
  health services
normalization concept,
  4–13
offenders with ID, 209
patient profiles, 253–4
pros and cons of different
  models, 255–7
service users' and carers'
  experiences, 262–7
specialized. See specialized
  mental health services
transition from childhood to
  adulthood, 124, 265
Severe Impairment Battery,
  56
severe myoclonic epilepsy of
  infancy. See Dravet
  syndrome
sex offenders, 209
therapeutic interventions,
  212–14
sexual abuse, 100
sexuality, 235
sexually transmitted diseases,
  235
Short Dynamic Risk Scale
  (SDRS), 210
Shultz Mini-Mental State
  Exam, 49
side effects, medication, 144,
  235
sirolimus (rapamycin), 245

skills training
  alcohol misuse, 216
  offending behavior,
    215, 216–17
Smith–Magenis syndrome, 197
social context
  behavioral phenotypes, 198
  mental ill-health, 163
social phobia, 91
social skills training, firesetting
  behavior, 214
specialized mental health
  services, 252, 283
  client groups suited to, 256
  clinical outcomes, 254–5
  historical context, 5
  international trends, 7, 9
  patient profiles, 253–4
  service users' experiences,
    264–5
  staff attitudes to mainstream
    services, 282
  strengths and limitations,
    256
specific learning disorders
  (SLD), 29
spiritual beliefs, 236
staff (paid carers)
  impact of problem
    behaviors, 269–74
  perceptions of causes of
    aggression, 271–3
  positive aspects of caring,
    271
  qualities of good, 266
  service users' experiences,
    264–5
  training, 273
Staff Positive Contributions
  Questionnaire (SPCQ),
  271
Standardized Assessment of
  Personality (SAP),
  109–15
START model, 8
state-dependent intellectual
  impairment, 244
Static-99, 210
stereotypy, behavioral
  interventions, 175–6
stigmatization
  psychological impact,
    163, 163–4
  service provision and, 282
stimulant medications, 134,
  141, 187

stress, 99
  acute reactions, 100–1
  adjustment disorders,
    101–2
  in carers and families,
    270
  problems in autism, 120
  reactions in ID, 99–102
substance abuse, 235
subtyping of IDD, 26–7
suicide, 81
Suitability for Psychotherapy
  Scale, 152
swallowing difficulties,
  234

terminology for ID, 15,
  19–21
  DSM-5, 15, 18–20, 30
  ICD-10, 16
  proposed for ICD-11,
    19, 20–1, 30
Therapy Expectation Measure,
  165
timeout, 174
transference, 156
transition from childhood to
  adulthood, service
  provision, 124, 265

trauma, psychological, 100,
  102, See also post-
    traumatic stress disorder
traumatic brain injury,
  epilepsy and ID, 244
traumatic distress,
  bereavement-related, 103
tricyclic antidepressants, 141,
  143, 187
tuberous sclerosis complex,
  245, 247
22q11.2 deletion syndrome
  (velocardiofacial
  syndrome), 68, 143
212 Multi-Centre Risk Study,
  210

United States (US), service
  provision, 4–5, 8
Usher syndrome, 68

valproic acid/divalproex, 84, 238
vascular dementia, 57
velocardiofacial syndrome
  (VCFS), 68, 143
vigabatrin, 247, 249
Violence Risk Appraisal Guide
  (VRAG), 210
vision problems, 232

vitamin-D deficiency, 57
volition, expression of, 273
voltage-gated potassium-
  channel complex
  antibodies, 246

West syndrome, 247
Williams syndrome
  behavioral phenotype,
    198, 198–9
  pharmacotherapy, 143
Wolfensburger, W., 3
World Health Organization
  (WHO)
  Atlas on ID (2007), 2
  classification of ID, 16
  ICD-10 revision working
    group (IAGRMR), 15, 18,
    20–1, 27
World Psychiatric Association
  (WPA)
  Intellectual Disability
    section (WPA-SPID),
    17–28
  medication guidelines,
    145

Zung Self-Rating Depression
  Scale, 48

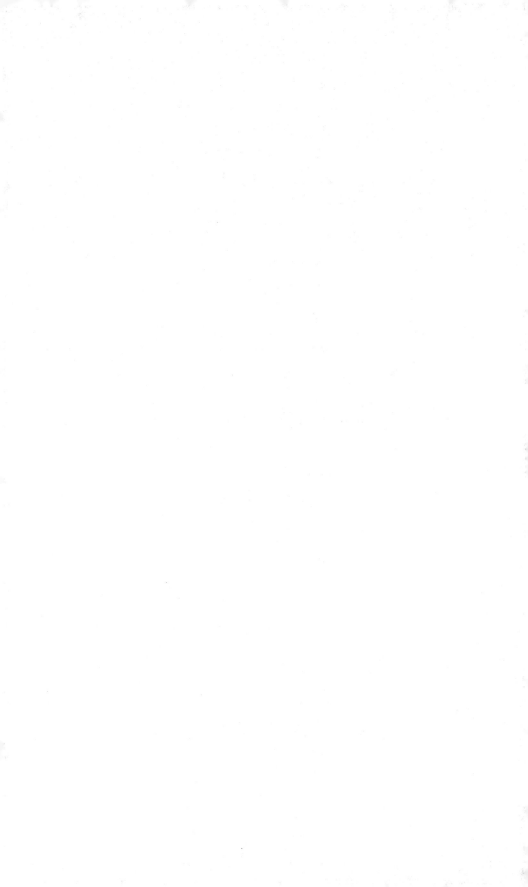

Printed in the United States
By Bookmasters